BRUNNSTROM'S
CLINICAL KINESIOLOGY

BRUNNSTROM'S
CLINICAL KINESIOLOGY

REVISED BY

L. DON LEHMKUHL, PH.D.

ASSOCIATE DIRECTOR FOR RESEARCH, DEPARTMENT OF PHYSICAL THERAPY
THE INSTITUTE FOR REHABILITATION AND RESEARCH
ASSISTANT PROFESSOR OF PHYSIOLOGY AND REHABILITATION
BAYLOR COLLEGE OF MEDICINE
HOUSTON, TEXAS

LAURA K. SMITH, PH.D.

PROFESSOR, DEPARTMENT OF PHYSICAL THERAPY
SCHOOL OF ALLIED HEALTH SCIENCES
THE UNIVERSITY OF TEXAS MEDICAL BRANCH
GALVESTON, TEXAS

FOURTH EDITION

F. A. DAVIS COMPANY Philadelphia

Library of Congress Cataloging in Publication Data

Brunnstrom, Signe.
  Brunnstrom's Clinical kinesiology.

  Bibliography: p.
  Includes index.
  1. Kinesiology.   I. Lehmkuhl, L. Don, 1930–
II. Smith, Laura K., 1923–   . III. Title.
IV. Title: Clinical kinesiology.   [DNLM: 1. Movement.
2. Muscles.   WE 103 B897c]
QP303.B78   1983   612'.74   82–25249
ISBN 0–8036–5529–0

PREFACE TO
THE FOURTH EDITION

We are pleased to have the opportunity to continue the work of Signe Brunnstrom whom we admire as the master clinician, teacher, researcher, and author. Miss Brunnstrom's precise and enthusiastic application of mechanical, neurophysiologic, and behavioral principles of human motion can be seen in the photograph and appreciated in the brief biographical sketch following the preface to the first edition of *Clinical Kinesiology*.

Building upon the solid foundation of content contained in the earlier editions of this widely used textbook, we have expanded the first two chapters on Mechanical Principles and Aspects of Muscle Physiology into four chapters. Additional and more current information on kinematics, kinetics, and the physiologic basis for producing and controlling posture and movement are presented, along with an expanded coverage of mechanical and physiologic interactions during movement. Many new illustrations have been added to these first four chapters to assist in clarifying the concepts presented. Several of the chapters have been restructured and the order of topics changed to permit certain concepts to be covered earlier than done previously. For example, general principles of equilibrium and stability discussed in Chapter 10 of the third edition have been integrated into Chapters 1 and 2 of this edition. Other major changes and additions include:

- Addition of metric units of measurement; most of the examples of forces, distances, torques, and masses are expressed in both English and metric units. Our original intent was to use only metric units; however, the practicalities of transition require variable use of both systems. We hope that this step will ease the transfer of common usage to metric units within our lifetime. Future revisions will undoubtedly go further with this effort.

- Substitution of the terms "proximal attachment" and "distal attachment" for the terms "origin" and "insertion," respectively, to reinforce the concept that muscle contraction may produce movement at either or both of its attachments.
- Emphasis on joint areas, with increased information on arthrokinematics, palpation of soft-tissue structures, ranges of joint motions, forces that occur at joints in activity, and additional joint areas such as the costo-vertebral and temporomandibular joints.
- Description of kinematic and kinetic measurements of joints and muscles in functional activities.
- Inclusion of practical examples of the clinical applications of mechanical and neurophysiologic principles in all new and rewritten sections of the text, so as to continue the emphasis so well conveyed by Signe Brunnstrom.

With the exception of illustrations reproduced from other published works, the new illustrations appearing in this fourth edition are the work of Charles Moens, a medical illustrator on the staff of the University of Texas Medical Branch in Galveston, Texas. After being provided with crude sketches by the authors and listening to an explanation of the concepts to be portrayed, Mr. Moens created illustrations that highlight the functional concepts while preserving important anatomic detail. In the words of Charles Moens, "Art permits us to see things in an understanding manner."

L. Don Lehmkuhl
Laura K. Smith

PREFACE TO
THE FIRST EDITION

Kinesiology—broadly defined as the science of human motion—has ramifications reaching into many fields of study, such as anatomy, physiology, mechanics, physics, mathematics, orthopedics, neurology, pathology and psychology. To be of practical value, a textbook dealing with such a vast subject must be geared to the specific needs of the groups for which it is intended, in the present case the members of medical, paramedical and physical education professions. Because the background requirements and the curricula for students who prepare to enter these professions include subjects closely related to kinesiology, the task at hand was to supplement, not duplicate, the contents of other courses. A certain amount of overlap between courses in anatomy and kinesiology was inevitable. However, throughout the preparation of this book an effort was made to present a minimum of anatomical details while emphasizing the function of skeletal and neuromuscular structures. Both the text and the illustrations aim at developing the student's skill in palpating anatomical structures in the living, a skill which is invaluable in dealing with patients.

Much of the contents of this book has been used over the years by the author in teaching kinesiology to students of physical therapy and occupational therapy. The writing of the book originated with a teaching grant from the Office of Vocational Rehabilitation which enabled the author to prepare a mimeographed laboratory manual to serve as a study aid for students of physical therapy and occupational therapy at College of Physicians and Surgeons, Columbia University. The original manual was then revised and enlarged to include material on certain aspects of pathological motor behavior. The clinical aspects of kinesiology were given emphasis to meet the needs of workers in the field of rehabilitation of the physically handicapped.

Although basic kinesiology is concerned with normal motion of individuals with intact neuromuscular systems, the inclusion of selected pathological cases seemed justifiable and desirable. The effect of loss of specific muscles or muscle groups on movement is particularly well demonstrated in individuals having certain types of peripheral nerve injuries; since the paralysis in this group is specific, illustrations have been drawn mainly from these patients. The motor behavior of patients with upper motoneuron lesions was not included because, to be of value, such a discussion would have to be too lengthy to fit into the framework of this publication.

The section on erect posture, although brief, is intended to present the most important mechanical principles governing the balance of body segments in the upright position. These principles may also serve as a rationale for evaluating the difficulties arising from disorders of the lower extremities, as in persons with paraplegia, lower extremity amputations, poliomyelitis, and the like. By implication, some understanding of the basic principles of bracing and of lower extremity prosthetics should also be derived, although the latter subjects have not been dealt with specifically.

Originally, the author did not intend to discuss human locomotion, but did so at the request of professional personnel who felt that, without a chapter on locomotion, a textbook of kinesiology would be incomplete. Justice cannot be done to this subject in one short chapter, hence the locomotion chapter must be looked upon as an introduction only. For the benefit of those who wish to go deeper into the study of locomotion, references to scientific material are given.

In preparing this book, the author was many times tempted to discuss the application of kinesiology to various therapeutic training procedures employed by physical therapists and occupational therapists. Such follow up of the basic material, however, does not belong in this publication—special courses are offered to deal with therapeutic applications.

The book has fulfilled its purpose if the reader gains a basic knowledge and appreciation of human motion and if, to some extent, it opens scientific vistas which call for further exploration and investigation.

ACKNOWLEDGMENTS FOR THE FIRST EDITION

The author is happy to acknowledge the valuable assistance she has received from colleagues and professional friends in the preparation of this book, and to extend to them her sincere thanks for their efforts and interest:

To Dr. Herbert O. Elftman, Associate Professor of Anatomy, College of Physicians and Surgeons, Columbia University, for reading the manuscript and for giving so generously of his time and effort. Thanks to his constructive criticism, errors have been corrected, questionable statements clarified, and much irrelevant material eliminated. It has been a privilege, indeed, to have Dr. Elftman take an active interest in this publication.

To Dr. Robert E. Darling, Professor of Physical Medicine and Rehabilitation, for his support and encouragement.

To Professor Mary E. Callahan, Director, Courses for Physical Therapy, and to Professor Marie Louise Franciscus, Director, Courses for Occupational Therapy, for their interest and assistance. To Professors Ruth Dickinson, R.P.T., and Martha E. Schnebly, O.T.R., co-instructors in Kinesiology, who have tested and evaluated the material under actual teaching conditions, and who have assisted in numerous ways.

To Dr. T. Campbell Thompson, for the permission to use photographs taken at Hospital for Special Surgery.

The author also wishes to extend her thanks to the young man who patiently served as a model for a great many photographs in this book and to Mr. Crew, of the Crew Photo Studio, Carmel, New York, for his splendid cooperation.

SIGNE BRUNNSTROM

BRIEF BIOGRAPHICAL SKETCH OF SIGNE BRUNNSTROM

Signe Brunnstrom graduated from Uppsala College in Sweden and received her physical therapy education at the Royal Gymnastic Central Institute in Stockholm, from which she was graduated in 1919.

She was in the private practice of physical therapy in Lucerne, Switzerland, from 1921 to 1928 when she came to the United States. She served at the Hospital for the Ruptured and Crippled and at other hospitals in the New York area, and from 1938 to 1941 was Instructor in Physical Therapy at New York University.

During World War II she was a physical therapist at the Station Hospital, Sheppard Field, Texas, and chief physical therapist at the U.S. Naval Hospital, Mare Island, California.

Following World War II she took part in the locomotion study at the University of California, and from 1947 to 1949 she was a research associate in the Suction Socket Study sponsored by the Veterans Administration and New York University. In 1950 to 1951 she served in Athens, Greece, as a Fulbright Consultant in Rehabilitation.

Her contributions to locomotion and exercise, particularly for patients with cerebrovascular accidents, have been outstanding. Throughout the world patients with amputations have been beneficiaries of her work in developing training methods for the use of artificial limbs.

Miss Brunnstrom has produced several motion pictures and has authored many books and articles in the areas of teaching patients with amputations and with strokes to regain function. In addition, she shared her special knowledge and skills with other clinicians by organizing and presenting workshops on the evaluation and treatment of patients with disorders of motor control.

In July 1965, she became the recipient of the first Marian Williams Award for research in physical therapy, presented at the Annual Conference of the American Phys-

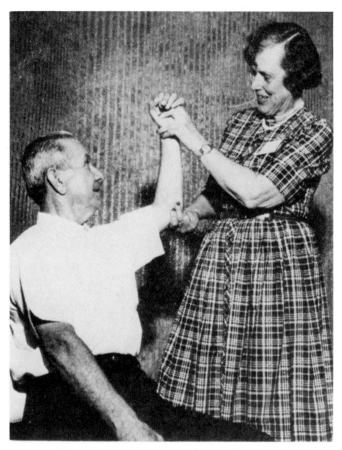

Signe Brunnstrom demonstrates technique with a patient. (From Physical Therapy 45(11): 1083, 1965, with permission.)

ical Therapy Association in Cleveland, Ohio. And in 1971, she retired from her position as an Instructor in Physical Therapy at the College of Physicians and Surgeons, Columbia University, and Consultant for the Veterans Administration, but continued to present workshops for several years until poor health prevented such strenuous activity. As of this writing, Miss Brunnstrom resides in a nursing home in Connecticut.

CONTENTS

xvii

xviii

1

MECHANICAL PRINCIPLES: KINEMATICS

Kinesiology, the study of motion, developed from the fascination of human beings with animal motion: How does a person walk? How do fish swim? How do birds fly? What are the limits of muscular strength? From this quest the science of motion evolved, combining theories and principles from anatomy, physiology, psychology, anthropology, and mechanics. The application of mechanics to the living human body is called *biomechanics*. Mechanics may be further subdivided into *statics*, which is concerned with bodies at rest or in uniform motion, and *dynamics*, which treats bodies that are accelerating or decelerating. Since most of the motion with which physical and occupational therapists deal therapeutically is slow and lacks rapid accelerations, the concepts from mechanics applicable to clinical practice can be gained using principles from statics.

The purpose for studying *clinical kinesiology* is to understand the forces acting on the human body and to manipulate these forces so that human performance may be improved or injury may be prevented. Although humans have always been able to see and feel their postures and motions, the forces affecting motion (gravity, muscle tension, external resistance, and friction) are never seen and seldom felt. Where these forces act in relation to positions and movements of the body in space is fundamental to the ability to produce human motion and to modify it.

KINEMATICS

The human body can assume many diverse positions that appear difficult to describe or classify (Fig. 1-1). *Kinematics* is the science concerned with describing the posi-

1

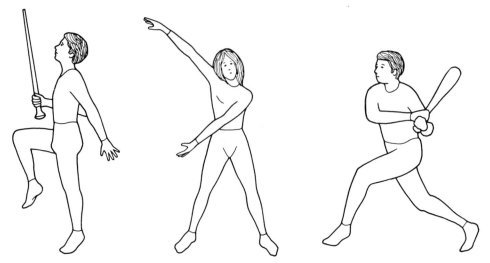

FIGURE 1-1. Examples of the variety of joint and segment positions that the human body can assume.

tions and motions of the body in space and which permits an exact description of these diverse positions of the body.

Planar Classification of Position and Motion

To define joint and segment motions and to record the location in space of specific points on the body, a reference point is required. In kinesiology, the three-dimensional rectangular coordinate system is used to describe anatomic relationships of the body. The standard *anatomic body position* is defined as standing erect with the head, toes, and palms of the hands facing forward and with the fingers extended. Three imaginary planes are arranged perpendicular to each other through the body, with their axes intersecting at the center of gravity of the body (a point slightly anterior to the second sacral vertebra). These planes are called the *cardinal planes* of the body (Fig. 1-2). Each of the three planes is divided into four quadrants by two of the three perpendicular axes x, y, and z.

Frontal Plane

The frontal plane (coronal or XY plane) is parallel to the frontal bone and divides the body into front and back parts. Motions that occur in this plane are defined as *abduction* and *adduction*. Abduction is a position or motion of the segment away from the midline, regardless of which segment moves. Abduction of the hip (Fig. 1-3) occurs when either the thigh segment approaches the pelvic segment or the pelvic segment approaches the thigh, as in tilting to the side while standing on one leg. Adduction is

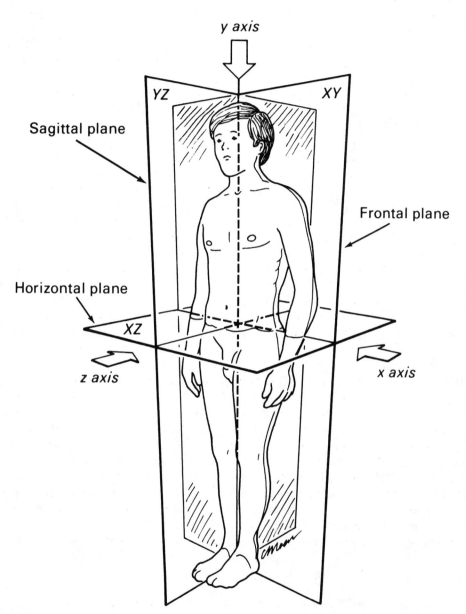

FIGURE 1-2. The three cardinal planes and axes of the body standing at ease. (A person is considered to be in the standard anatomic position when standing with the palms facing forward.)

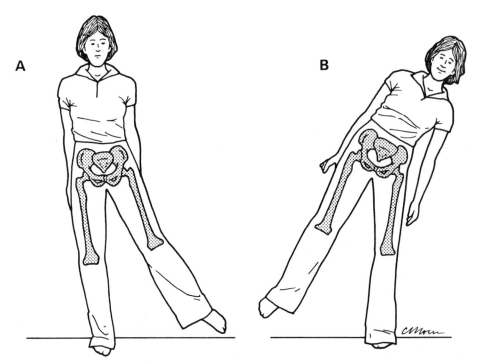

FIGURE 1-3. Abduction of the left hip: (A) femur abducted on the pelvis and (B) pelvis abducted on the femur.

a position or motion toward the midline. Motions of abduction and adduction occur around the z axis.

Sagittal Plane

The sagittal plane (mid-sagittal or YZ plane) is vertical and divides the body into right and left sides. Photographically, this is a side view. Joint motions occurring in the sagittal plane are defined as *flexion* and *extension*. Flexion indicates that the angle of a joint becomes smaller or that the two segments approach each other; for example, flexion of the elbow may be accomplished by flexion of the forearm on the arm or by flexion of the arm on the forearm, as in a pull-up. *Extension* occurs when the angle of a joint becomes larger. If extension goes beyond the anatomic reference position, it is called *hyperextension*. Motions of flexion and extension pivot around the x axis.

Horizontal Plane

The horizontal plane (transverse or XZ plane) divides the body into upper and lower parts and is like a view from above. Rotations occur in this plane around the vertical y axis. *Internal rotation* (inward or medial rotation) is a transverse rotation oriented to the anterior surface of the body. Internal rotation of the hip brings points marked on the anterior surface of the pelvis and femur closer together regardless of which one of the segments moves. *Pronation* is the term used for internal rotation of the forearm. *External rotation* (outward or lateral rotation) is in the opposite direction and is oriented to the posterior surface of the body. *Supination* is the term used at the forearm and is the reference position for the anatomic position.

Special Cases

Sagittal, frontal, and horizontal planes may be laid through points other than the center of gravity of the body, but these are *secondary planes*. For example, it may be convenient to lay three planes through the center of a joint, such as the hip joint, for determination of body points in relation to such a joint.

Definitions for motions of the digits require placing the coordinate system on the extremity. In the hand, the sagittal plane is centered through the *third segment*; in the foot, the sagittal plane is centered through the *second segment*. Motion or position away from the reference segment is called abduction, and motion toward the segment is called adduction. At the wrist, the motion of abduction is frequently referred to as *radial deviation* (toward the radius), and adduction is referred to as *ulnar deviation*. Upward motion at the ankle is usually called *dorsiflexion*, and downward motion is referred to as *plantar flexion*.

The thumb is also a special case since it is normally rotated 90 degrees from the plane of the hand. Thus, motions of flexion and extension occur in the frontal plane, and abduction and adduction are in the sagittal plane.

TYPES OF MOTION

The shape and congruency of articulating joint surfaces determine the movements permitted at various joints. Movements are described as occurring around an axis or a pivot point, identified in mechanical terminology as *rotary motion, angular motion, or rotation*. Rotary motions take place about a fixed or relatively fixed axis. These motions are called rotary since every point on a segment adjacent to the joint follows the arc of a circle, the center of which is the joint axis. Thus, in flexion and extension of the elbow, the bones of the forearm (or the bone of the upper arm or both) rotate about the axis of the elbow joint. Individual points on the segment move at different velocities, the velocity of each point being related to its distance from the axis of motion. Thus, if the arm swings forward and backward at the shoulder, the velocity (in cm per sec) of the hand is greater than that of the elbow and far greater than that of a point on the upper portion of the arm which lies close to the center of rotation. (Note, however, that the angular velocity, i.e., degrees per sec, is the same for all points on the rotating segment.)

In mechanics, the term *translatory motion* is used to describe movement of a body in which *all of its parts* move in the same direction with equal velocity. Thus, any point on the body could be used to describe the path of the total body. Translatory motion may either be in a straight line (linear) or follow a curve (curvilinear). There are few examples of true translatory motions in the human body; these usually involve passive transport of the body in a vehicle such as a wheelchair, stretcher, or car. In walking, the trunk and the body as a whole move in a forward direction, but this is not a true translatory motion since the body segments move with different velocities. Nevertheless, it is an example of how multiple rotary motions of limb segments can produce a "relative" translatory movement of the body as a whole. In the upper extremity, combinations of rotary motions at the shoulder, elbow, radio-ulnar, and wrist joints permit the hand to move freely in space, taking a translatory path.

DEGREES OF FREEDOM

The ability of the body to transform stereotyped angular motions of joints into more efficient curvilinear motion of parts can be appreciated by using the concept of *degrees of freedom* of motion. The expression was coined by Reuleaux (1875) for use in engineering and was adapted to biomechanics by Otto Fisher (1907). Joints have been classified according to the number of planes in which their segments move or the number of primary axes they possess.

Joints that move in one plane possess one axis and have *one degree of freedom*. Examples are the interphalangeal and elbow joints, which possess motion of flexion and extension around a transverse (x) axis, and the radio-ulnar joints, which permit supination and pronation around a longitudinal (y) axis. Any one point on the moving segment is restricted to a predetermined arc of motion in a single plane.

If a joint has two axes, the segments can move in two planes and the joint is said to possess *two degrees of freedom of motion*. Examples are the metacarpal-phalangeal joints of the hand and the radio-carpal joint of the wrist, which permit flexion-extension around a transverse axis and abduction-adduction around a sagittal axis.

Actually, motions may take place about any number of *secondary* axes through the center of the joint to combine various degrees of the main motions. For example, motion may take place about an oblique axis so that flexion-adduction occurs in one direction and extension-abduction in the opposite direction.

Ball-and-socket joints such as the hip joint, which permit flexion-extension, abduction-adduction, and transverse rotation, are said to possess *three degrees of freedom*. Movements take place about three main axes, all of which pass through the joint's center of rotation (in the case of the hip joint, the axes pass through the center of the head of the femur). At the hip, the axis for flexion-extension has a transverse direction; the axis for abduction-adduction has a sagittal direction; and the axis for transverse rotation courses longitudinally from the center of the hip joint to the center of the knee joint. The gleno-humeral joint of the shoulder is another example of a joint with three degrees of freedom.

By well-coordinated, successive combinations of the movement components, a *circumduction* motion is performed during which the moving segment follows the surface of a cone and the tip of the segment traces a circular path. Circumduction is characteristic of joints with two and three degrees of freedom but cannot take place in joints with one degree of freedom.

By definition, three degrees of freedom of motion are the maximum number that a *single* joint can possess. It is through the summation of the degrees of freedom of two or more joints that parts of the body may gain sufficient degrees of freedom to produce smooth translations of the body and curvilinear motions.

KINEMATIC CHAINS

A combination of several joints uniting successive segments constitutes a *kinematic chain*. Successively, the more *distal segments can have higher degrees of freedom than do proximal ones*. For example, from the thoracic wall to the finger, 19 degrees of freedom can be found (Steindler, 1955). Such freedom of motion constitutes the mechanical basis for performance of skilled manual activities and the versatility of the upper extremity. In the lower extremity and trunk, the 25 or more degrees of freedom between the pelvis and the toe not only permit the foot to adjust to an irregular or slanting surface but also allow the body's center of gravity to be maintained within the small base of support (see Chapter 2).

Limitation of normal joint motion (such as joint fusion, soft tissue tightness, or pain) reduces the degrees of freedom of the segments, and normal motion is not possible. The large number of degrees of freedom in a kinematic chain is an advantage, however, in minimizing the disabling effects of single joint restrictions. More motion above or below the restriction can be used to accomplish a function. For example, the person who cannot supinate or pronate the forearm can compensate by using trunk, shoulder, and wrist motions to accomplish tasks such as eating or writing. Walking can be accomplished quite well by a person whose hip joint is fused in extension. The lower extremity is advanced by flexing the pelvis and lumbar spine. Rotation, however, is an essential motion of the hip joint during walking. Compensation for loss of this rotation can occur in the lumbar spine, the knee, and even the foot. Because of the great forces that occur in weight-bearing, these compensations above and below restrictions of motion can, in time, lead to hypermobility, instability, and pain in other joints.

Open and Closed Kinematic Chains

In an open kinematic chain, the distal segment terminates free in space, whereas in a closed kinematic chain, the distal segment is fixed. Closed kinematic chains are commonly used in machines; open chains are more common in the human body, as exemplified by the vertebral column and the limbs. A number of closed chains are also found in the human body, such as the pelvic girdle (where the segments are united by the two sacro-iliac joints and the symphysis pubis) and the thorax (where each rib with its vertebral and sternal connections forms a ring). Steindler (1955) describes the closed chain (which he calls the kinetic chain) as "one in which the terminal joint meets with some considerable resistance which prohibits or restrains its free motion."

Planar classifications of motion imply that the proximal segment is fixed and the distal segment moves. Although this open-chain type of motion is important in human motion, it is only *one* type. Equally important are closed-chain motions that occur when the distal segment is fixed and the proximal segment moves, and when *both* segments move. Examples include sitting down in a chair (Fig. 1-4). Here the leg moves forward on the fixed foot (dorsiflexion), the thigh approaches the leg (knee flexion), and the thigh approaches the pelvis (hip flexion). Walking and stair-climbing are examples of alternation of closed-chain motion during the support phase of the extremity and open-chain motion during the swing phase. When a person uses the arm rests of a chair to assist in coming to the standing position (or performs a pushup in a wheelchair), the hand is fixed and the forearm moves from a position of wrist extension toward wrist flexion, the arm moves away from the forearm (elbow extension), and the arm moves toward the trunk (shoulder adduction). Other clinical examples of closed-chain motion in the upper extremity include crutch-walking and elevating the body using an overbed trapeze.

ARTHROKINEMATICS

Arthrokinematics is concerned with the movement of the articular surfaces in relation to the direction of movement of the distal extremity of the bone (osteokinematics). Although human joints have been compared with geometric shapes and mechanical joints such as the hinge, pivot, plane, sphere, and cone, the exquisite motions and capabilities of animal joints exceed any joint that humans have made. Normally, human joints retain their functional capacities beyond the organic life span of the human being (70 to 100 years). The phenomenal superiority of human joints as compared to man-made joints not only is due to the physiologic capacities of biologic joints such as low coefficient of friction, presence of sensation and proprioceptive feedback, and dynamic growth responses to wear and use, but also is due to the mechanical complexities of human joints.

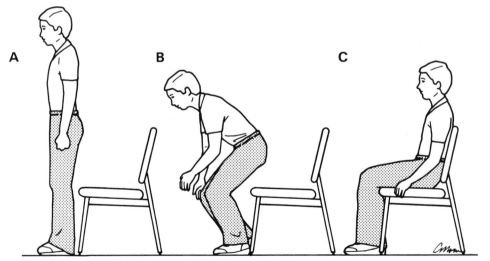

FIGURE 1-4. Closed kinematic chain motion of the ankle, knee, and hip joints as the subject moves from the standing to the sitting position.

OVOID AND SELLAR JOINT SURFACES

The surfaces of movable joints are not flat, cylindric, conic, or spheric; they are *ovoid* (egg-shaped), a shape in which the radius of curvature varies from point to point (MacConaill and Basmajian, 1969). Matching ovoid surfaces of two articular surfaces form a convex-concave paired relationship (Fig. 1-5). The concave-convex joint relationship may range from "nearly planar," as in the carpal and tarsal joints, to "nearly spheroid," as in the gleno-humeral and hip joints. In engineering, the convex curvature is called the male component, and the concave curvature is called the female component. The center of rotation is in the convex component at some distance from the joint surface. Thus, the direction of movement of the *joint surfaces* is different than would be expected in a mechanical hinge joint. If the bone with the convexity is

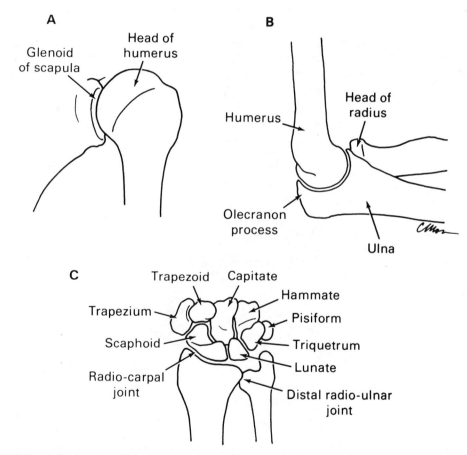

FIGURE 1-5. Examples of concave-convex relationships of joint surfaces redrawn from radiographs. *(A)* Gleno-humeral joint of the shoulder (anterior-posterior view). *(B)* Humero-ulnar joint of the elbow (lateral view). *(C)* Radio-carpal and intercarpal joints of the wrist (anterior-posterior view).

moved on the bone with the concavity, the convex surface moves in the *opposite* direction to the bone segment (Fig. 1-6). If the opposite bone segment is moved (concave on convex), the concave surface moves in the *same* direction as the bone segment. Thus, arthrokinematically, the planar motion of shoulder abduction is either a downward motion of the humeral head on the glenoid fossa when the humerus is moving, or an upward movement of the glenoid on the humerus when the scapula is moving. Likewise, flexion at the metacarpal-phalangeal *joint surfaces* is either a downward movement of the female surface (phalanx) or an upward movement of the male surface (metacarpal).

These joint surface relationships are of extreme importance when motion of the joint is limited and exercise is being used to increase motion. If, for example, interphalangeal joint flexion is limited (as may occur with scar tissue formation of the skin, capsule, tendon, or ligaments), the normal downward movement of the *phalanx* into a position of flexion (Fig. 1-6, C) cannot occur. Since the concave base of the phalanx cannot move down, a force applied distally on the phalanx may pry the joint so that some structures are overstretched and others are compressed (Fig. 1-7, C). This could result in further injury to joint structures. Attention should be paid to gaining downward movement of the phalanx by applying the force close to the joint and in line with normal joint surface movements (Fig. 1-7, B).

Some joints have both convex and concave surfaces on each articulating bone (Fig. 1-8). These are called *sellar* (L., saddle) joints since they resemble the matching of a

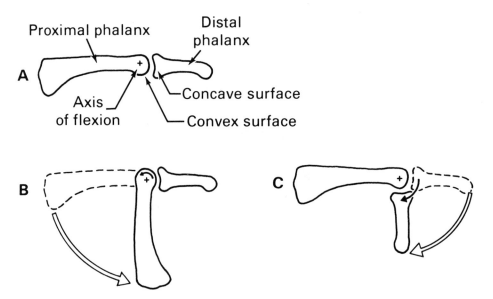

FIGURE 1-6. Lateral view of the proximal interphalangeal joint of the index finger in extension (A) and in flexion (B, C). When the bone with the convex joint surface moves into flexion (B), the joint surface moves in an *opposite* direction to the motion of the shaft of the bone. When the bone with the concave joint surface moves into flexion (C), the joint surface moves in the *same* direction as the shaft of the bone.

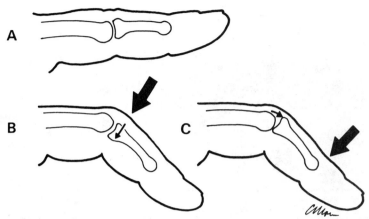

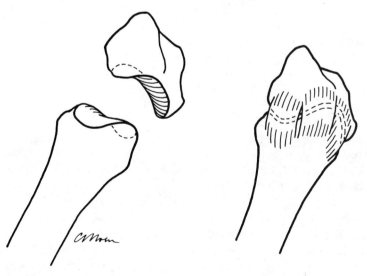

FIGURE 1-7. A normal interphalangeal joint in extension (A) and in flexion (B), showing the base of the middle phalanx moving down on the head of the proximal phalanx, and eventually under the head. (C) Application of a distal stretching force to a joint with limited motion. The base of the middle phalanx is pried away from, and compressed against, the proximal joint surface in an abnormal manner.

FIGURE 1-8. Sellar joint with concave and convex surfaces on each bone (carpal-metacarpal joint of thumb).

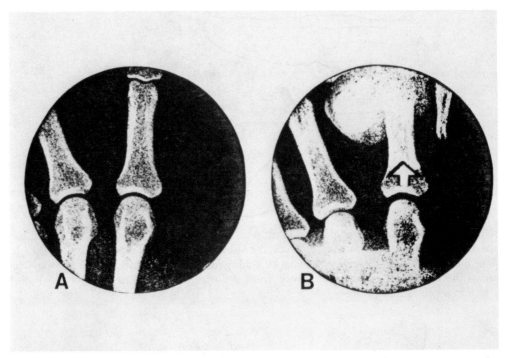

FIGURE 1-9. Radiograph of the metacarpo-phalangeal joint of the index finger at rest *(A)* and at the limit of long-axis extension *(B)*. The relationship of the articulating surfaces of the bones in *B* should be compared with their relationship with the joint at rest. Arrow indicates direction of pull by examiner. (From Mennell, JM: *Joint Pain: Diagnosis and Treatment Using Manipulative Techniques.* Little, Brown & Co, Boston, 1964, p 33, with permission.)

rider in a saddle. Examples of sellar joints are the carpal-metacarpal joint of the thumb, the elbow, the sterno-clavicular joint, and the ankle. The same principles of movement of the joint surfaces apply to the sellar types.

CONGRUENCY

Joint pairs match each other perfectly only in one position of the joint. This point of congruency (coinciding exactly) is called the *closed packed* position (MacConaill and Basmajian, 1969). In addition to the congruency of the joint surfaces in the closed packed position, the maximum area of surface contact occurs and the ligaments and the capsule become taut. The joint is mechanically compressed and cannot be distracted (separated). In all other positions, the joint surfaces do not fit perfectly but are incongruent and called *loose packed*. The ligamentous and capsular structures are slack, and the joint surfaces may be passively distracted several millimeters.

The closed packed position occurs in full extension at the elbow, wrist, interphalangeal, hip, and knee; dorsiflexion at the ankle; and flexion at the metacarpal-phalangeal joints. In these positions, the joint has additional rigidity with a reduction

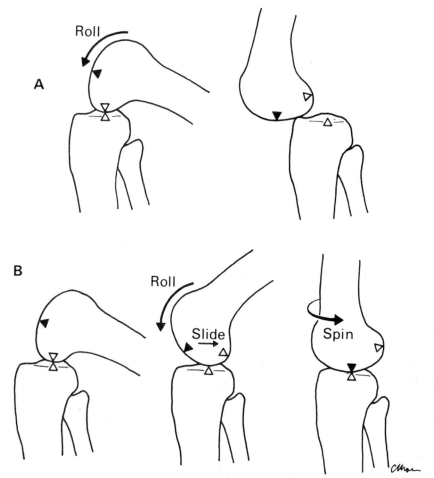

FIGURE 1-10. Movements of joint surfaces. *(A)* Pure rolling or hinge motion of the femur or the tibia would cause joint dislocation. *(B)* Normal motion of the knee demonstrates a combination of rolling, sliding, and spinning in the last 20 degrees of extension (terminal rotation of the knee).

in the need for muscle forces to provide stability. When the metacarpal-phalangeal joints are in 90 degrees of flexion, lateral motion (abduction) cannot occur and muscle force is not required to keep the fingers together during gripping. This "locking" mechanism occurs in the knee with complete extension (screw-home mechanism or terminal rotation) and permits humans to stand upright with little or no contraction of the muscles of the knee.

ACCESSORY MOTIONS

In addition to angular motions such as flexion or abduction, joint surfaces can be moved *passively* a few millimeters in translatory motion. These small motions are

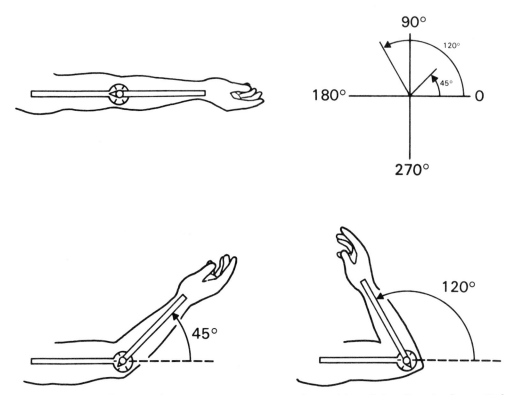

FIGURE 1-11. Application of a goniometer to measure the position of the elbow in the sagittal plane. The stationary arm of the goniometer is aligned parallel to the long axis of the subject's arm. The moving arm of the goniometer is aligned parallel to the long axis of the forearm, and the axis of the goniometer is placed over the axis of the elbow joint.

called *accessory movements* (Maitland, 1970) or joint play (Mennell, 1964). An example is distraction or separation of joint surfaces at the metacarpal-phalangeal joint (Fig. 1-9). In addition to distraction, the surfaces of freely movable joints may undergo lateral glide, anterior-posterior glide, and rotation. Accessory motions cannot be performed voluntarily by the subject, but rather require relaxation of muscles and the application of passive movement by an examiner. These small motions are essential for normal pain-free joint function and are performed by therapists in both the evaluation and treatment of joint motion problems. The importance of the presence of accessory motions can be appreciated in the arthrokinematic example of gleno-humeral joint abduction. If the necessary distal movement of the head of the humerus on the glenoid fossa is not present, elevation of the hand would be severely restricted— "frozen shoulder." The greater tuberosity may strike the acromion process instead of sliding beneath it. Striking the acromion process (and adjacent soft tissues) would produce additional injury and pain.

Mennell defines the condition of loss of normal joint play (movement) that is accompanied by pain as *joint dysfunction*. He describes a vicious cycle that occurs:

"1) When a joint is not free to move, the muscles that move it cannot be free to move it, 2) muscles cannot be restored to normal if the joints which they move are not free to move, 3) normal muscle function is dependent on normal joint movement, and 4) impaired muscle function perpetuates and may cause deterioration in abnormal joints."

MOVEMENTS OF JOINT SURFACES

When a joint moves, three types of motion can occur between the two surfaces: (1) rolling or rocking, (2) sliding or gliding, and (3) spinning. In a pure rolling motion such as a ball rolling on a table, each subsequent point on one surface contacts a new point on the other surface. In sliding and spinning, the same point on one surface contacts new points on the mating surface. *Most normal joint movement has some combination of rolling, sliding, and spinning.* The knee joint shows this most clearly. If there were only a rolling of the condyles of the femur on the tibial plateau, the femur would roll off the tibia and the knee would dislocate (Fig. 1-10, A). Instead, when the femur is extended on the fixed tibia as in rising from a seated to a standing position, the femoral condyles *roll and slide* so that they are always in contact with the tibial condyles (Fig. 1-10, B). In the last part of the knee extension, the femur spins (internally rotates on the tibia), and the knee is in the closed packed position.

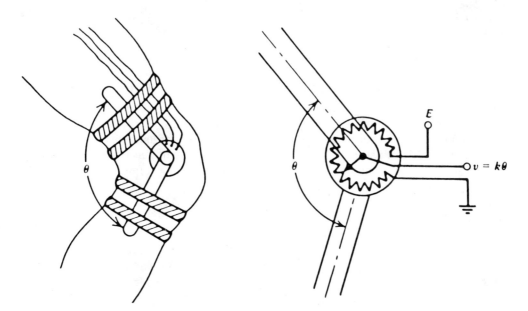

FIGURE 1-12. Mechanical and electric arrangement of a goniometer located at the knee joint. Voltage output is proportional to the joint angle and can be recorded on a moving strip chart. (From Winter, DA: *Biomechanics of Human Movement.* John Wiley & Sons, New York, 1979, p 12, with permission.)

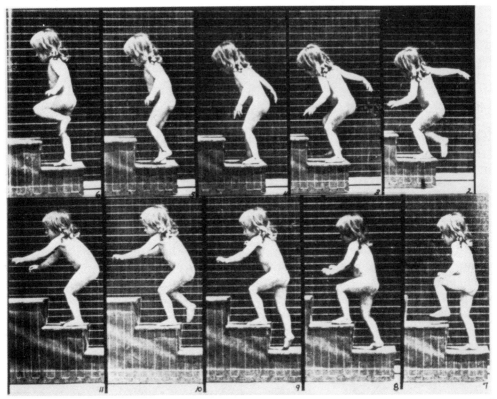

FIGURE 1-13. Serial photographs of child ascending steps, showing the changes in position of various joints. The action proceeds from right to left in each row of photographs. (From Muybridge, E: *The Human Figure in Motion.* Dover, New York, plate 190, reprinted in 1955 from original volume published in 1887, with permission.)

The combination of roll, slide, and spin thus permits a large range of motion while using a small articular surface. If joints possessed only one of these motions, the range of motion would be limited or joint surfaces would need to be larger to accomplish the same range of motion.

JOINT AXES

Because of the incongruity of joint surfaces and the motions of roll, slide, and spin, animal joint axes are complex. The axis does not remain stationary, as in a mechanical hinge joint, but moves as the joint position changes. The joint center usually follows a curved path (see page 290). The largest movement of the axes occurs in the knee, elbow, and wrist. In addition, the joint axes are seldom perpendicular to the long axes of the bones but are frequently oblique. This is particularly noticeable when the little finger is flexed into the palm. The tip of the finger points to the base of the thumb

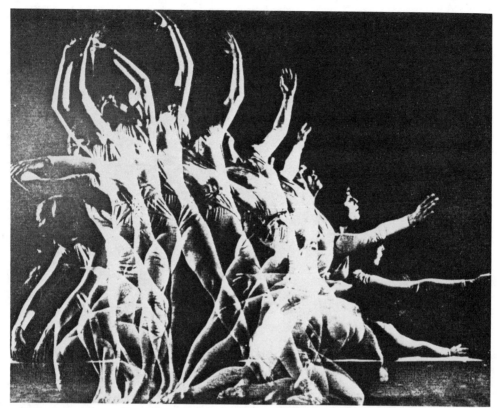

FIGURE 1-14. Pattern of motion of a dancer moving from one position to another. The superimposed images were produced by multiple exposures of one photographic negative. (From Jensen, CR and Schultz, GW: *Applied Kinesiology*, ed 2. McGraw-Hill, New York, 1977, p 183, with permission.)

rather than to the base of the fifth metacarpal. When the elbow is extended from full flexion with the forearm in supination, the forearm laterally deviates 0 to 20 degrees. This is called the "carrying angle" and is usually larger in females than in males.

These oblique axes and changing positions of the joint centers create problems and necessitate compromise when mechanical appliances and joints are applied to the body, as in goniometry, orthotics, and exercise equipment. Mechanical appliances usually have a fixed axis of motion that is perpendicular to the moving part. When the mechanical and anatomic parts are coupled, perfect alignment can occur at only *one point* in the range of motion. At other points in the range of motion, the mechanical appliance may bind and cause pressure on the body part, or it may force the human joint in abnormal directions. Thus, the placement of mechanical joints is critical where large ranges of motion are desired. Search continues for mechanical joints that more nearly approximate the complexity of human joints.

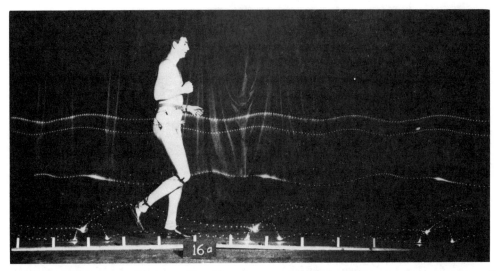

FIGURE 1-15. Interrupted light studies. The photograph was obtained by having a subject walk in front of the open lens of a camera in a dimly lit room while wearing small light bulbs located at the hip, knee, ankle, and foot. A slotted disk was rotated in front of the camera, producing a series of white dots at equal time intervals. These dots trace the motion of the part to which the light was attached. At one point in the study, a bright light was flashed to produce an image of the entire subject on the film. (From Inman, VT, Ralston, HJ, and Todd, F: *Human Walking.* Williams & Wilkins, Baltimore, 1981, p 12, with permission.)

Methods for Studying Motion of Body Segments

GONIOMETRY

Goniometry is an application of the coordinate system to a joint in order to measure the degrees of motion present in each plane. The goniometer, which is a protractor with two arms hinged at the origin, represents the plane. It is placed parallel to the two body segments to be measured and with the axis of the joint and the axis of the goniometer superimposed (Fig. 1-11). Thus, the position of the segments in the plane can be recorded. When joints have motions in several planes, as in the shoulder (flexion, abduction, and rotation), the goniometer is moved to each plane and axis for measurement. Average ranges of normal motion are listed in Appendix B at the end of this book, along with references on technique and positioning.

Even though degrees of joint motion may be measured, there is a great communication problem because two systems of recording exist. The system presented here uses 0 degrees as the reference point for the standard anatomic position (extension, adduction, and neutral rotation). Motions or positions of flexion, abduction, and internal and external rotation are recorded as they move toward 180 degrees. The second system uses 180 degrees as the reference point for the standard anatomic position and

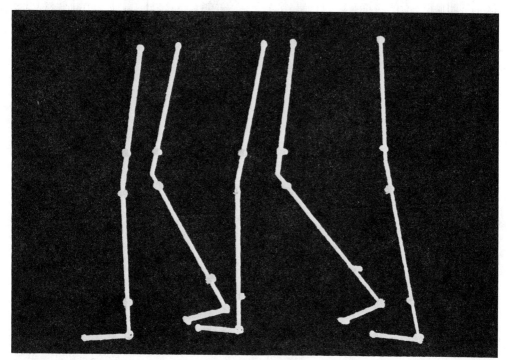

FIGURE 1-16. Computer-generated stick figures of a subject walking. Data for producing the stick figures came from tracking the movement of six light-emitting diodes (LED) taped to the subject's leg.

records flexion, abduction, and the rotations as they approach 0 degrees. Thus, the same position of the elbow would be reported in the first system as 120 degrees and in the second as 60 degrees. This not only is confusing when the system being used is not identified but can have serious consequences in interpretation of patient records.

ELECTROGONIOMETRY

Electrogoniometry is a technique for continuously and automatically recording joint movement. Figure 1-12 shows a simple electrogoniometer in which motion of one arm of the goniometer with respect to the other changes the voltage output of a potentiometer mounted over the axis of rotation of the goniometer. The output signal is amplified and recorded on a strip chart to provide a permanent record of the rate and amount of angular motion occurring at the joint. When the output of the potentiometer is suitably calibrated, the recorded signal can be read as degrees of motion.

PHOTOGRAPHIC TECHNIQUES

Photographic techniques were developed late in the 19th century for obtaining serial "stopped-action" photographs of animals and humans in motion. Figure 1-13 shows a

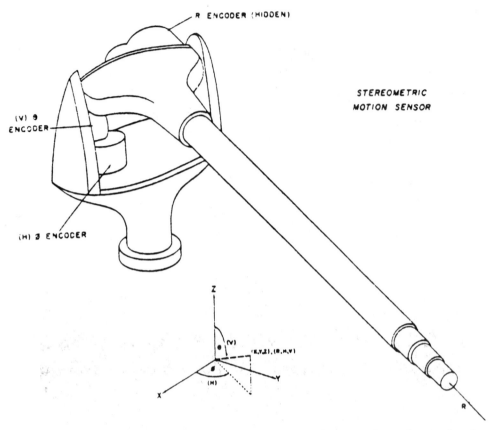

FIGURE 1-17. Design of stereometric motion sensor showing location of encoders used to determine spheric coordinates of points recorded during movement of the telescoping arm.

set of photographs published by Muybridge in 1887 that capture the changes in position of different parts of the body as a child ascends a stairway. Exposing a photographic negative several times in succession while a subject moves to a different position yields a series of "stopped-action" images superimposed on one another, as in Figure 1-14. The amount of displacement of a particular part (or parts) of the body can be measured from photographs taken under controlled conditions (Fig. 1-15). Since the time between each adjacent pair of white dots in Figure 1-15 is equal, a greater distance between dots indicates that the part was moving at a faster velocity. Many studies have been performed during the past 30 years to quantify the patterns of motion of body parts in able-bodied subjects and persons with impairments of neuromuscular function caused by disease or injury (Eberhart and Inman, 1951; Drillis, 1958; Murray, Drought, and Kory, 1964; Lamoreux, 1971; Soderberg and Gabel, 1978; Inman, Ralston, and Todd, 1981).

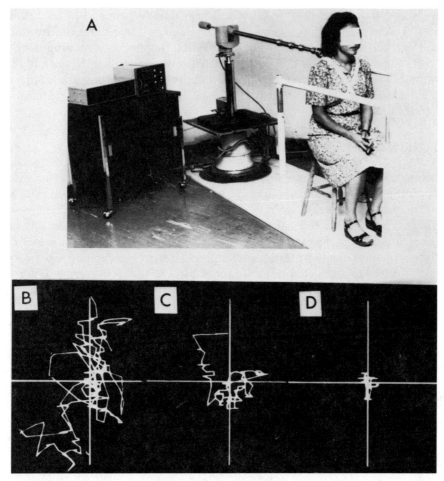

FIGURE 1-18. Biostereometric motion sensor being used to quantify postural stability of seated patient *(A)* at: 10 weeks *(B)*, 12 weeks *(C)*, and 20 weeks *(D)* after traumatic injury to the brain. Each tracing depicts the motion occurring in the horizontal plane during a 2-min test period.

SELSPOT APPARATUS

The *SELSPOT apparatus* (Lindholm, 1974; Florence et al, 1978; Larsson, Sandlund, and Oberg, 1978) provides a means for automatically recording movement with the aid of small sources of light attached to the body parts. In many respects, this is similar to photographic techniques, but a photosensitive transducer (photocell) is used instead of film. A special television camera containing the photocell is focused on the light-emitting spot. Movement of the lightspot image over the photocell generates an electric signal that is easy to record on magnetic tape and to analyze with a computer. The movement of several lightspot sources can be tracked by the same photocell and the output displayed on a television monitor as a moving stick figure (Fig. 1-16). The stick figure is generated by electronically connecting each of the dots representing the original light sources affixed to the body. Computer programs can be used to automatically detect and display the angle at each joint and to compute angular velocities of motion.

BIOSTEREOMETRIC MOTION SENSOR

The *biostereometric motion sensor* is another recently developed device for automatically recording and analyzing motion of body parts (Sheffer et al, 1978). The sensor (Fig. 1-17) consists of a lightweight telescoping rod with one end attached to a point permitting horizontal and vertical rotation about a pivot. Encoders detect any motion of the telescoping rod and generate an electric signal, which quantifies the motion and which is recorded on magnetic tape for later processing by a computer. The free end of the rod is attached to a selected point on the subject so that it is carried along in any motion of the part. Thus, movement of the body part is automatically tracked and recorded. Figure 1-18 illustrates the use of the biostereometric motion sensor as a means of measuring the postural sway of a patient recovering from traumatic injury of the brain. The dramatic reduction in extent of trunk excursions (compare Fig. 1-18, B with Fig. 1-18, D) while attempting to sit upright on a stool reflects improvement in control of the muscles that maintain posture of the seated subject.

CHAPTER 2

MECHANICAL PRINCIPLES: KINETICS

Kinetics, a branch of dynamics, *deals with forces that produce, arrest, or modify motions of bodies.* In applying principles of kinetics, the clinician is particularly concerned with the forces exerted by gravity, muscles, friction, and external resistances.

THEORIES OF MOTION

For more than 1500 years, the theories of Aristotle (384–322 BC) satisfactorily explained the cause of animal and human motion. The natural state was considered to be rest. Motion required a *mover* such as a horse pulling a wagon. When the mover stopped, the motion also stopped. Aristotelian theorists, however, had to give special properties to air and water in order to explain the movement of the arrow after it left the bowstring and the movement of the boat when the oars were out of the water. The missing element of this theory was the effect of the force of *friction* on motion. Even now, it is difficult to create a friction-free environment or to envision what motion would be like in the absence of friction. Galileo (1564–1642) by experimentation and deduction concluded that an external force was required to *change* the velocity of motion but that no force was needed to maintain motion. A very smooth block set in motion on a very smooth surface would continue in motion indefinitely if it did not meet resistance. Galileo's discoveries and those of others contributed to Newton's (1642–1727) development of the three laws of motion that form the current basis for mechanics and biomechanics.

Equilibrium

Fundamental in Newtonian mechanics is that the *natural state is equilibrium* (L. *aequilibrare*, to balance). In a state of equilibrium, the *sum of the forces* acting on the body is balanced or equal. A hockey puck resting on an ice rink is in equilibrium since the weight or force of the puck is balanced by an equal force on the rink. After the puck has been struck, it will again be in equilibrium and will move in a particular direction and at a particular velocity until other forces are impressed upon it. Friction between the ice–puck interface will slow the velocity of the puck, and collision with a stick or wall will change the direction and speed. Newton's first law, the law of inertia, states, *"Every body persists in its state of rest or of uniform motion in a straight line unless it is compelled to change that state by forces impressed on it"* (Resnick and Halliday, 1960). In simpler terms, it can be said that a force is required to start a motion, to change direction or speed of a motion, and to stop a motion.

Translatory applications of this law can be disastrous when a person is being transported in a wheelchair, on a stretcher, or in an automobile and the vehicle is stopped suddenly. Since the person is not attached to the vehicle, the body continues forward until stopped by another force. Fractured femurs are common injuries to patients who are thrown out of wheelchairs in this manner. Seat belts or restraining straps are recommended, and frequently required, to prevent injuries caused by abrupt stops of wheelchairs and stretchers, as well as of automobiles.

Clinical applications of the law of equilibrium affecting angular motion at a joint are found in the lower extremity during the swing phase of walking. Not only is a force required to start the leg moving (hip flexors), but also a force is required to stop the leg (hamstring muscles). The magnitude of this stopping force can be appreciated when walking barefooted in the dark and striking the toes against a rock, chair leg, or bedpost. Persons with above-knee amputations, on the other hand, do not have muscles to stop the swing of the prosthetic leg. The problem of permitting the leg to swing without overswinging requires careful adjustment of the frictional forces in the joint of the artificial knee.

MASS AND ACCELERATION

The same force or forces acting on different bodies will cause the bodies to move differently. The property of a body that resists change in motion or equilibrium is defined as *inertia*. Newton's second law of motion states: *The acceleration (a) of a body is proportional to the magnitude of the resultant forces (F) on it and inversely proportional to the mass (m) of the body.* As an equation, this is written:

$$a \propto \frac{F}{m}$$

More simply stated, a greater force is required to move (or stop the motion of) a large mass than a small one.

Application of this law is demonstrated in the movement of body segments in response to muscle contraction. When a muscle contracts, it shortens and produces the same amount of force at its proximal and distal attachments (origin and insertion). Thus, *either one or both* segments may move. This can be seen in a subject performing a sit-up. Since the hip flexor muscles (iliopsoas) attach to the trunk and to the femur, the part with the least mass will move when the muscles contract forcefully. Individuals with relatively light mass in their lower extremities have difficulty in performing a sit-up because the lower extremities will elevate before the trunk. Stabilization of the lower extremities is needed to perform the desired motion. Other clinical applications of the law of inertia are seen with changes in the mass of segments. When the mass is increased, as in walking with heavy boots or a cast on the leg, greater muscle force is needed to start and stop the leg swing. In patients with muscle weakness (inability to develop adequate muscle force), one of the important considerations is to keep the mass of appliances (such as splints and adapted equipment) as light as possible in order to reduce the muscle force requirements.

Weight

The basic equation describing the relationship among acceleration, force, and mass can also be written as $F = ma$. With this equation, the concept of *weight* can be differentiated from mass. Weight (W) is the effect of the acceleration of gravity (g) on a mass. Thus, the equation for weight is $W = mg$. Weight, then, is a force and is expressed in pounds, Newtons, or dynes. Mass is expressed in slugs, kilograms, or grams (Tables 2-1, 2-2). The weight of a body varies with its location from the center of the earth, whereas the mass (inertia) always remains the same. Although this difference has little importance in clinical kinesiology, it is of major importance in space kinesiology and the understanding of humans' ability to move and perform work in a gravity-reduced environment such as the moon. When an astronaut in space reaches forward or attempts to push a lever or door, the body will move in the opposite direction from the work because there is insufficient weight to stabilize the body. In order to stabilize the body, toe-holds and clamps are needed. One clinical environment in which the weight of a subject is reduced is the therapeutic pool. Here, very weak muscles can move body parts and be exercised. As in space, the therapist may need to grasp fixed objects in order to stabilize oneself or the patient so that the desired motions can be carried out.

TABLE 2-1. Systems Commonly Used to Express Weights and Measures

System	Mass	Force	Distance	Torque	Time
B.E.	slug	pound	foot	lb-ft	sec
MKS	kg	Newton	meter	N-m	sec
cgs	gram	dyne	cm	dyne-cm	sec

B.E.=British Engineering (foot, pound, sec); MKS=meter, kilogram, second; cgs=centimeter, gram, second

TABLE 2-2. Conversion Factors

Mass

1 slug (sg)	= 14.59 kilograms (kg)
1 gram (gm)	= 0.001 kilogram (kg)

Force

1 pound (lb)	= 4.448 Newtons (N)
1 dyne	= 0.00001 Newton (N)
1 pound (lb)	= 2.2 kilograms (kg)*

Distance

1 foot (ft)	= 30.48 centimeters (cm)
1 inch (in)	= 2.54 centimeters (cm)
1 centimeter (cm)	= 0.01 meter (m)

Torque (bending moment)

1 pound-foot (ft-lb)	= 1.356 Newton-meters (N-m)
1 dyne-centimeter (dyne-cm) =	0.0000001 Newton-meter (N-m)

*The kilogram is a unit of mass, but it is commonly used as a unit of force instead of the correct unit, Newton.

Forces

A simple way to define force is to say that it is a push (compression) or a pull (tension). Therapeutically, four primary sources of force are of major concern to the therapist:

1. *Gravity* or weight of body parts and attachments such as splints, casts, eating utensils, books, or weights.
2. *Muscles*, which can produce forces on the bone segments by active contraction or by being passively stretched.
3. *Externally applied resistances* such as exercise pulleys, manual resistance, doors, or windows.
4. *Friction*, the ever-present friend and foe.

Application of these primary forces may, in turn, lead to three secondary consequences of considerable clinical importance:

1. Joint compression.
2. Joint distraction.
3. Pressure (force per unit area) on body tissues.

The understanding of where, how, and to what degree these forces act permits their manipulation to increase motion, restore function, and relieve pain.

FORCE CONVENTIONS AND DEFINITIONS

Forces are vector quantities since they have both magnitude and direction, as opposed to scalar quantities, which have magnitude only (e.g., 6 books or 12 oranges). Vectors are visualized graphically by a *line of action*, an arrowhead showing *direction*, and a *point of attachment* (Fig. 2-1). The line of action is drawn to an arbitrary scale to show the magnitude of the force. The tail of the vector is the point of attachment and represents the application of the force to another body. The arrowhead is called the *sense* and indicates the direction of the force. Vectors are located in space by placement on the coordinate system. Vectors whose directions are to the right or up are given a positive sign (+), and vectors with a direction to the left or down are given a negative sign (−).

Action and Reaction

Each of the forces acting on a body or part *arises from another* body. Thus, forces do not act in isolation but rather as an *interactive* pair where the two bodies come in contact. A weight held in the hand creates a 10-lb (44.5 N) force on the hand, and the hand resists the weight with a 10-lb force. A muscle pulls on a bone, and the bone reacts with an equal and opposite force as seen in Figure 2-1. Newton's third law of motion states that *for every action, there is an equal and opposite reaction*. Thus, whenever two bodies are in contact, they exert equal and opposite forces on each other.

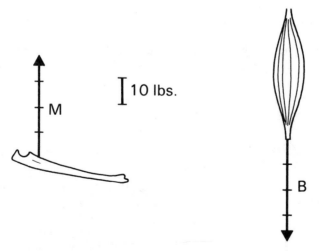

FIGURE 2-1. Vector representation of the force of the brachialis muscle (M) contraction on the bone, and of the force of the bone (B) on the muscle.

Free Body Diagram

Newton's third law of action and reaction is used as a method to visualize and calculate forces. One body is shown, and the other bodies that touch it or affect it are replaced by force vectors (Figs. 2-3, B; 2-8, I and II). In engineering, this is called the *free body diagram*. The body or segment of interest is drawn in isolation, and the other bodies or forces acting upon it are represented by their force vectors.

COMPOSITION OF FORCES

Frequently, several forces act simultaneously on a body (Fig. 2-2). In order to simplify and better visualize the magnitude and direction of such multiple forces, the process of composition of forces is used. By adding or subtracting two or more forces, their combined effect can be shown by a single *resultant force*. This resultant force is the simplest force (or force system) that can produce the same effect as all the forces acting together. If two or more forces act along a line or parallel lines, the forces can be added to find the single resultant force. In Figure 2-3, the weights of the leg and the exercise apparatus form a linear force system that causes distraction of the knee joint. The magnitude of the distracting force can be found by graphic composition of forces (drawing the force vectors to scale) or by algebraic composition of forces (see Fig. 2-3, D) using the formula that the resultant force (R) is equal to the sum of the individual forces (R = ΣF). In both methods, the resultant force is the same and has the same effect on the femur as the three original forces.

Similar procedures can be used to find the resultant force in a linear force system when the forces act in opposite directions, as occurs when applying a 25-lb (111.2 N) traction force to the cervical structures with the subject sitting upright (Fig. 2-4). In this case, the upward force on the cervical spine is only 15 lb (66.7 N).

Forces Acting at Angles

The resultant force of vector forces in the same plane acting at angles to each other cannot be found by simple addition or subtraction, but must be found graphically or

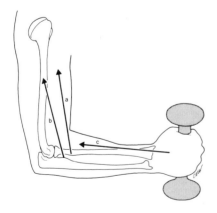

FIGURE 2-2. Vector representation of forces developed by the biceps brachialis (a), brachialis (b), and a combination of the brachio-radialis, extensor carpi radialis longus, and extensor carpi radialis brevis muscles (c) when the subject lifts an exercise weight with the hand and forearm.

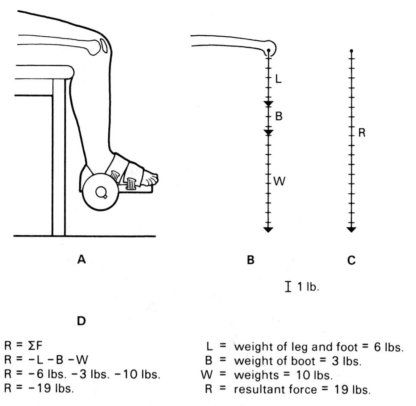

A   B   C

I 1 lb.

D

R = ΣF   L = weight of leg and foot = 6 lbs.
R = −L −B −W   B = weight of boot = 3 lbs.
R = −6 lbs. −3 lbs. −10 lbs.   W = weights = 10 lbs.
R = −19 lbs.   R = resultant force = 19 lbs.

FIGURE 2-3. Forces acting at the knee joint when the subject is sitting with an exercise-boot and weight on the foot: (A) Anatomic diagram. (B) Free body diagram of the forces on the femur. (C) Graphic composition of the resultant force. (D) Algebraic composition of the resultant force (negative sign indicates that the direction of the force is down).

trigonometrically. If two forces are pulling from the same point, the resultant force can be found graphically by constructing a parallelogram (Fig. 2-5). The resultant force is the diagonal of the parallelogram, not the sum of the two forces. Note that as the angle between the two forces increases, the resultant force decreases, reaching a minimum when the forces are on the same line and acting in opposite directions, when the angle becomes 180 degrees. Conversely, as the angle between the forces becomes smaller, the resultant force increases. When the angle becomes zero, the forces are on the same line, and the resultant force is the sum of the two forces. Thus, in the leg traction example, if the patient moves toward the head of the bed, the angle between the ropes will become smaller, and the traction force will increase. If the patient moves toward the foot of the bed, the angle between the ropes will become larger, and the traction force will decrease. The same effects would occur if someone moved the fixed pulleys on the bed post farther apart or closer together.

Other examples of forces acting at angles to each other occur in muscles where parts may have different lines of pull. Examples include contraction of the upper and

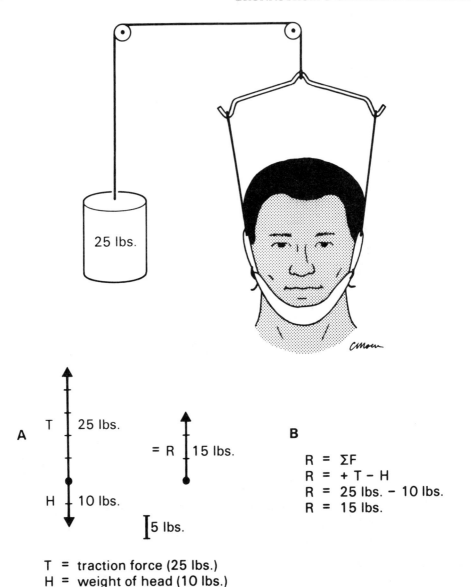

T = traction force (25 lbs.)
H = weight of head (10 lbs.)

FIGURE 2-4. Graphic (A) and algebraic (B) solutions for the force applied to the head and neck structures when an upward force of 25 lb is applied to the head, which weighs 10 lb.

lower trapezius to result in adduction of the scapula, and contraction of the two heads of the gastrocnemius with a resultant force on the tendon of Achilles.

When more than two forces are acting, the resultant force can be obtained graphically by forming a *polygon*. One force vector is drawn to scale and placed in its proper direction. Subsequent vectors are drawn in the same manner, and the tail of each

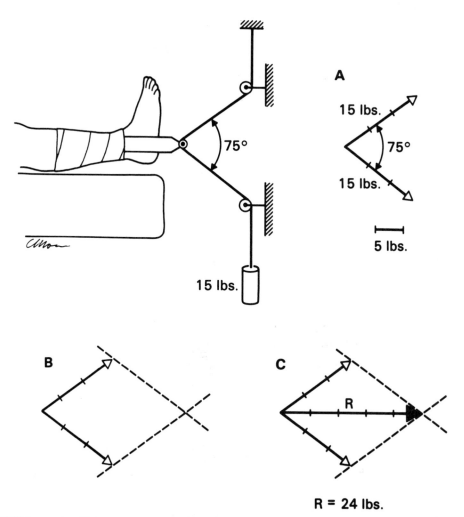

FIGURE 2-5. Parallelogram method to find the resultant traction force on the leg. *(A)* The force vectors acting on the leg are drawn to scale. *(B)* Lines are drawn parallel to each force vector from the sense of the other vector to form a parallelogram. *(C)* The resultant force is the diagonal from the origin of the forces. The magnitude can be found by measuring the length of the action line.

vector is placed at the tip of the previous vector (Fig. 2-6). This process forms a polygon that is open on one side. *The resultant force closes the polygon.* Measurement of the magnitude and the angle of the resultant force shows the single effect of the diverse forces.

In actuality, the parallelogram method for two forces is a special case of the polygon method. Instead of drawing a parallelogram, one could draw the second force tail to tip on the first. Closing the triangle forms the resultant force. Algebraic solutions of

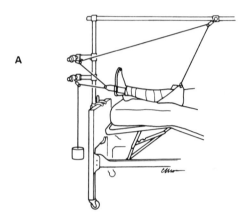

A

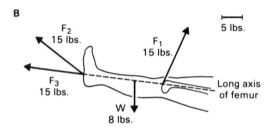

B

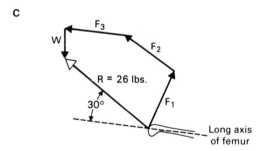

C

FIGURE 2-6. Polygon method for composition of forces using Russell's traction, which applies a distraction force on the femur (A). Fifteen lb of weight are suspended on the weight carrier. The leg, foot, and foot piece weigh 8 lb. (B) Scale diagram of the forces acting on the femur. (C) The force vectors are connected serially according to their angle and direction. The open side of the polygon is the single resultant force. In this case, the traction force on the femur is 26 lb and is acting at a 30-degree angle from the long axis of the femur. Realignment of the pulleys is needed to bring the resultant force in line with the long axis of the femur.

the resultant force for the triangle and polygon can be found using the cosine law of trigonometry (LeVeau, 1977).

LEVERS

A machine that operates on the principle of a rigid bar being acted upon by forces which tend to rotate the bar about its pivot point is called a lever. In biomechanics, the principles of the lever are used to visualize the more complex system of forces that produce rotary motion in the body. By reducing these forces to their simplest form of *three resultant forces*, approximate magnitudes of forces and displacement of segments can be found, and the basis for therapeutic manipulation of forces can be better understood.

The three forces of the mechanical lever are the axis A (or pivot), the weight W (or resistance R), and the moving (or holding) force F (Fig. 2-7). The perpendicular distance from the pivot point (or center of rotation) to the line of action of the weight is called the weight arm. The perpendicular distance from the holding force to the axis is called the force arm.

Mechanical advantage (MA) of the lever refers to the ratio between the length of the force arm and the length of the weight arm. The equation is:

$$MA = \frac{\text{Force arm length}}{\text{Weight arm length}}$$

The ratios for the lever systems shown in Figure 2-7 would be: I = 1, II = 2, and III = 0.5. The higher the number, the greater the mechanical advantage. An increase in the length of the force arm or a decrease in the length of the weight arm (or resistance arm) results in greater mechanical advantage, thus facilitating the task to be performed.

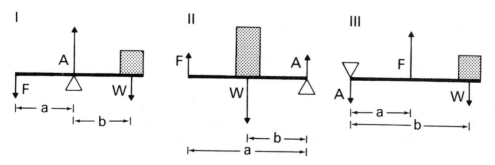

FIGURE 2-7. Vector diagrams of the first-, second-, and third-class levers. Classification is according to the positions of the weight and force in relation to the axis. A = axis or fulcrum; W = weight or resistance; F = moving or holding force; a = force arm distance; b = weight or resistance arm distance.

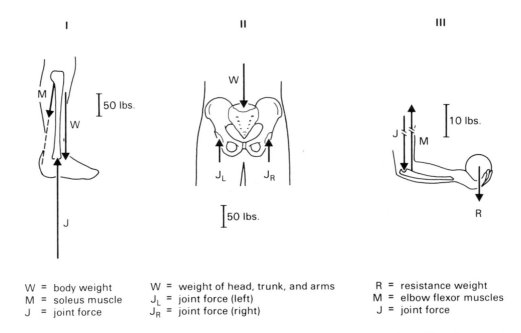

W = body weight   W = weight of head, trunk, and arms   R = resistance weight
M = soleus muscle   J_L = joint force (left)   M = elbow flexor muscles
J = joint force   J_R = joint force (right)   J = joint force

FIGURE 2-8. Anatomic examples of the three lever systems: (I) Forces at the ankle when standing on one foot. (II) Forces on the pelvis when standing on both feet. (III) Forces on the forearm
when holding a weight in the hand (weight of the forearm neglected). The break in vectors (J
and M in III) indicates their magnitude is not drawn to scale.

In angular motions or postures of the body, the bone or segment is the lever, and the
axis is usually at the joint. Muscle contraction is the holding or moving force, and the
resistance is the weight of the part, body segments, or applied resistances (Fig. 2-8).
Different positions of these forces on the lever arm give different advantages for motion and work. The operation of levers provides *either force or speed advantages.*

First-Class Lever

First-class levers, such as the seesaw or balance scale, may be used to gain either force
or distance, depending on the relative lengths of the force arm and the weight arm.
This principle is used in the forearm trough of the ball bearing feeder (Fig. 2-9) by
moving the axis proximally or distally. In the body, the first-class lever system is
frequently used for maintaining postures or balance (see Fig. 2-8, I). An example is
found at the atlanto-occipital joint (axis), where the head (weight) is balanced by neck
extensor muscle force. The same principle occurs at the intervertebral joints in sitting
or standing, where the weight of the trunk is balanced by the erector spinae muscle
forces acting on the vertebral axis. This type of lever arrangement is commonly used
in orthotics to apply a support or correctional force to body parts (Fig. 2-10), and is
frequently called the *three point* system for applying a force.

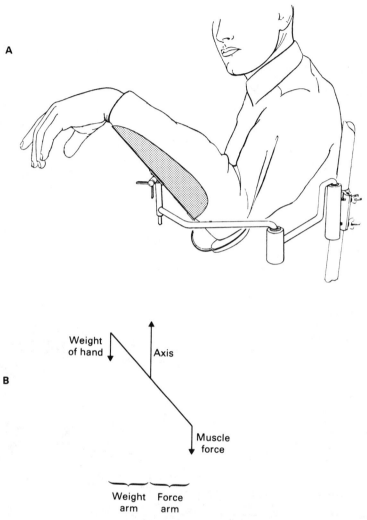

FIGURE 2-9. Ball bearing forearm orthosis (feeder) used by patients who have severe muscle weakness of the elbow and shoulder (A). The trough is an example of a first-class lever system (B). With careful placement of the axis to gain the proper weight arm and force arm distances, patients with very little muscle strength can feed and groom themselves. (Adapted from Licht, S and Kamenetz, H: *Orthotics Etcetera*. Elizabeth Licht, Publisher, 1966, p 219.)

Second-Class Lever

Second-class levers provide a force advantage such that large weights can be supported or moved by a smaller force. The wheelbarrow and the use of a crowbar for prying are mechanical examples of this type of leverage. In the body, there are limited examples of the second-class lever. The forces on the floor when a person is standing

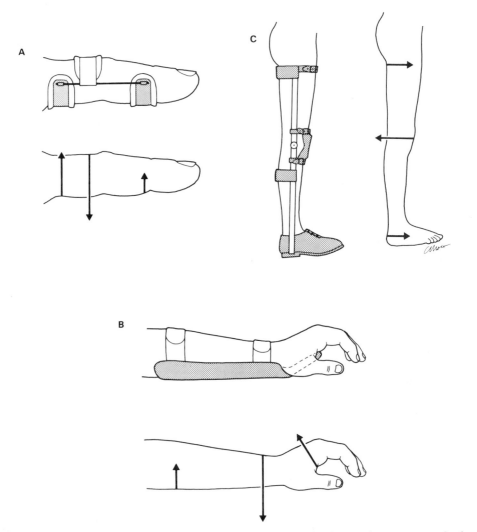

FIGURE 2-10. Examples of static positioning orthoses and the forces they exert on the body part. *(A)* Interphalangeal extension splint. *(B)* Cock-up splint to maintain wrist extension. *(C)* Knee ankle foot orthosis (KAFO) to prevent knee flexion.

on both feet would be an example, as would the forces at the hip joints in bilateral stance (see Fig. 2-8, II). The only muscle example is the pull of the brachio-radialis and the wrist extensors to maintain the position of elbow flexion. Normally, however, these muscles do not act in this isolated manner. Some patients with muscular dystrophy who have paralysis of the biceps brachii and brachialis muscles can use the brachio-radialis and wrist extensors to hold the elbow in a position of flexion. If anything heavy is held in the hand, however, the system changes to a third-class lever, and the brachio-radialis and wrist extensor muscle forces cannot maintain the position.

Third-Class Lever

The third-class lever is more common in the body. In this type of leverage, the weight arm is always longer than the force arm, and the mechanical advantage may be 0.1 or even lower. This arrangement is designed for producing *speed* of the distal segment and for moving a small weight a long distance. Thus, in the human body, a small amount of shortening of a muscle such as the brachialis causes a large arc of motion of the hand. This type of leverage is found in most open-chain motions of the extremities: the deltoid acting on the gleno-humeral joint, the flexor digitorum profundus and superficialis at the interphalangeal joints, the extensor carpi radialis at the wrist, the anterior tibialis at the ankle joint, and the biceps-brachialis at the elbow (see Fig. 2-8, III).

All three types of levers demonstrate that *what is gained in speed or distance is lost in force* and, conversely, *what is gained in force is lost in speed.*

Static Equilibrium

More important than memorization of the lever systems is recognition of the commonalities of the placement, directions, and magnitudes of the three forces. Review of the force vector diagrams in Figures 2-7, 2-8, 2-9, and 2-10 shows that *all* have a *large central force in one direction flanked by two smaller forces in the opposite direction.* The central force is equal in magnitude to the sum of the magnitudes of the two other forces when the three forces are parallel. In the first-class lever system (Fig. 2-7), A = F + W or A − F − W = 0. The single *resultant* force for this system would be zero, since the direction (sign) of A is positive and the directions of F and W are negative. The system is in equilibrium (at rest or in uniform motion) when the *resultant of all the forces acting on the system is zero.* In the fundamental equation of mechanics, F = ma, F represents the resultant of *all* forces acting on the body. Thus, if the sum of these forces equals zero ($\Sigma F = 0$), there would be no acceleration. *Statics,* then, is a special case of dynamics when there is no acceleration. The simpler formulas of statics can be used to illustrate the placement and magnitude of the forces that occur in the body in the majority of therapeutic situations. For example, it can be shown that in standing, the force between the joint surfaces (e.g., the force on the tibia when standing on one leg) is greater than the superincumbent body weight (weight of segments above the joint). Referring to Figure 2-8, I, we see that the center-of-gravity line (W) of the body falls not through the ankle joint, but slightly anterior to the lateral malleolus. The axis of motion (or potential motion) is the ankle joint (J). The person is prevented from falling forward at the ankle (dorsiflexion) by contraction of the soleus muscle (M) whose proximal attachment is on the tibia and distal attachment is on the calcaneus. Using a body weight of 150 lb (667.2 N) and positive signs for upward forces and negative signs for downward forces, the equation would be:

$$\Sigma F = 0$$
$$- M + J - W = 0$$
$$- M + J - 150 \text{ lb} = 0$$
$$J = 150 \text{ lb} + M$$

The compression force on the ankle is 150 lb *plus* the force the muscle must exert to maintain the position. Calculation of the magnitude of the muscle and joint forces, however, requires the use of lever arm distances and torque.

Torque

Torque (τ), or moment of a force, is the product of a force times the perpendicular distance from its line of action to the axis of motion (or potential motion). The equation is $\tau = F(\perp d)$. Torque is the expression of the effectiveness of a force in turning a lever system. A common example is represented by attempts to open a door that is stuck. One may push or pull at the center of the door with all the force that can be mustered and not open the door. If, however, this same force is applied as far as possible from the door hinges (axis), the force will be more effective in opening the door (increased length of the force arm). Using a simple mechanical lever, such as the seesaw, a 50-lb (222.4 N) child can balance a 100-lb (444.8 N) child *if* the lever arm distance for the 50-lb child is twice the length of the lever arm distance for the 100-lb child. Extending this principle further, the resistance of the 100-lb child could be balanced by fingertip pressure *if* the force lever arm were very long. This principle is used by therapists in testing the strength of muscles (manual muscle testing) and in applying manual resistive exercise. For example, in testing the strength of the elbow flexors, the therapist would prefer to apply resistance at the wrist rather than in the middle of the forearm. In each case, the *torque* produced by the patient's elbow flexors would be the same. The *force* that the therapist applied, however, would be approximately one half less at the wrist than at the mid-forearm because of the longer resistance arm. This lower force provides the therapist with better control and discrimination of the torque produced by the patient.

In Figure 2-11, the subject is shown holding an exercise weight in the hand with the shoulder in three positions of flexion. At the shoulder, the torque produced by the weight varies with the *perpendicular distance from the line of action of the force (weight) to the joint center.* The perpendicular distance is then the resistance arm. Thus, the torque produced by the weight increases as the hand is brought away from the body, and reaches the maximum at 90 degrees of shoulder flexion. The torque then decreases again as shoulder flexion continues. *Only* when the line of action of a force is perpendicular to the lever arm is the distance the same as the actual lever arm. (The procedure for resolution of forces on page 41 provides for use of a perpendicular component of the force whereby the actual lever arm length can be used.)

Clinically, torque reduction is emphasized in lifting and carrying in order to prevent strain or injury to the person lifting. For example, in the two- or three-person lift

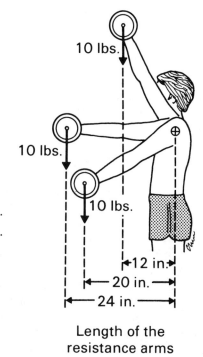

$$\tau \quad = F \times \perp d$$
$$\tau_{60°} = 10 \text{ lbs. x 20 in.} = 200 \text{ in.lbs.}$$
$$\tau_{90°} = 10 \text{ lbs. x 24 in.} = 240 \text{ in.lbs.}$$
$$\tau_{150°} = 10 \text{ lbs. x 12 in.} = 120 \text{ in.lbs.}$$

FIGURE 2-11. Variation of the resistance torque at the shoulder when a 10-lb weight is held in the hand and the shoulder is flexed to 60, 90, and 150 degrees.

and transfer of a patient from bed to stretcher or wheelchair, instructions include *sliding* the patient close to the edge of the bed (and to the bodies of the lifters) before attempting to lift the patient. The next instruction is to lift and quickly *roll* the patient toward the lifters' chests. The moves of first sliding and then rolling the patient bring the patient's center of gravity closer to the center of gravity of the lifters, thus reducing the torque and likelihood of injury from excessive strain.

At equilibrium when no motion or acceleration of the body is occurring, the torque of the resistance force will equal the torque of the holding force: force times the force arm equals resistance times the resistance arm. In the lever examples in Figure 2-7, the equation would be F × a = W × b for each type of lever. The general equation is derived from Newton's first law. If a body is in equilibrium, the *sum of the resultant forces equals zero and therefore the sum of the torques must also be balanced and equal to zero.* The equation for torque at equilibrium is $\Sigma\tau = 0$.

The conventions used to indicate direction of torques are positive (+) and negative (−) signs. If the torque produces (or tends to produce) a clockwise (CW) motion of the lever or coordinate system, the sign is positive. If the torque tends to produce a counterclockwise (CCW) motion, the sign is negative. In Figure 2-7, placing the axes (A) of the levers at the origin of the coordinate system would cause the equations to be properly written as:

$$I - (F \times a) + (W \times b) = 0$$
$$II + (F \times a) - (W \times b) = 0$$
$$III - (F \times a) + (W \times b) = 0$$

In all three cases, however, the formula would reduce to $F \times a = W \times b$. A force acting at the origin of the coordinate system such as the axis (A) in the above examples has *no effect in turning* the lever or system since the distance to the axis is zero. This force, therefore, does not appear in *torque* equations. Thus, placement of the origin of the coordinate system at the origin of an unknown force conveniently eliminates one unknown value from torque equations.

In the shoulder flexion diagram (see Fig. 2-11), the torque of the resistance varied with the weight arm distance and was at a maximum of 20 ft-lb when the extremity was horizontal. At equilibrium, the shoulder flexor muscles also must produce an equal torque at each position ($\Sigma\tau = 0$). The force arm of the muscles is, however, only a few inches long. Thus the muscles must exert great forces (more than 10 times that of the weight) to hold the weight at the 2-ft distance. If the elbow is flexed, the torque produced by the weight is reduced along with the muscle torque and, therefore, the force that the muscle must produce is also decreased.

Attention to torque alterations and the effect on forces is important in orthotic applications. Shortening of a lever arm will increase the force applied to body parts and therefore increase the pressure on those parts. Conversely, lengthening of a lever arm can decrease forces. An example of such changes can be seen in the dynamic outrigger handsplint used to assist in opening the hand (Fig. 2-12).

The equilibrium equation for torque ($\Sigma\tau = 0$) permits the finding of the magnitude of muscle and joint forces that cannot be measured directly. If the forces are all perpendicular to the lever arm (as in the parallel force systems in Figs. 2-7 and 2-8, II and III) and the distances that the forces act from each other are measured, then the magnitude of the unknown joint and muscle forces can be found easily. Even when the forces are not precisely parallel (as in Fig. 2-8, I), the equation is useful to demonstrate *concepts and approximations* both of the tremendous forces that the normal healthy body can sustain and of the minimal muscle and joint forces needed to provide functional use of the body. As an example, the ankle problem has been redrawn in Figure 2-13 with the use of approximate lever arm distances of 1 inch (2.5 cm) from the ankle joint center for the weight line and 2 inches (5.1 cm) from the joint center for the distal attachment of the soleus. The force vectors are placed on the coordinate system with the joint force (J) coinciding with the origin. Using the formula that the $\Sigma\tau = 0$ solves for the magnitude of the soleus muscle force at 75 lb (333.6 N). Using the formula that the $\Sigma F = 0$ solves for the magnitude of the joint force at 225 lb (1000 N).

If the person illustrated in Figure 2-13 swayed forward slightly so that the gravity line fell 2 inches (5 cm) in front of the ankle center, the soleus muscle would need to produce 150 lb (667 N) of force to prevent the person from falling (maintain equilibrium). The joint force would then increase to 300 lb (1334 N). This problem can be as easily solved by placing the soleus force at the origin of the coordinate system and solving first for J. The problem is not as easy to solve if the body weight vector were placed at the origin, since the equation would then contain *two* unknown forces.

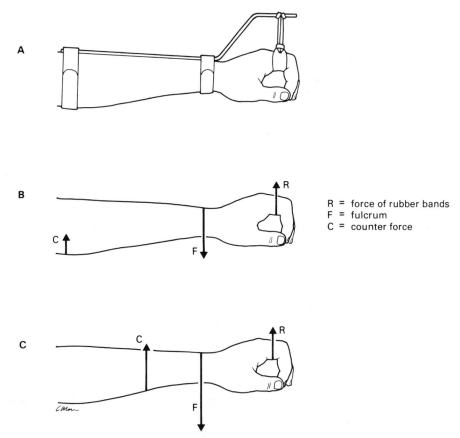

FIGURE 2-12. (A) Forearm splint for assisting finger extension. (B) Forces exerted on the forearm and hand. (C) Increase in counterforce "C" (and consequently in "F") when the forearm lever arm is reduced in length.

Resolution of Forces

Many of the forces that occur in or on the body are applied at angles to the segment rather than in a linear or parallel system, as in previous examples. Figure 2-14 shows an example in which the forces (W, M, and J) are neither parallel to each other nor perpendicular to the lever arm. *Resolution of a force* into two component forces is used (1) to visualize the effect of such angular forces on the body, (2) to determine the torque produced by the forces, and (3) to calculate the magnitude of unknown muscle and joint forces. The process is based on the principle that any number can be represented by two or more different numbers (e.g., 7 can be represented by 6 + 1 or 5 + 2). Thus, any vector can be represented by two or more vectors. Resolution of a force vector is the division of the vector into two or more *component vectors* whose combined magnitudes and directions produce the same effect as the original force

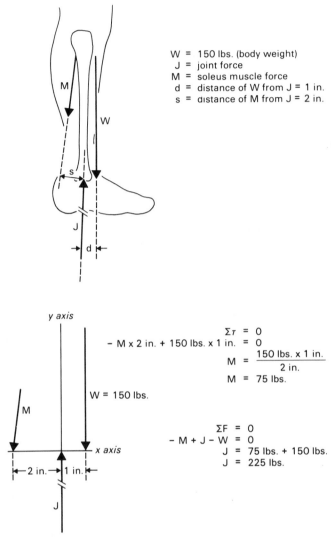

W = 150 lbs. (body weight)
J = joint force
M = soleus muscle force
d = distance of W from J = 1 in.
s = distance of M from J = 2 in.

$\Sigma \tau$ = 0

– M x 2 in. + 150 lbs. x 1 in. = 0

$$M = \frac{150 \text{ lbs. x 1 in.}}{2 \text{ in.}}$$

M = 75 lbs.

ΣF = 0

– M + J – W = 0

J = 75 lbs. + 150 lbs.

J = 225 lbs.

FIGURE 2-13. Diagram and equations for the forces on the tibia during unilateral stance with approximate calculations of the magnitudes of the muscle (M) and joint compression (J) forces.

(Fig. 2-15). In biomechanics, *two rectangular components* are drawn from the point of the original force so that *two right triangles are formed,* with the original force as the common hypotenuse. The rectangular (right angle) components are formed, first, by drawing a line of action *perpendicular* to the x (or y) axis of the coordinate system and, second, by drawing a line of action *parallel* to the x (or y) axis. The magnitudes of the two component forces are found by drawing lines parallel to the component forces that *intersect at the sense of the original force.*

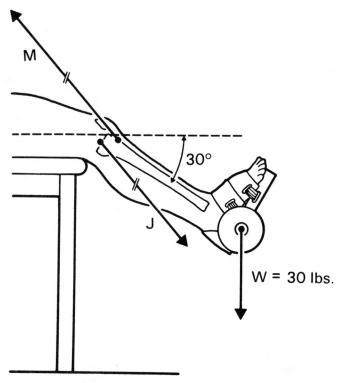

FIGURE 2-14. Forces acting on the leg (tibia) when the seated subject has an exercise weight on the foot and the knee is in 30 degrees of flexion. The weight of the leg and foot have been omitted in this example.

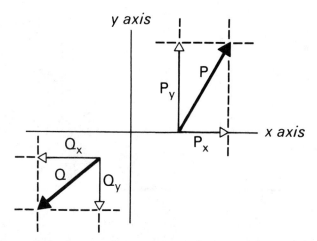

FIGURE 2-15. Resolution of force vectors P and Q into two components (Py, Px and Qy, Qx) whose combined magnitude and direction will produce the same effect as the original force.

In Figure 2-16, the coordinate system has been placed on the leg so that the x axis coincides with the long axis of the tibia. The quadriceps muscle force (M) and the resistance force (W) have been resolved into their rectangular components. The *perpendicular component* (M, or W,) is called the *rotary component* or the *rotary force*. It is that part of the original force (M or W) that is effective in causing rotary motion of the segment around the axis (or maintaining a posture or resisting a motion). In the example, the quadriceps muscle (M), with a line of pull at an acute angle to the tibia, must produce a relatively large force in order to create a sufficient rotary component (M,) to maintain the knee in extension. Conversely, the weight (W) acting at an acute angle to the long axis of the segment resists extension of the knee—not with the full force of 30 lb, but with the smaller rotary component W,. Only when the weight acts at a 90-degree angle (perpendicular) to the segment is the rotary force the same magnitude as the weight. Since the rotary component is perpendicular to the long axis, the measurement of distances to calculate torque ($\tau = F \perp d$) is simplified. Torque of the

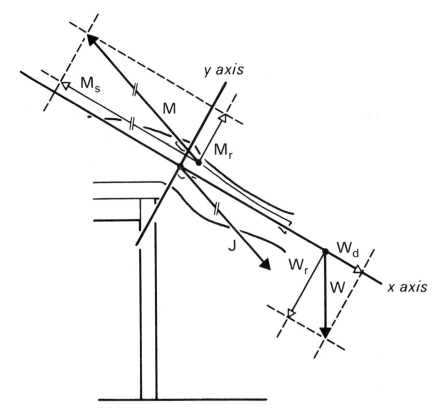

FIGURE 2-16. Resolution of the resistance (W) and muscle (M) forces from Figure 2-14 into rectangular components. The rotary components (W, and M,) are *perpendicular* to the long axis of the segment. The stabilizing component of the muscle force (M$_s$) and the distracting component of the weight (W$_d$) are *parallel* to the long axis of the segment. (The weight of the leg and foot have been omitted from this diagram.)

weight (or muscle force) can be found by multiplying the rotary component (W_r) by the actual weight arm distance of the lever.

The *parallel component* of the original force causes either *compression* or *distraction* of the joint surfaces, depending on the direction of the component. In the example shown in Figure 2-16, a large part of the tension produced by the quadriceps muscle (M) is directed toward the femur and is causing the tibia to be compressed against the femur. This component (M_s) is called the *stabilizing* component of the muscle force (M). On the other hand, the parallel component of the weight (W_d) causes separation of the joint surfaces and is called the *distracting component*. The magnitudes of both the distracting and stabilizing components of the force can vary from 0 to 100 percent of the total force, depending upon joint position, but the magnitudes are inversely related, with one approaching 0 as the other approaches 100 percent.

Examples of the effect of different angles of application of a force are illustrated in Figure 2-17 with the rubber band finger extension sling. If the band is attached proximally (to an outrigger), the force applied to gaining extension will not be the full force of the band (A) but rather only the perpendicular rotary component. The parallel component (F_s) is causing joint compression. If the point of attachment is moved forward, the rotary component increases (B). Only when the sling is attached at a right angle (C) is the full force of the rubber band applied to gaining extension. If the patient later develops the ability to increase the range of extension (D), but the outrigger has not been adjusted, the rotary component of the force will again decrease and the parallel component will cause a distraction at the joint.

Laws of the Right Triangle

The rectangular components of the force are used to take advantage of the laws of the right triangle so that the magnitudes of the torques and unknown muscle and joint forces can be calculated. The rectangular components (with their parallel sides) form two right triangles, with the original force as the hypotenuse (Fig. 2-18). The ratios of the sides and hypotenuse of the right triangle are always the same for a specified angle. The relationship is expressed by the Pythagorean theorem: the square of the hypotenuse of a right triangle is equal to the sum of the squares of the two sides. The ratio of the sides to the angle is expressed by the trigonometric functions sine (sin), cosine (cos), and tangent (tan). Table 2-3 lists the values of common trigonometric functions. For example, the value of 0.500 for the sine of a 30-degree angle means that the opposite side is one half the length (magnitude) of the hypotenuse. Thus, if the values of one side and one angle are known (or two sides), the remaining sides and angles can be found.

Calculation of Muscle and Joint Forces

The forces that occur in muscles and between joint surfaces cannot usually be measured directly in the living human subject. This information can be gained indirectly by use of the equilibrium formulas ($\Sigma F = 0$ and $\Sigma \tau = 0$), composition and resolution

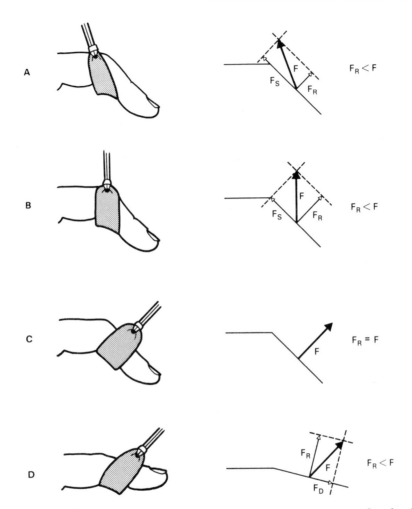

FIGURE 2-17. Resolution of the force (F) of a sling (attached to an outrigger hand splint) for gaining interphalangeal joint extension. In *A* and *B*, the line of pull is incorrect; in *C*, the outrigger is adjusted to gain the correct perpendicular line of pull; in D, the range of motion has increased and the line of pull is again incorrect.

of forces, and the trigonometric ratios of the right triangle. An example of this process is illustrated in Figure 2-19, which demonstrates how to find the magnitude of the unknown quadriceps muscle and knee joint compression forces when the subject is sitting and extending the knee with a 30-lb weight on the foot (Fig. 2-14). In Figure 2-16, this example has been placed on the coordinate system with the origin coinciding with the unknown joint force, and in Figure 2-19, each of the three forces (W, M, and J) has been resolved into perpendicular components. The diagram has been labeled and the measured weight, angles, and distances recorded. The magnitudes of the muscle force (M = 380 lb) and joint force (J = 350 lb), as well as the direction of the joint force

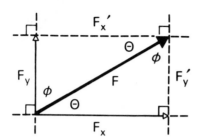

F = original force
$F_x \; F_y$ = rectangular components of F
$F_x' \; F_y'$ = parallels to $F_x \; F_y$
$\theta \; \phi$ = acute angles formed by F with F_x and F_y
$\square$ = 90°

Relationships

Pythagorean theorum	Angles	Sides
$F^2 = F_x{}^2 + F_y{}^2$	90° + θ + ϕ = 180°	$F_x = F_x'$
$F = \sqrt{F_x{}^2 + F_y{}^2}$	θ + ϕ = 90° 90° − θ = ϕ	$F_y = F_y'$

Trigonometric Functions

$$\sin \theta = \frac{F_y}{F} \qquad F_y = F \sin \theta$$

$$\cos \theta = \frac{F_x}{F} \qquad F_x = F \cos \theta$$

$$\tan \theta = \frac{F_y}{F_x}$$

FIGURE 2-18. Resolution of a force into rectangular components with the geometric relationships of the sides and angles of the resulting right triangles.

(α = 17 degrees), are found using the equilibrium formulas and trigonometric ratios. The following equations are arranged to show a step-by-step solution to the same problem. They illustrate the details of the relationships and provide solutions or explanations to parts of the problem, such as the rotary force of the weight, the torque of the resistance or the muscle force.

The rotary component (W_r), of the 30-lb weight must first be found; use resolution of forces:

W_r = W cos 30°
W_r = 30 lb × 0.866
W_r = 26 lb

To find the torque produced by the weight (τ_w), use the formula for torque:

τ_w = W_r × d
τ_w = 26 lb × 20 in
τ_w = 520 in-lb

TABLE 2-3. Useful Trigonometric Functions and Ratios of Common Angles (for Other Angles, the Reader Should Refer to Tables of Natural Trigonometric Functions)

ANGLE	SIN	COS	TAN
0°	0.000	1.000	0.000
10°	0.174	0.985	0.176
20°	0.342	0.940	0.364
30°	0.500	0.866	0.577
45°	0.707	0.707	1.000
60°	0.866	0.500	1.732
70°	0.940	0.342	2.747
80°	0.985	0.174	5.671
90°	1.000	0.000	∞

To find the torque that the muscle must produce (τ_m), use the equilibrium formula:

$$\Sigma\tau = 0$$
$$\tau_w - \tau_m = 0$$
$$\tau_m = \tau_w$$
$$\tau_m = 520 \text{ in-lb}$$

To find the force in the muscle (M), the rotary component M_r must first be found. To find the magnitude of the rotary component of the muscle (M_r), use the formula for torque:

$$\tau_m = M_r \times s$$
$$M_r = \tau_m \div s$$
$$M_r = 520 \text{ in-lb} \div 4 \text{ in}$$
$$M_r = 130 \text{ lb}$$

To find the muscle force (M), use trigonometric functions of the right triangle:

$$\sin 20° = M_r \div M$$
$$M = M_r \div \sin 20°$$
$$M = 130 \text{ lb} \div 0.342$$
$$M = 380 \text{ lb}$$

To find the magnitude of the joint force (J), use the equilibrium formula:

$$\Sigma F = 0$$
$$-J + M - W = 0$$
$$-J = -380 \text{ lb} + 30 \text{ lb}$$
$$J = 350 \text{ lb}$$

To find the angle of application for J, one of the components of J must be found. If, at equilibrium, the sum of the forces is zero, then the sum of the rectangular components must also be zero. To find the magnitude of J component, use the equilibrium formula $\Sigma F_x = 0$ or $\Sigma F_y = 0$.

$$\Sigma F_y = 0$$
$$-J_r + M_r - W_r = 0$$
$$-J_r = -M_r + W_r$$
$$-J_r = -130 \text{ lb} + 26 \text{ lb}$$
$$J_r = 104 \text{ lb}$$

To find the angle of the joint force, use trigonometric functions and find the degree of the angle in a table of sines and cosines.

$$\text{Sin } \alpha = J_r \div J$$
$$\text{Sin } \alpha = 104 \text{ lb} \div 350 \text{ lb}$$
$$\text{Sin } \alpha = 0.297$$
$$\alpha = 17°$$

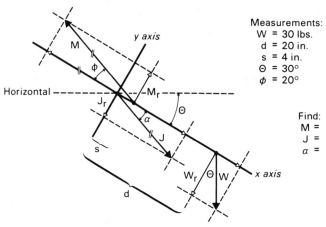

Measurements:
W = 30 lbs.
d = 20 in.
s = 4 in.
Θ = 30°
ϕ = 20°

Find:
M =
J =
α =

A

$$\Sigma_T = 0*$$
$$W \cos \Theta \, (d) - M \sin \phi \, (s) = 0$$
$$30 \text{ lbs. } (0.866) \, 20 \text{ in.} - M \, (0.342) \, 4 \text{ in.} = 0$$
$$-M = \frac{-520 \text{ in.lb.}}{1.37 \text{ in.}}$$

$$\boxed{M = 380 \text{ lbs.}}$$

B

$$\Sigma F = 0$$
$$-J + M - W = 0$$
$$-J = -380 \text{ lbs.} + 30 \text{ lbs.}$$

$$\boxed{J = 350 \text{ lbs.}}$$

C

$$\Sigma Fy = 0$$
$$-J_r + M_r - W_r = 0$$
$$-J_r + M \sin \phi - W \cos \Theta = 0$$
$$-J_r = -380 \text{ lbs. } (0.342) + 30 \text{ lbs. } (0.866)$$
$$-J_r = -130 \text{ lbs.} + 26 \text{ lbs.}$$
$$J_r = 104 \text{ lbs.}$$

D

$$\sin \alpha = \frac{J_r}{J}$$

$$\sin \alpha = \frac{104 \text{ lbs.}}{350 \text{ lbs.}}$$

$$\sin \alpha = 0.297$$

$$\boxed{\alpha = 17°}$$

FIGURE 2-19. Trigonometric solution for the magnitude of the muscle and joint forces as well as the angle of the joint force when the seated subject is holding a 30-lb weight on the foot and the knee is at 30 degrees of flexion (see Fig. 2-14). Force vectors are placed on the coordinate system and resolved into components as in Figure 2-16. Angles and distances are determined and labeled. The problem is solved using the two equilibrium formulas and a trigonometric ratio. The angle and the distance of the patellar tendon attachment were measured from radiographs. The angle of knee flexion and the distance of the weight from the joint center were measured on the subject.

---

*This is a vector equation that estimates the value and is used to simplify the calculations. For greater precision, one should use the sum of the forces in the x and y axes, along with the Pythagorean theorem to solve for J. Using the simpler solution causes J to be underestimated by 8 lbs, but the computed angle remains the same.

If this problem were repeated with the knee in full extension, the rotary component of the weight (W_r) would be larger, thus increasing the torque of the weight (τ_w) as well as the torque of the muscle (τ_m), the muscle force (M), and the joint force (J). Conversely, if the angle between the horizontal and the tibia were increased to 60 degrees, the values of W_r, τ_w, τ_m, M, and J would all be less.

Note that the weight of the leg and foot was omitted in this problem (see Fig. 2-19). The weight of the leg and foot (w) is approximately 9 lb acting at its center of gravity 8 inches from the origin of the coordinate system in a vertical direction. When this force is added, the corrected equilibrium equations are:

$$\Sigma\tau = 0$$

A. $30 \text{ lb } (0.866)\ 20 \text{ in} + 9 \text{ lb } (0.866)\ 8 \text{ in} - M\ (0.342)4 \text{ in} = 0$

$$M = 425 \text{ lb}$$

B. $\Sigma F = 0$

$$-J = 425 \text{ lb} - 30 \text{ lb} - 9 \text{ lb} = 0$$

$$J = 385 \text{ lb}$$

For examples of calculations in other activities, positions, and joint areas and for calculation of forces in dynamics, the reader is referred to *Biomechanics of Human Motion* (Le Veau, 1977).

CLINICAL APPLICATIONS OF STATICS

Weight and the Center of Gravity

The action line of the force vector of the weight of a body is *always* vertical and is located at the *center of gravity* of the body. The center of gravity is defined as the single point of a body about which every particle of its mass is equally distributed ($\Sigma\tau = 0$). If the body were suspended (or supported) at this point, the body would be perfectly balanced. Each body behaves as if its entire mass were acting or being acted upon at its center of gravity.

Stable, Unstable, and Neutral Equilibrium

If the center of gravity of a body is disturbed slightly and the body tends to return the center of gravity to its former position, the body is said to be in *stable equilibrium*. Examples would include attempting to turn a brick over or pushing on a person who is sitting in a rocking chair. If the center of gravity does not tend to return but seeks a new position, the body falls. The body was then in a state of *unstable equilibrium*, such as might occur if a person sitting on a narrow-based stool leaned forward. *Neutral equilibrium* is demonstrated by a rolling ball or a person being propelled in a wheelchair. When the center of gravity is displaced it remains at the same level, that is, it neither falls nor returns to its former position.

The degree of stability or mobility of a body depends on four factors: (1) the *height of the center of gravity above the base of support*, (2) the *size of the base of support*, (3) the *location of the gravity line within the base of support*, and (4) the *weight of the body*. Stability is enhanced by a low center of gravity, a wide base of support, the gravity line at the center of the support, and heavy weight. The size of, and the positions taken by, a football lineman promote stability and resistance to being overthrown. Mobility, on the other hand, is enhanced by a high center of gravity, narrow base of support, and light weight as exemplified by the positions and moves of football running backs.

CENTER OF GRAVITY

The concept of center of gravity of a solid object, such as a brick or a ball, is not difficult to visualize. The human body, however, has many irregularly shaped segments. As the positions of the segments change, so does the center of gravity of the body as a whole. A patient with muscle weakness can collapse in a fraction of a second if the gravity line is allowed to move outside the base of support. Knowledge of where and how the force of gravity acts on the body (and its segments) is important clinically to facilitate motion, alter exercise loads, balance parts, and prevent falls.

The *center of gravity of the adult human in the anatomic position has been found to be slightly anterior to the second sacral vertebra* (Braune and Fischer, 1889), or approximately 55 percent of a person's height (Hellebrandt et al, 1938). The horizontal plane through this point can be found experimentally using a long board supported at one end by a bathroom scale and supported at the other end by blocks (Fig. 2-20). Triangular strips of wood are placed between the plank and the supports to act as "knife edges." The distance between the edges is measured. Then the subject who has been previously weighed lies down on the board with all of the body positioned between the knife edges to form a second-class lever system. The values for (1) the scale reading, (2) the subject's weight, and (3) the distance between the knife edges can be entered into the equilibrium formula $\Sigma\tau = 0$ to find the distance from the axis (A) that the weight is centered. This distance is the center of gravity in the horizontal plane and can be marked on the subject with chalk before the subject moves from the board.

The center-of-gravity mark will usually fall near the level of the anterior-superior spines of the ilium. Variations in body proportions and weight distribution will cause alterations in the location of this point. It is usually found to be slightly higher in males than in females, since males tend to have broader shoulders and females, broader hips. The center of gravity of infants and children will be relatively higher because of their proportionally larger heads and trunks. Patients with above-knee amputations will have a high center of gravity and may be in unstable equilibrium in a conventional wheelchair unless compensatory weights are placed on the footrests.

Any change from the anatomic position will cause the center of gravity to move. If the arms are folded on the chest or raised overhead, the center of gravity will rise. If the subject flexes the head, trunk, and hips, the center of gravity moves toward the

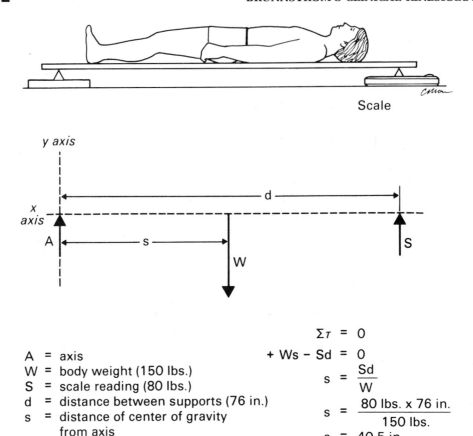

$$\Sigma_T = 0$$
$$+ Ws - Sd = 0$$

A = axis
W = body weight (150 lbs.)
S = scale reading (80 lbs.)
d = distance between supports (76 in.)
s = distance of center of gravity
　　from axis

$$s = \frac{Sd}{W}$$

$$s = \frac{80 \text{ lbs.} \times 76 \text{ in.}}{150 \text{ lbs.}}$$

$$s = 40.5 \text{ in.}$$

FIGURE 2-20. Experimental method for finding the center of gravity in the horizontal plane when the subject is in the anatomic position. The vector diagram is placed on the coordinate system with the axis (A) at the origin and the board on the x axis. The weight of the board is eliminated from the equation by placing the scale on zero before the subject lies down.

feet. The relatively high center of gravity in humans places the erect person in a position of unstable equilibrium. Only a small force is needed to cause displacement of the body and to initiate walking. Falling of the body is prevented by an intact and automatic neuromuscular system, which places a base of support (the extended leg) under the center of gravity. Thus, walking can be described as a sequence of disturbing and catching the center of gravity. Uncertainty in the person's ability to control and balance the body may cause the subject to protectively lower the center of gravity, even though this may require greater energy or promote further loss of balance. For example, the novice snow skier will sit back rather than lean forward. People who attempt to walk in a dark and unfamiliar place will usually tend to flex at the hips and knees, as will patients who are unsure or frightened. *The therapist is responsible for providing both the physical and psychologic support* to help patients learn to take advantage of their center of gravity in performing motor tasks safely and effectively.

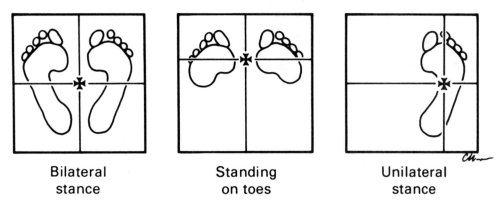

| Bilateral
stance | Standing
on toes | Unilateral
stance |

FIGURE 2-21. Sagittal and frontal plane projections of the center of gravity to the base of support in the erect subject.

Base of Support

For stability, the center of gravity of a body *must project within the base of support*. The frontal and sagittal plane projections of the center of gravity to the base of support in an upright subject can also be found by using the board-and-scale method. A piece of paper is lightly taped to the board. The subject who has been previously weighed stands on the paper facing the axis, and the feet are outlined on the paper with a pen. The calculations are made using the formula in Figure 2-20, and the distance from the axis is marked on the paper to locate the frontal plane projection. To locate the sagittal plane projection, the paper with the outlined feet is turned 90 degrees on the board. The subject places the feet into the outline and stands in the same posture as before, and the calculations are repeated. Intersection of the two lines indicates the projection of the center of gravity to the base of support. The projection is found near the center of the outlined base of support, if the subject has been standing erect with weight evenly distributed on both feet. When the subject is facing the axis and leans forward (or rises up on the toes), the center of gravity will move forward, but it will always remain within the base of support (Fig. 2-21). When the subject is facing at a right angle to the axis (sagittal plane) and bears more weight on one leg, the center of gravity will shift toward that foot. If the subject stands on one leg, the center of gravity projects within the weight-bearing foot. Balance on this smaller base of support increases the demand on the neuromuscular system, as can be seen by the increased muscle contractions about the ankle and knee. Lateral balance on one leg becomes a major task because the safety zone for stability of side-to-side sway is limited.

A common problem of patients with hemiplegia* is the inability to move the center of gravity of the body over the foot of the involved lower extremity. These patients will

---

*Hemiplegia (Gr. *hemi-*, half, plus *plege*, a stroke). Paralysis or paresis of one side of the body, usually caused by interruption of blood flow to a region of the brain containing nerve cells that control movement of muscles.

state that they "can move the bad leg forward but cannot move the good leg!" Since they are supporting their weight on the "good" (unaffected) extremity, it is, of course, impossible to pick it up and move it forward. Only after patients learn to bear the body weight on the affected extremity can they move the unaffected extremity forward. Another problem that hemiplegic patients have with moving their center of gravity over the base of support is in coming to the standing position from a chair. As illustrated in Figure 2-22, the center of gravity of the seated subject falls beneath the chair. In order to stand up, the center of gravity of the body must first be moved forward so that it projects beneath the feet. Patients with hemiplegia, however, frequently push the body backward and upward when trying to stand up. Instead, they should be taught to move forward over the feet to bring the center of gravity over the new base of support. When this occurs, the patient is in a position to stand up.

Increased stability is gained by broadening the base of support. In the presence of diminished muscle strength or poor coordination, crutches, canes, and walkers may provide stability for the patient. The patient must learn, however, to shift the center of gravity of the body so that the assistive device or a lower extremity can be lifted and moved forward. A wide base of support is also advantageous in lifting and carrying. This principle is exemplified by weight-lifters as well as therapists transferring the paralytic patient from bed to wheelchair. In preparation for the lift and transfer, therapists will place their feet in a wide anterior-posterior stance so that the weight can be placed primarily on one foot at the initiation of the lift and shifted to the other foot at the end of the lift. Although the patient's weight may be moved the distance of a meter, the therapist provides stability to the system by containing the weight between both feet. If the therapist kept the feet together and "walked" the patient to the wheelchair, the patient and the therapist would be in a condition of unstable equilibrium, leading to a fall of the patient or an injury to the therapist.

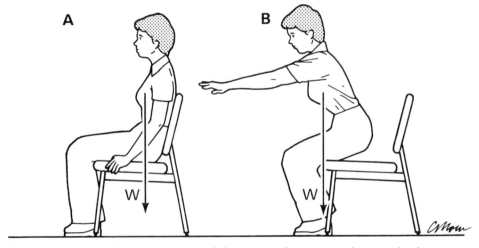

FIGURE 2-22. Sagittal plane projections of the center of gravity in the seated subject *(A)*. In order to stand up, the subject must move the center of gravity of the body forward over the base of support formed by the feet *(B)*.

Centers of Gravity and Weights of Segments

The center of gravity of the body as a whole is the sum of the centers of gravity of individual segments ($\Sigma\tau = 0$). Knowledge of the location of the segmental centers of gravity and the approximate weight of the segments is clinically useful in adjusting exercise loads, applying traction, and balancing parts of the body.

Approximate locations of the individual centers of mass and weight of body segments are given in Figure 2-23 and Table 2-4. Body segment parameters have been determined on cadavers by Braune and Fisher (1889), Dempster (1955), and Clauser and associates (1969). For specific details, the reader is referred to the original studies or to the reviews by LeVeau (1977) and Drillis and associates (1964).

The center of gravity of the extended upper extremity is just above the elbow joint, and that of the extended lower extremity is just above the knee joint. The arm, forearm, thigh, and leg are larger proximally, and thus their individual centers of gravity

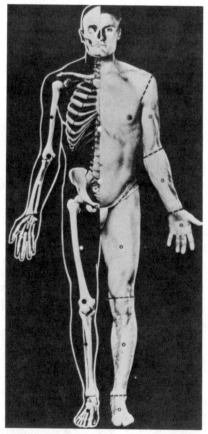

FIGURE 2-23. Location of center of gravity in major body segments of a man weighing 150 lb. See also Table 2-4. (From Williams, M and Lissner, HR: *Biomechanics of Human Motion.* WB Saunders, Philadelphia, 1962, p 14, with permission.)

TABLE 2-4. Average Weight of Body Segments and Anatomic Location of Center of Gravity of Individual Body Segments of a Man Weighing 150 lb

Segment Weights and Percentage of Total Body Weight	Approximate Anatomic Location of Centers of Gravity
Head: 10.3 lb (6.9%)	*Head.* In sphenoid sinus, 4 mm beyond anterior inferior margin of sella. (On lateral surface, over temporal fossa on or near nasion-inion line.)
Head and neck: 11.8 lb (7.9%)	*Head and neck.* On inferior surface of basioccipital bone or within bone 23 ± 5 mm from crest of dorsum sellae. (On lateral surface, 10 mm anterior to supratragic notch above head of mandible.)
Head, neck, and trunk: 88.5 lb (59.0%)	*Head, neck, and trunk.* Anterior to eleventh thoracic vertebra.
UPPER LIMB. Just above elbow joint.	
Arm: 4.1 lb (2.7%)	*Arm.* In medial head of triceps, adjacent to radial groove; 5 mm proximal to distal end of deltoid insertion.
Forearm: 2.4 lb (1.6%)	*Forearm.* 11 mm proximal to most distal part of pronator teres insertion; 9 mm anterior to interosseus membrane.
Hand: 0.9 lb (0.6%) Upper limb: 7.3 lb. (4.9%) Forearm and hand: 3.3 lb. (2.2%)	*Hand* (in rest position). On axis of metacarpal III, usually 2 mm deep to volar skin surface. 2 mm proximal to proximal transverse palmar skin crease, in angle between proximal transverse and radial longitudinal crease.
LOWER LIMB. Just above knee joint.	
Thigh: 14.5 lb (9.7%)	*Thigh.* In adductor brevis muscle (or magnus or vastus medialis) 13 mm medial to linea aspera, deep to adductor canal. 29 mm below apex of femoral triangle and 18 mm proximal to most distal fibers of adductor brevis.
Leg: 6.8 lb (4.5%)	*Leg.* 35 mm below popliteus, at posterior part of posterior tibialis; 16 mm above proximal end of Achilles tendon; 8 mm posterior to interosseus membrane.
Foot: 2.1 lb. (1.4%) Lower limb: 23.4 lb. (15.6%) Leg and foot: 9.0 lb. (6.0%)	*Foot.* In plantar ligaments, or just superficial in adjacent deep foot muscles; below proximal halves of second and third cuneiform bones. On a line between ankle joint center and ball of foot in plane of metatarsal II.
ENTIRE BODY. Anterior to second sacral vertebra.	

From Williams, M and Lissner, HR: *Biomechanics of Human Motion.* WB Saunders, Philadelphia, 1962, p 15, with permission.

lie closer to the proximal end. This point is approximately ⁴/₉ (45 percent) of the length of the segment, measured from the proximal end.

A change in the position of individual segments causes a change in the position of the center of gravity of the extremity and the body as a whole. When the extremity is flexed, the center of gravity moves proximally and to a point on a line between individual segment centers (Fig. 2-24). Deliberate movement of the center of gravity of segments is frequently used in therapeutic exercise to alter the resistive torque (weight times its perpendicular distance to the axis of motion) of an extremity. Shoulder flexion against gravity is easier to perform when the elbow is flexed than when the elbow is extended. The sit-up is easiest to perform when the arms are at the sides and becomes progressively more difficult as the arms are folded on the chest or the hands placed behind the head. Changing the torque of the lower extremities provides a method for altering the difficulty of abdominal muscle exercises. In the supine position, these muscles contract to stabilize the pelvis when the legs are raised. The resistance that the abdominal muscles must meet is reduced by flexing the lower extremities before lifting the legs, and the resistance is further reduced by raising only one leg. The magnitude of the decrease in torque is illustrated in Figure 2-24. Although the weight of the single extremity is the same in both positions, the center of gravity has moved from 15 inches (37 cm) from the hip joint axis to 8 inches (20 cm); therefore, the torque has been reduced from 360 in-lb (40.6 N) to 192 in-lb (21.7 N). This decrease in torque not only reduces the stabilization force required on the abdominal

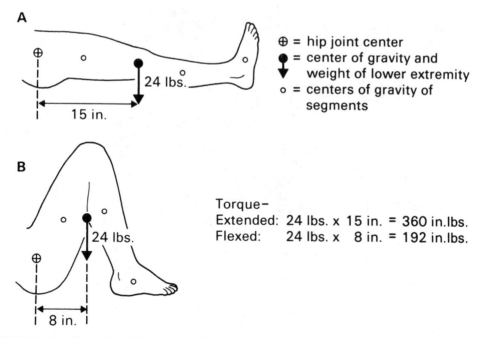

FIGURE 2-24. Alteration of the torque of the lower extremity by changing position of individual segments.

muscles, but also reduces the force that the hip flexor muscles must produce to raise the leg.

The center of gravity of the head, arms, and trunk (HAT as described by Elftman, 1955) is located anterior to the border of the 11th thoracic vertebra and just below the xiphoid process of the sternum. The weight of HAT is approximately equal to 60 percent of the body weight. In Figure 2-25, note the increased distance from the hip joint to the line of the center of gravity of HAT as forward inclination is increased. This position requires increasingly more force in the back and hip extensor muscles to support the weight of the trunk. In patients with paralysis of the hip musculature (paraplegia and quadriplegia), control of the center of gravity of HAT is essential for stability in sitting and standing. Although momentary sitting balance may be achieved, the patient is in a position of unstable equilibrium. Stability of HAT for functional use of the hands then requires an additional external force. In a wheelchair, this may be gained by leaning against the back rest or holding onto parts of the chair (Fig. 2-26). Wheelchair fitting requires consideration not only of stability of the trunk in the sitting position, but also of control and stability in other positions of function. As illustrated in Figure 2-26, a high-back chair can provide greater stability when sitting, but the high back may prohibit hooking the elbow or wrist around the handles to control the trunk when reaching forward.

Applied Weights and Resistances

Clinically, the external resistances encountered by the body include the forces produced by casts, braces (orthoses), books, plates of food, pulleys, dumbbells, crutches,

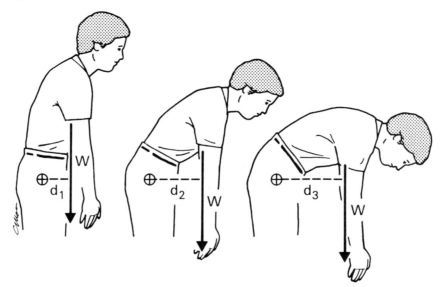

FIGURE 2-25. Distance (d_1, d_2, d_3) from the center of hip joint to center-of-gravity line of head, arms, and trunk (HAT) increases as forward inclination increases.

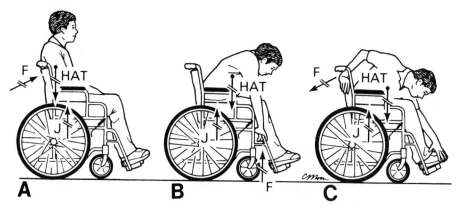

FIGURE 2-26. Methods of stability and control of the center of gravity of head, arms, and trunk (HAT) in a patient with a cervical spinal cord transection, where J = the force supporting the body at the center of the base of support and F = a counterforce needed to maintain equilibrium. *(A)* Sitting with support of back rest. *(B)* Leaning forward on passively "locked" elbows and using scapular muscles. *(C)* Hooking wrist around handle bar and using elbow flexors to lower and raise trunk.

doors, exercise equipment, or manual resistance by a therapist. Although these forces may be small, they are usually applied distally on the extremity and, therefore, exert relatively large torques that the muscles must match. Knowledge of the behavior of these forces and their rectangular components permits their manipulation and adaptation for therapeutic purposes. For example, if the objective is to give resistive exercise to a particular muscle, a resistive torque should be selected that most nearly matches the torque which the muscle is capable of developing. If, however, the objective is to assist functional use of a weak muscle, the resistance torque should be made as small as possible.

Applied weights such as dumbbells or books behave in the same manner as weights of body segments. The maximum resistance torque of the weight occurs when the extremity or segment is horizontal. In this position, the perpendicular distance from the action line of the force to the axis of motion is the longest (see Fig. 2-11); or alternatively, the rotary component of the weight is equal to the weight vector. At all other points in the range of motion, the resistance torque is less. The two alternative methods for calculating torque are shown in Figure 2-27. The first method uses the magnitude of the force (weight or muscle contraction) times the measured perpendicular distance from the line of action of the force to the axis of motion (see Fig. 2-11). The second method uses the method of resolution of forces (see page 41) to find the rotary component of the force times the measured distance from the point of attachment of the force to the axis of motion. In each method, the *distance is perpendicular* to the force or the rotary component, and the resulting torque will be the same. The method selected is one of convenience as to ease in obtaining measured distances and angles.

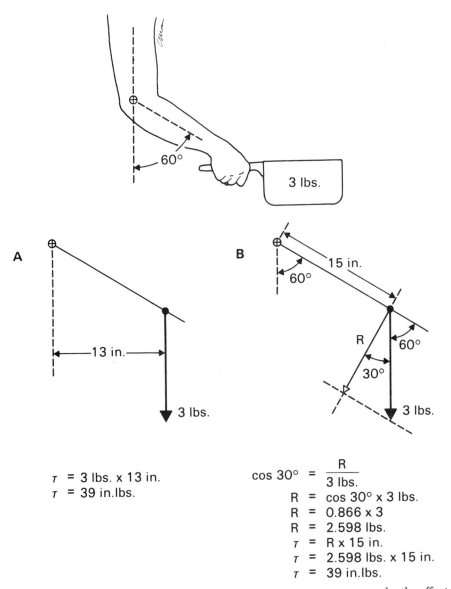

$$\tau = 3 \text{ lbs. x } 13 \text{ in.}$$
$$\tau = 39 \text{ in.lbs.}$$

$$\cos 30° = \frac{R}{3 \text{ lbs.}}$$
$$R = \cos 30° \times 3 \text{ lbs.}$$
$$R = 0.866 \times 3$$
$$R = 2.598 \text{ lbs.}$$
$$\tau = R \times 15 \text{ in.}$$
$$\tau = 2.598 \text{ lbs. x } 15 \text{ in.}$$
$$\tau = 39 \text{ in.lbs.}$$

FIGURE 2-27. Alternative methods for calculating torque using, as an example, the effect on the elbow of a 3-lb weight held in the hand. (A) The force times the perpendicular distance *from its action line* to the axis of elbow motion. (B) The *rotary component* of the force times the distance from its attachment to the axis of motion. The same methods may be used for other forces such as muscle contraction and applied resistances. In this example, if it were desired to find the torque in several positions of the elbow, (B) would be more convenient.

Distractive Component of Weights

Weights applied to the extremities frequently exert traction on joint structures, which may or may not be therapeutically desirable. The magnitude of the traction force is the distractive component of the resistive force and is found by resolution of forces (see page 41). Thus, if the elbow in Figure 2-27 were in extension, the weight would be acting entirely as a distracting force and would not have a rotary component. Such a distracting component may be desired to promote more normal arthrokinematics. Codman's pendulum exercises for reducing limitation of shoulder motion are based on this effect (Zohn and Mennell, 1976). The subject holds a weight in the hand, bends over, and flexes at the hips, thus placing the shoulder in a position of flexion. The extremity is swung as a pendulum so that the hand describes larger and larger circles within the pain-free range. The distracting component of the weight promotes the downward movement of the head of the humerus on the glenoid fossa so that shoulder flexion and abduction may occur.

In some pathologic conditions, the effect of the distracting component of a weight is unwanted since it may cause pain and further damage to joint structures. For example, in ligamentous injuries to the knee, weights attached to the foot for the purpose of applying strengthening exercises to the knee extensor muscles may be contraindicated (see Figs. 2-3 and 2-14). In such cases, a resistance method should be used that has *only a rotary component*. This is accomplished by applying the resistance force perpendicular to the long axis of the segment, as can be done manually by the therapist or by using equipment designed to eliminate the distractive component of the resistive force.

Externally applied forces, which may occur with manual resistance, exercise pulleys, crutch-walking, propelling a wheelchair, or opening a door, do not act in a vertical direction as do weights attached to the body. Instead, the forces exert effects that vary according to their particular angle of application. In pulley systems, the angle of application changes in different parts of the range of motion (Fig. 2-28). Each change in the angle (or direction) of the force causes a change in the magnitude of the rotary component of the force. Consequently, the resistance torque will also vary in different points of the range of motion.

Pulley

Pulleys are frequently used in exercise and traction equipment to change the direction of a force or to increase or decrease the magnitude of a force.

SINGLE FIXED PULLEY. The line of action of a force may be changed by means of a pulley (Fig. 2-29). A force F, acting in a downward direction, is used to move a weight in an upward direction. Such a single fixed pulley does not provide any mechanical advantage to the force, but only changes its direction. This principle is illustrated by the cervical traction example (see Fig. 2-4).

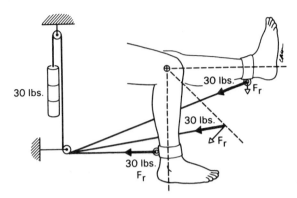

FIGURE 2-28. Vector diagram of the decreasing magnitude of the rotary component (F_r) or resistive force to knee extension in a pulley system when the knee is at (1) 90 degrees, (2) 45 degrees, and (3) 0 degrees of flexion. The rotary component (F_r) of the 30-lb force in the pulley system is found using the formula $\cos \Theta = F_r/30$ lb, or $F_r = \cos \Theta \times 30$ lb:

	Knee angle	Θ	$\cos \Theta \times 30$ lb	=	F_r
(1)	0°	60°	0.5 × 30 lb		15 lb
(2)	45°	30°	0.86 × 30 lb		24 lb
(3)	90°	0°	1.0 × 30 lb		30 lb

MOVABLE PULLEY. If a weight is attached to a movable pulley (Fig. 2-30), half of the weight is supported by the rope attached to the stationary hook, and half by the rope on the other side of the pulley. Therefore, the mechanical advantage of the force F is 2. The rope, however, must be moved twice the distance that the weight is raised, and what is gained in force is lost in distance. The fixed pulley in the illustration serves only to change the direction of the force but gives no mechanical advantage. The movable pulley is not represented in the body but may be convenient to use for exercise equipment. The leg traction systems in Figures 2-5 and 2-6 are examples. The pulley at the foot can be considered "movable" and the pulleys on the bed post fixed. Since the pulley at the foot receives the force from two parts of the rope, this pulley in turn exerts greater than 15 lb of traction on the leg. In the exercise system in Figure 2-28, the two fixed pulleys change only the direction of the force. Some systems, how-

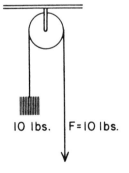

10 lbs. F=10 lbs.

FIGURE 2-29. Fixed pulley. Change of direction of force, but no mechanical advantage.

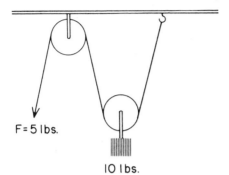

F = 5 lbs.

10 lbs.

FIGURE 2-30. Movable pulley. Mechanical advantage for force.

ever, have a movable pulley on the weight pan, as in Figure 2-30, which reduces the exercise force to one half of the weight.

DEFLECTION OF TENDON. The tendon of a muscle may be deflected from its straight course by a bony prominence or by other means. Such a pulley arrangement in the human body, unlike the mechanical single pulley, may also provide mechanical advantage to the muscle by lifting the tendon away from the joint axis. The tendon of the quadriceps, for example, not only changes its direction of pull as a result of the interposed patella, but its leverage also improves.

Another type of pulley system involving the tendons of the long finger flexors is found on the flexor side of the finger joints. When the flexor digitorum profundus and superficialis contract, their tendons rise somewhat from the joint axes, excessive rising being prevented by a pulley-like loop. This loop simultaneously causes a deflection of the tendons (Fig. 2-31). The line of action of the tendon over the joint is represented by a straight line from loop to loop, or from loop to attachment on the bone.

Muscle Forces and Leverage

Anatomically, muscles may be diverted by a pulley mechanism around a condyle; in biomechanics, however, the muscle force vector is straight. The line of action is usually from the immediate point of attachment of the muscle to the bone and extends into space according to the magnitude of the force (see Figs. 2-13, 2-14). The vector may, however, be placed at some point along the line of pull of the muscle. In either case, the vector is straight and does not follow the anatomic directions of the entire muscle.

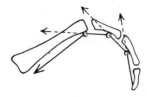

FIGURE 2-31. Pulley-like arrangement, deflecting tendon of flexor digitorum profundus. (Redrawn from *Gray's Anatomy*.)

Mechanically, the greater the perpendicular distance between the action line of the muscle and the joint center (force arm distance), the greater the torque produced by the muscle at that joint. This principle is sometimes called the *leverage factor* of muscles. Bony processes thus play an important role in providing force arm distances for the muscles and in increasing the angle of attachment of tendon to bone. The neck of the femur places the hip abductor muscles several inches away from the hip joint. The condyles of the phalanges increase the force arm distances of the finger flexors. The patella raises the line of pull of the quadriceps muscle from the knee joint axis. Small changes in these processes, as may occur with disease, injury, or surgery, can cause marked changes in the torque that a muscle can produce.

The first step in analyzing leverage factors of muscles is to identify at any single joint all the axes about which rotary movements occur. Following this, the relationship (distance) of each muscle action line to each axis can be visualized, and the movement capabilities of those muscles will be clarified. If a muscle crosses one joint that permits one degree of freedom of movement, and if this muscle runs directly between its attachments (i.e., its direction is not changed by bony processes or other means), its line of action is comparatively simple to define. Complexity of analysis of the line of action increases in instances where muscles possess widespread attachments and where joints permit increased degrees of freedom of movement.

The leverage principle is an important consideration in a muscle whose force arm distance changes as movement occurs, for its torque output will also vary at different points in the range of motion. A prime example of changing leverage in a muscle is the biceps brachii acting as an elbow flexor (Fig. 2-32). When the elbow is in extension, the action line of the muscle is closest to the joint center. As the elbow is flexed toward 90 degrees, the action line moves away from the joint center and then begins to return as the elbow reaches 120 degrees of flexion. Thus, *for the same force of muscle contraction, the biceps muscle would produce the most torque at 90 degrees of elbow flexion.* The muscle would be least effective as an elbow flexor when the elbow was in extension. Although the leverage factor affects the torque output of all muscles, the effect varies with the muscle, joint, and motion. The biceps brachii, brachio-radialis, and hamstring muscles show this effect more than muscles such as the triceps brachii, deltoid, or gastrocnemius-soleus where the perpendicular distance to the joint axis shows minimal changes throughout the range of motion.

In joints with large ranges of motion, however, muscles can produce *inverse actions.* That is, a muscle may be able to produce opposite actions from different positions in the range of motion depending on where the line of action falls in relation to the axes of motion. Inverse actions occur with the adductor muscles at the hip joint. When the hip is flexed, the adductor muscles can act as hip extensors (as in climbing a ladder). Conversely, when the hip is in extension, the adductor muscles may act as hip flexors. In the upper extremity, the wrist extensors cross the elbow joint and are attached on the lateral epicondyle of the humerus. When the elbow is in extension, the wrist extensors pass posteriorly to the elbow joint axis, and the muscles act as elbow extensors. When the elbow is flexed, however, the line of action of the wrist extensors in considerably anterior to the elbow axis, and these muscles become elbow flexors.

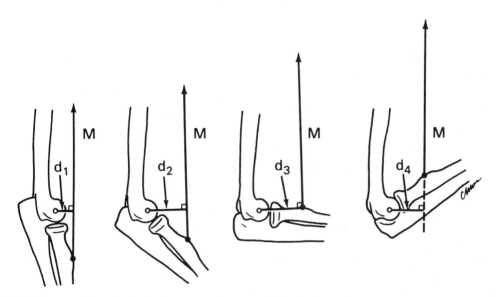

FIGURE 2-32. Changes in the force arm distance (d) for the biceps brachii muscle in four positions of elbow flexion. The maximum muscle torque would occur at the greatest lever arm distance (d_3, when attachment of the muscle to bone is perpendicular).

Mechanical Disadvantage of Muscles

Muscle attachments and action lines lie close to joint axes, and most muscle tendons attach to bones at an acute angle. Consequently, muscles have short force arm distances and a mechanical disadvantage relative to the more distally placed resistances. Muscles must generate large forces to match or overcome the resistance torques. As an example, the subject illustrated in Figure 2-33 is shown pressing down with the hand on a scale that registers 20 lb (89 N). In order to maintain this position and to keep the elbow from flexing, the triceps brachii muscle must exert a force of 222 lb (987 N)! Although presented as a problem of statics, the forces at the elbow are similar to those that would be found in dynamic activities such as sanding wood, cutting a tough steak, or pushing up from an armchair.

If, in Figure 2-33, the olecranon process of the ulna were reduced in length by only 1/4 inch (0.6 cm) and if the muscle could still generate 222 lb of force, the force recorded by the scale would be reduced from 20 to 15 lb. In the hand, changes in force arm distances of even a few millimeters can affect function markedly. This occurs frequently in rheumatoid arthritis, where the extensor digitorum tendons may move down between the metacarpal heads.

Joint Forces

Forces occur in joints secondary to the primary forces of muscle contraction, gravity, external resistance, and friction. Understanding the causes and the results of these

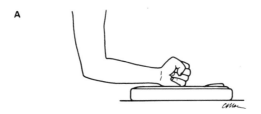

A

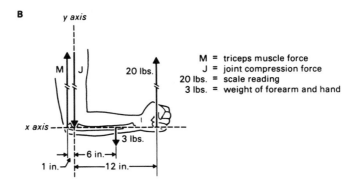

B   y axis

M = triceps muscle force
J = joint compression force
20 lbs. = scale reading
3 lbs. = weight of forearm and hand

M   J   20 lbs.

x axis

3 lbs.

6 in.
1 in.   12 in.

C Calculation of triceps muscle force:

$$\Sigma \tau = 0$$
$$+ (M \times 1 \text{ in.}) + (3 \text{ lbs.} \times 6 \text{ in.}) - (20 \text{ lbs.} \times 12 \text{ in.}) = 0$$
$$+ M = \frac{+ 240 \text{ in.lb.} - 18 \text{ in.lb.}}{1 \text{ in.}}$$
$$M = 222 \text{ lbs.}$$

D Calculation of joint compression force:

$$\Sigma F = 0$$
$$+ 222 \text{ lbs.} - J - 3 \text{ lbs.} + 20 \text{ lbs.} = 0$$
$$- J = - 239 \text{ lbs.}$$
$$J = 239 \text{ lbs.}$$

FIGURE 2-33. Example of the magnitudes of muscle and joint forces that occur with a moderate distal resistance. *(A)* Subject sitting and pressing down on a scale that records a force of 20 lb. *(B)* Diagram of the forces on the forearm and the lever arm distances placed on the coordinate system with the joint force (J) at the origin. *(C)* Equilibrium formula and calculations of the force of the triceps brachii muscle (M). *(D)* Equilibrium formula and calculations to find the joint compression force (J).

joint forces forms a major basis for the rationale of therapeutic exercise and physical rehabilitation. The primary forces may produce joint distraction, as when holding a suitcase in the hand, applying traction (see Fig. 2-4), or placing exercise weights on a dependent extremity (see Fig. 2-3). In these cases, tension is placed on the ligaments and joint capsules.

Most activities, however, produce compression of joint surfaces. Compression is readily appreciated in weight-bearing joints in sitting, standing, or walking. What is not always appreciated by able-bodied persons is the magnitude of joint compression forces that occur with these activities, as well as those that occur with active muscle contraction and functional activities. In rotary motions or postures of the body, one end of the bone (near its joint surface) serves as the fulcrum or axis of the lever system (see Figs. 2-7, 2-8). The joint force (J) is the reaction force of the mating joint surface. In the elbow extension problem (see Fig. 2-33), J represents the force on the distal end of the humerus. The calculations show this joint force to be 239 lb (1063 N)! In joint pathologies such as arthritis, function is lost because such large compressive forces cause excruciating pain. To illustrate this effect, the elbow problem in Figure 2-33 can be calculated assuming that the subject can tolerate only a 20-lb force at the joint. Placement of the origin of the coordinate system at the muscle force (M) permits calculation of the small amount of force (F) the subject could exert on the scale:

$$\Sigma_T = 0$$
$$(20 \text{ lb} \times 1 \text{ in}) + (3 \text{ lb} \times 7 \text{ in}) - (F \times 13 \text{ in}) = 0$$
$$F = \frac{20 \text{ in-lb} + 21 \text{ in-lb}}{13 \text{ in}}$$
$$F = 3.1 \text{ lb}$$

Although the amount of joint compression force developed in this parallel force system is large, it is frequently even greater because most muscles attach at an acute angle to the bone rather than at a right angle (see Fig. 2-16). In order to produce an effective rotary component, the muscle must generate a relatively large force, which in turn creates a large stabilization component. Thus, in most instances *when muscles contract, joint surfaces are strongly compressed.*

STRETCHING VERSUS JOINT MOBILIZATION

Passive stretching in an attempt to increase joint motion after fractures, surgery, or joint pathologies has long been considered contraindicated by many therapists and orthopedists. Biomechanically, there are sound reasons for this caution. When force is placed on the distal end of a bone, that force is exerted on a long lever arm and has a high mechanical advantage over the limiting or injured joint structures. This force can be amplified 10 to 20 times in the joint area. If, for example, in passive stretching of a knee or an elbow, the therapist pulled with a force of only 10 lb (4.5 kg) applied 10 inches (25 cm) from the joint center, this would be the same as applying a force of 50 lb 2 inches from the joint center or 100 lb 1 inch away. Forces of these magnitudes readily cause additional trauma to healing tissues. In addition, such distally placed forces do not reproduce normal joint motions; instead, they may cause levering of joints and abnormal motions (see Fig. 1-7).

On the other hand, mobilizations or passive movements of *joint surfaces* following normal accessory motions are frequently indicated in pathologic conditions to relieve pain and restore normal joint motions. Some biomechanical commonalities of the basic mobilization techniques are that:

1. The direction of the applied force follows the normal arthrokinematics of that joint.
2. The magnitude of the force is *carefully* controlled to be gentle and compatible with the underlying pathology. "No forceful movement must ever be used and no abnormal movement must ever be used" (Mennell, 1964).
3. Motions of the joint surfaces are small, ranging from barely perceptible to a few millimeters in distance.

Achievement of such precision and control is gained by using *very short* force arms. In most instances, the force is applied at the head (or base) of the bone that forms the joint.

CHAPTER 3

SOME ASPECTS OF MUSCLE PHYSIOLOGY AND NEUROPHYSIOLOGY

Movement is a fundamental characteristic of human behavior. *Movement is accomplished by contraction of skeletal muscles acting within a system of levers and pulleys formed by bones, tendons, and ligaments.* The individuality of each person is expressed by the pattern of contractions that produce facial expression, body posture, performance of fine motor skills such as typing or playing a musical instrument, and performance of gross motor activities such as walking and running. The able-bodied individual has a remarkable ability to develop just the right amount of muscle contraction to perform an endless variety of motor tasks—from dabbing just the right amount of eyeliner on the rim of the eyelids to carrying a full load of textbooks to class.

Every muscle or group of muscles exhibits properties that permit it to meet, within wide limits, the requirements placed upon it. These properties demonstrate a compromise among various needs. For example, speed of movement is a desirable quality, but so is economy of energy in maintaining posture. Muscles must shorten sufficiently to provide a full range of movement at the joints across which they are situated, yet they must generate sufficient power to move a load at each end of the range. Muscles must sometimes function for long periods without fatiguing and at other times must provide maximal efforts of great force for only a few seconds. The fine control of muscle contraction over a wide range of lengths, tensions, speeds, and loads is accomplished by an elaborate system of nerve cells. One division of the system is designed to provide accurate and timely information (in the form of sensory nerve impulses) about the status of each part of the body and the state of the surroundings. This information is used by another division of the system, in conjunction with information previously stored in the brain, to initiate instructions (in the form of motor nerve impulses) to muscles to produce desired movements. Thus, the end product—*desired movement*—*is achieved through the collaborative interaction of a large number of anatomic, physiologic, bio-*

chemical, and biomechanical factors, including the ability of muscles to develop graded amounts of active tension, the ability of the cardiovascular and respiratory systems to provide the ingredients that fuel the contractile process, and the ability of the nervous system to perceive what is happening and to regulate the rate and amount of contraction needed to accurately move certain body parts while stabilizing other parts.

The study of movement is the concern of many disciplines. The anatomist-physiologist studies motor function to describe which structures are responsible for producing movements at particular joints and the neural circuits used to control the particular muscles; the anthropologist studies motor function among different species and cultures as an indicator of evolutionary development; the physical educator is called upon to teach healthy persons how to perform relatively complex motor skills that serve as the foundation for various sports and recreational activities; members of health professions study motor function to detect the specific impairments that limit functional performance of an individual patient and to assist in finding solutions to identified problems. The more one understands about the characteristics and basic principles of operation of the systems that support and sustain motor behavior, the more effective one can be in assessing impairments of motor function and suggesting possible solutions to clinical problems. The material in this chapter may serve as a brief review for those who have previously studied the anatomy and physiology of the neuromuscular system. For those who have not had the benefit of such courses, sufficient detail is being included about the most important concepts and vocabulary to provide a basis for understanding the subject matter on clinical kinesiology that follows. A standard textbook on human physiology should be consulted for a more complete explanation of how the neuromuscular system functions.

STRUCTURE OF SKELETAL MUSCLE

Muscle Fibers

Examination of a sample of skeletal muscle (Fig. 3-1, A) reveals that it is composed of bundles of *fibers*. Each bundle is called a *fasciculus* (Fig. 3-1, B). The diameter of a muscle fiber is of the order of 50 to 100 micrometers (μm)* and its length from a few millimeters (mm) to 60 or 70 centimeters (cm). Each fiber (Fig. 3-1, C) is composed of a covering or membrane called the sarcolemma and a gelatin-like substance called sarcoplasm in which hundreds of contractile *myofibrils* and other important structures, such as mitochondria and the sarcoplasmic reticulum (Fig. 3-2), are imbedded. Mitochondria serve as tiny factories where metabolic processes occur. The function of the sarcoplasmic reticulum will be discussed later. The myofibril (Fig. 3-1, D) can be likened to a long train of boxcars, with each boxcar called a *sarcomere* (the portion between two Z disks). An interesting feature about the muscle fibers is the appearance of cross-striations, which is characteristic of skeletal muscle. For this reason, skeletal muscle is

---

*1 micrometer $= 10^{-6}$ meter

SKELETAL MUSCLE

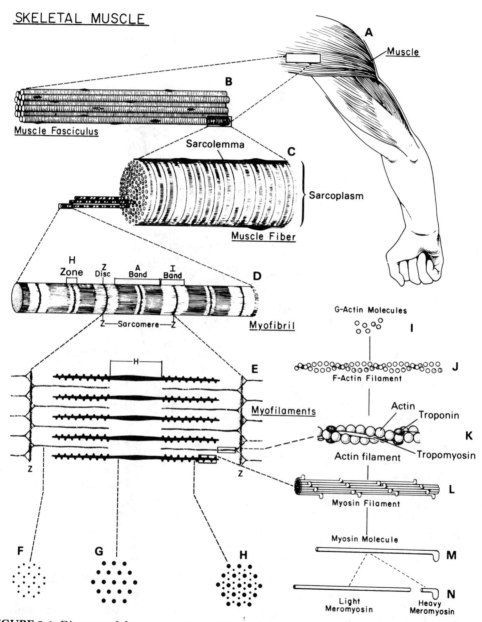

FIGURE 3-1. Diagram of the organization of skeletal muscle from the gross (A) to the molecular (E) level. F, G, and H are cross sections at the levels indicated. (Adapted from Bloom, W and Fawcett, DW: *A Textbook of Histology,* ed 10. WB Saunders, Philadelphia, 1975, p 306.)

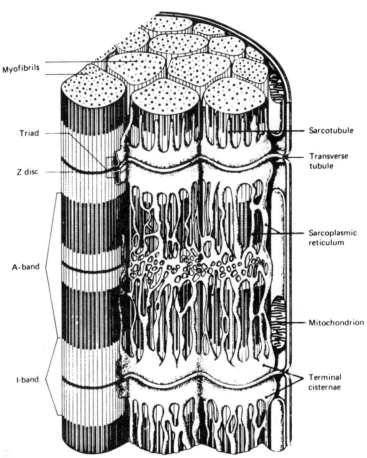

FIGURE 3-2. Endoplasmic reticulum of a skeletal muscle fiber. Sketch of the fine structure of part of a muscle fiber based on an electron micrograph. At the right-hand side of the sketch is the cell membrane; at the level of each Z disk it invaginates, sending transverse tubules across the interior of the fiber. Between the Z disks and parallel to the myofibrils runs the sarcoplasmic reticulum, saclike enlargements of which (the terminal cisternae) adjoin the transverse tubules. A cross section through transverse tubule and adjacent terminal cisternae reveals a configuration known as a triad (upper left). (From Bloom, W and Fawcett, DW: *A Textbook of Histology,* ed. 8. WB Saunders, Philadelphia, 1969, with permission.)

often called "striated" muscle. These striations are bands of alternately more and less light-refractive materials. When viewed under a microscope, the refractive materials are seen to be alternately lighter (isotropic or I band) and darker (anisotropic or A band; see Fig. 3-1, D). Each myofibril, in turn, contains many *myofilaments*, which are fine threads of two protein molecules called *actin* (thin filaments) and *myosin* (thick filaments; Fig. 3-1, E).

As illustrated in Figure 3-1, H, the A band contains *both* actin and myosin filaments, whereas the I band (Fig. 3-1, F) contains only actin filaments. Each I band is bisected transversely by a Z disk into which one end of the actin myofilaments is attached. A bands have a relatively isotropic middle zone called the H zone, which contains only myosin filaments (Fig. 3-1, G). As will be described in more detail later, the muscle develops tension and shortens through electrochemical reactions between actin and myosin filaments.

The thin filaments of the I bands are comprised of actin, tropomyosin, and troponin. The basic building block of actin is a globular molecule of actin (called G actin) about 5.5 nanometers (nm)* in diameter (Fig. 3-1, I). In muscle, the G-actin molecules are polymerized (linked together) to form a long fibrous strand (called F actin), and two strands are twisted about each other (Fig. 3-1, J) to form part of the actin filament. Tropomyosin is also a filamentous protein about 40 nm long. Two strands of tropomyosin are twisted around the double coil of F actin in such a way as to lie in the hollows of the twisted actin (Fig. 3-1, K). Troponin is another globular protein; it binds to a specific region of the tropomyosin filament, to give one troponin globule per 40 nm of tropomyosin filament. The important function of troponin is believed to be based on its enormous avidity for calcium ions (Ca^{++}), a property that will be considered when discussing the activation of the contractile process. This complex array of G actin, F actin, tropomyosin, and troponin comprises the actin filaments in the sarcomere. Myosin filaments (Fig. 3-1, L) are thicker than actin filaments and are comprised of myosin molecules, which form a rod about 150 nm long and 1.5 to 2.0 nm in diameter (Fig. 3-1, M). Under certain conditions, the myosin molecule can be split into two fragments, one about twice the weight of the other. The lighter-weight fragment (light meromyosin) is a straight rod that is responsible for the self-aggregation properties of myosin. The heavier fragment (heavy meromyosin) is shaped like the lower one fourth of a hockey stick (Fig. 3-1, N). This fragment exhibits the qualities of an enzyme capable of splitting adenosine triphosphate (ATP) into adenosine diphosphate (ADP) plus phosphate (PO_4) plus energy. The significance of this reaction will be discussed in the section dealing with the energetics of muscle contraction. Within the sarcomere unit, the thick filaments have small projections of heavy meromyosin extending transversely from the long axis of the filament in a helical pattern, as illustrated in Figure 3-1, L, with a repeat distance of approximately 43 nm. Those transverse processes of the myosin filament are believed to interact with specific sites on the actin filament to produce relative motion between the two types of filament.

Structural Basis for Muscle Contraction and Relaxation

Observations of the relaxed and contracted states of a muscle with light and electron microscopes have shown that the length of each serially repeating sarcomere unit changes from a relaxed length of approximately 2.5 μm to about 1.5 μm when fully contracted and to about 3.0 μm when stretched (Fig. 3-3). The sarcomere is bounded on each end by the Z disk (see Fig. 3-1, D). The width of individual A bands does not change during contraction. On the other hand, the I band becomes more narrow, and

---

*1 nanometer = 10^{-9} meter

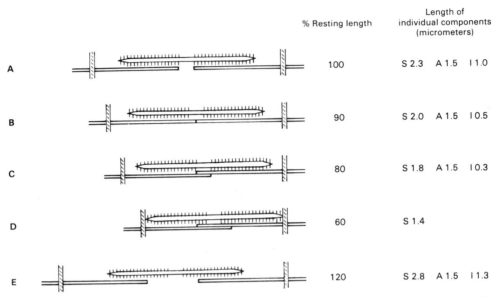

	% Resting length	Length of individual components (micrometers)		
A	100	S 2.3	A 1.5	I 1.0
B	90	S 2.0	A 1.5	I 0.5
C	80	S 1.8	A 1.5	I 0.3
D	60	S 1.4		
E	120	S 2.8	A 1.5	I 1.3

FIGURE 3-3. The structural basis for changes in muscle length: A sarcomere at resting length in A; showing changes in arrangement of filaments under various degrees of contraction, B through D; and when stretched, E. Relative changes in length of the sarcomere are indicated on the left, and the approximate lengths (in micrometers) of the sarcomere (S), A band, and I band are listed on the right. Note constancy of the A band length except under extreme nonphysiologic shortening. (Adapted from Schottelius, BA and Schottelius, DD: *Textbook of Physiology*, ed 17. CV Mosby, St. Louis, 1973, p 87).

the H zone of the A band is obliterated. These findings suggest that the *muscle contracts by the sliding of actin filaments toward each other in the central parts of the A bands. As the actin filaments move toward each other, the Z disks are pulled closer together so that the I bands shorten.* Although the amount of shortening of each sarcomere unit is small, for example, 0.5 to 1.0 μm, the *shortening of several thousands of sarcomere units linked in series like the boxcars of a train can produce an overall reduction in length of the muscle of several centimeters.* For example, a muscle fiber 10 cm in length, like many of those in the biceps brachii muscle, would have approximately 40,000 sarcomere units lined up end to end (1 cm = 10^4 μm; 10,000 μm/cm $\times$ 10 cm $\div$ 2.5 μm/sarcomere = 40,000 sarcomere units/10 cm). If each of the 40,000 sarcomere units shortened by 1 μm, the ends of the muscle fiber would be brought 4 cm closer together—a shortening of 40 percent.

This concept that actin and myosin filaments slide past each other during contraction is called the *sliding filament* theory of muscle contraction (Hanson and Huxley, 1953; Huxley, 1969). There is still uncertainty regarding the specific way in which actin filaments are drawn past the myosin filaments to develop muscle tension and shorten. Electron microscopy shows a regular array of transverse processes extending from each myosin filament (see Fig. 3-1, E) to link up with the six actin filaments surrounding it (see Fig. 3-1, H). When chemical energy is available following stimulation of the muscle fiber, an interaction occurs between the myosin transverse processes (cross-bridges) and active sites (partially shielded by troponin) on the actin filaments to cause movement of actin filaments into the H zone (see Fig. 3-3, B). The mechanical linkages between actin and myosin filaments that produce shortening of the sarcomeres and contraction of the muscle require two major processes: (1) *an electrical stimulus to trigger the coupling* and (2) *chemical reactions to provide energy for the development of active tension.*

EXCITATION OF NERVE AND SKELETAL MUSCLE FIBERS

The stimulus that produces muscle contraction originates in the nervous system and is conducted to each muscle fiber by a nerve fiber. Figure 3-4 illustrates the general anatomic features of the neural pathways for conducting nerve impulses from the brain to individual muscle fibers. Figure 3-4, A, depicts the two primary corticospinal pathways (one situated in the lateral portion of the spinal cord and one situated in the anterior portion) followed by axons of the upper motor neurons from the cerebral cortex to make synaptic contact with lower motor neurons situated in the ventral horn of the spinal cord gray matter. The lower motor neuron innervates and controls the activity of a set of muscle fibers in the muscle. Figure 3-4, B, illustrates a cross section of the spinal cord (sample taken from a thoracic segment of the cord) showing the location of major motor and sensory tracts. The name of the tract often indicates the general original and destination of the bundle of axons; for example, the spinocerebellar tract conveys sensory impulses from their point of entry into the spinal cord to the cerebellum. Figure 3-4, C and D, shows the general features of the connections between nerve and muscle and between nerve and nerve. An enlarged sketch of each major link in the pathway is included to show more anatomic detail, and the function of each of these links will be considered in more detail in subsequent portions of this chapter. The *stimulus is a wave of electrochemical activity that moves rapidly along nerve and muscle fibers and is associated with local changes in the electrical potential of each of the fibers.*

Membrane Potential

Differences in electrical potential exist across the membranes of all living cells. The fluids bathing both the inside and outside of each cell contain charged particles (ions) dissolved in solution. Metabolic processes occur in every cell to produce a net difference in the concentration of positive and negative ions between the inside and outside of each cell (Fig. 3-5, A). Two factors are responsible for the *ability of a cell to maintain a potential difference across its membrane:* (1) *the cell membrane is relatively impermeable to certain ions* (however, permeability of the membrane to an ion can be increased transiently by certain chemical substances released by nerve endings, as will be discussed later) and (2) *the cell can actively move ions across the membrane to*

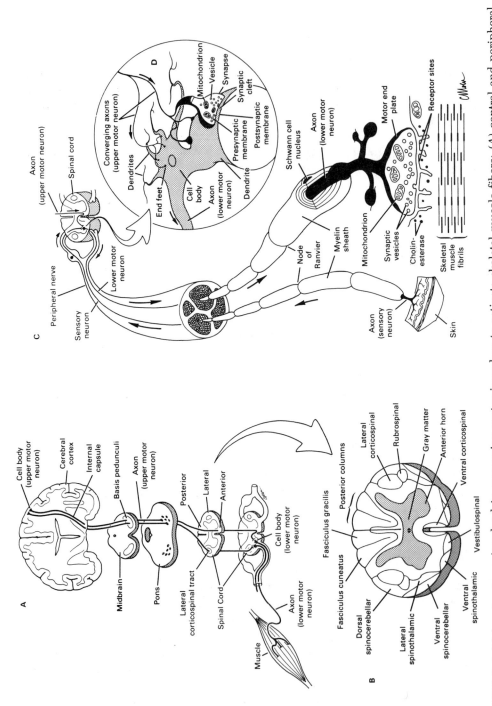

FIGURE 3-4. Major structures involved in conveying motor impulses to activate skeletal muscle fibers: (A) central and peripheral components, (B) cross section of spinal cord, (C) peripheral nerve fibers, (D) enlarged diagram of motor cell.

maintain the required resting potential. Nerve cells, muscle cells, and sensory receptors maintain a higher resting potential between the inside and outside of the membrane than other types of cells and therefore are *excitable* and capable of transmitting electrochemical impulses along their membranes.

Action Potential

Addition of a stimulus (electrical, mechanical, chemical, or thermal) of sufficient strength to an excitable cell can cause the cell membrane to become more permeable in the region where the stimulus was applied, resulting in a rapid exchange of positive and negative ions previously separated by the membrane (depolarization). This exchange establishes a difference in electrical potential between the active and inactive regions of the membrane, and a current flows between the two regions as illustrated in Figure 3-5. The flow of current between adjacent regions serves to excite the polarized region ahead, with the result that this region now contributes a greatly amplified electric signal, capable of spreading to the next region and exciting it also. Immediately after being depolarized, an active process begins in the cell membrane to re-establish the resting membrane potential—a process called *repolarization.* This advancing wave of depolarization and repolarization is called an *active potential.* The amplitude and shape of the action potential vary from one type of cell to another (Fig. 3-6). An action potential being transmitted over a nerve fiber is called a *nerve impulse,* and one being transmitted over a muscle fiber is called a *muscle impulse.*

Transmission of Impulses From Nerves to Skeletal Muscle Fibers: Myoneural Junction

The nervous system sends control signals in the form of action potentials to regulate the activity of muscle fibers. But the conversion of a nerve impulse to a muscle impulse occurs through a complicated process. The nerve fiber branches at its end to form a *motor end-plate,* which adheres tightly to the muscle fiber but which lies outside the muscle fiber membrane, as illustrated in Figure 3-4, C. This tight junction is a form of *synapse* (Gr. *synapsis,* a connection). It is also called a *myoneural* (Gr. *mye,* muscle) *junction.* The end-plate contains mitochondria that synthesize (manufacture) a special chemical substance called *acetylcholine,* the molecules of which are stored in small vesicles. The arrival of a nerve impulse at the myoneural junction causes the release of acetylcholine from some of the vesicles. When freed from storage in the vesicles, the acetylcholine diffuses rapidly across the short distance between the endplate and muscle fiber membrane. There, the acetylcholine interacts with *receptor sites* on the muscle fiber membrane to *increase permeability of the muscle cell membrane to ions in the fluid bathing the junction.* Movement of these ions into the muscle cell depolarizes the muscle fiber (postjunctional) membrane and triggers a muscle action potential that is propagated along the muscle fiber by an electrochemical mechanism similar to that responsible for the propagation of a nerve impulse.

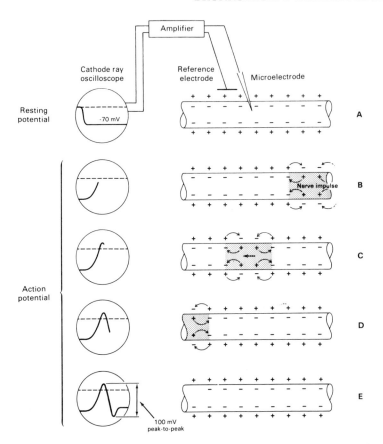

FIGURE 3-5. Generation of an action potential. A microelectrode can be introduced into an excitable cell to record the resting potential (A) and changes in transmembrane potential associated with the spread of the action potential along the cell membrane. The difference in electrical potential "seen" by the two electrodes (one outside and one inside the cell) is amplified electronically and displayed on the cathode ray oscilloscope on the left (B, C, D). Once a small region of membrane is depolarized, local electric currents flow which depolarize adjacent regions of the membrane. Very soon after being depolarized, the membrane becomes impermeable to most ions again, and the resting potential is re-established (repolarization; C, D). The dynamics of the passive and active migration of ions across the membrane actually result in some overshoot of the action potential above the zero line and below the average resting potential of −70 mV. Thus, the peak-to-peak amplitude of the action potential is of the order of 100 mV.

After causing the increase in permeability of the postjunctional membrane to ions, the acetylcholine is rapidly inactivated by an enzyme called *cholinesterase*. The cholinesterase is present in the fluid bathing the synaptic space and begins immediately to split the acetylcholine. The very short time that the acetylcholine remains in contact with the muscle fiber membrane, about 2 msec, is usually sufficient to excite the muscle fiber, and yet the rapid inactivation of acetylcholine prevents re-excitation after the muscle fiber has repolarized from the first action potential.

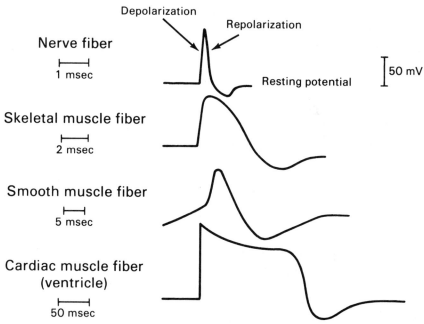

FIGURE 3-6. Examples of action potentials in different types of excitable cells. The amplitude and shape of the action potential vary from one type of cell to the next. The nerve impulse is a very rapid event lasting about 1 msec. The skeletal muscle impulse lasts about 5 to 10 times as long, and the cardiac muscle impulse lasts as long as 200 to 300 msec. Note the different time calibrations.

Conduction of the Muscle Impulse to the Interior of the Muscle Fiber: Endoplasmic Reticulum

The change in electrical potential in the immediate vicinity of actin and myosin filaments triggers the process that leads to shortening of each sarcomere. Thus, it is important for the muscle action potential to be conveyed throughout the entire muscle fiber as effectively as possible. As illustrated in Figure 3-2, the interior of a muscle fiber contains two interlaced systems of tubes that play an important role in excitation of muscle fibers and in the coupling of excitation to contraction. One of these is the *transverse tubular system* (T system), which speeds the transmission of the muscle action potential to all portions of the muscle fiber, and the other is the *sarcoplasmic reticulum* (SR), which has been implicated in the storage and release of calcium ions during the contractile process. Together, the two systems are calls the *endoplasmic reticulum.*

Excitation—Contraction Coupling

Energy must be supplied to myofilaments to cause movement of the actin filaments toward the center of the A bands. Energy for this purpose is *available* from molecules of adenosine triphosphate (ATP), which are coupled to the myosin cross-bridges. The energy is actually *provided* when molecules of ATP are split into adenosine diphosphate (ADP) and a phosphate group (PO₄) by the action of myosin. This enzymatic ATP-splitting property of myosin is called *myosin ATPase activity,* and the essentials of the splitting of ATP for energy are expressed by the equation:

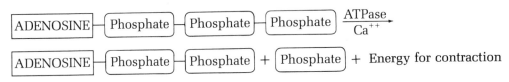

The ATPase activity of myosin is stimulated by Ca^{++}.

SLIDING FILAMENT THEORY OF MUSCLE CONTRACTION

Figure 3-7 depicts the sequential series of events that are hypothesized to explain how the sliding filaments develop tension and shorten. At rest (Fig. 3-7, A), Ca^{++} is stored in the sarcoplasmic reticulum, and the ATP molecules are coupled near the end of each cross-bridge (transverse projection of heavy meromyosin). *Potential reactive sites on the actin filament are covered by troponin.* As a pulse of depolarization descends the T tubules, quantities of Ca^{++} are released from storage sites in the sarcoplasmic reticulum. Some of these ions are bound by troponin, causing a *deformation in the shape of the troponin molecule* (Fig. 3-7, B). This appears to *uncover an active site on* the actin filament that attracts (electrostatically) the cross-bridge. Linkage between the myosin cross-bridge and an active site on the actin triggers the ATPase activity of myosin and results in splitting of the ATP. This produces transient flexion of the cross-bridge (Fig. 3-7, C), which *pulls the actin filament a short distance* before the linkage is broken and another molecule of ATP is coupled to the end of the cross-bridge (Fig. 3-7, D). Once recharged with ATP, the cross-bridge can react with another active site and pull the actin filament a little farther past the myosin filament. This recharging process occurs hundreds of times each second. The *strength of contraction* (active tension) *of the individual myofibril appears to depend on the average number of links between actin and myosin at any given instant. Energy must be spent to maintain active tension* even in the absence of overall shortening such as occurs when the muscle is attempting, unsuccessfully, to lift an excessively heavy load (absence of external work being accomplished).

Muscle Relaxation

Once depolarization of the muscle fiber has come to an end (5 to 10 msec), the intracellular concentration of Ca^{++} drops very quickly, and relaxation occurs. The rapid drop in intracellular Ca^{++} appears to be the result of an active "pumping" of calcium ions from the region of myofilaments into storage sites in the sarcoplasmic reticulum. The exact nature of these pumps is unknown, but metabolic energy is required to

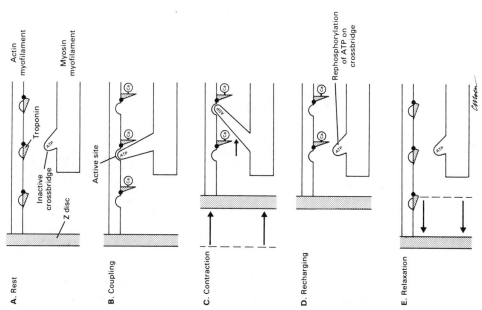

FIGURE 3-7. The sequential series of reactions between active sites on actin and myosin filaments that is hypothesized to pull the actin filament (and attached Z disk) past the myosin filament to produce shortening of the sarcomere. The recovery process is also depicted. Many repetitions of the cycle at a large percentage of the active sites are needed to produce a strong contraction. (A) Rest: Cross-bridges project from myosin myofilament but are not coupled with actin myofilament; ATP is attached near head of cross-bridge; troponin covers active sites on actin; calcium ions are stored in sarcoplasmic reticulum. (B) Coupling: Arrival of muscle action potential depolarizes sarcolemma and T tubules; calcium ions are released and react with troponin; change in shape of troponin-calcium complex uncovers active sites on actin; cross-bridge couples with adjacent active site, thereby linking myosin and actin myofilaments. (C) Contraction: Linkage of cross-bridge and active site triggers ATPase activity of myosin; ATP splits to ADP + PO$_4$ + energy; reaction produces transient flexion of cross-bridge; actin myofilament is pulled a short distance past myosin myofilament; Z disks are moved closer together. (D) Recharging: Cross-bridge uncouples from active site and retracts; ATP is replaced on cross-bridge; recoupling, flexion, uncoupling, retraction, and recharging process is repeated hundreds of times per second. (E) Relaxation: Cessation of excitation occurs; calcium ions are removed from vicinity of actin myofilament and returned to storage sites in sarcoplasmic reticulum; troponin returns to original shape, covering active sites on actin; actin and myosin myofilaments return to rest state.

transport Ca^{++} across the membrane into the sarcoplasmic reticulum. Active transport of Ca^{++} against a concentration gradient continues until the concentration of Ca^{++} in the intracellular fluid bathing the myofilaments reaches a very low level under resting conditions. Thus the *interaction between actin and myosin myofilaments is brought to a stop due to an insufficient concentration of intracellular Ca^{++}.* A summary of the events producing contraction and relaxation of muscle fibers is shown in the right-hand column of Figure 3-7.

ENERGY SOURCES FOR MUSCLE CONTRACTION

Muscle cells, like other living cells in the body, expend energy even when at rest to support metabolic processes required for the maintenance of life. When a muscle contracts, chemical energy derived from the breakdown of ATP is converted to mechanical energy, thereby increasing the need for more chemical energy. *The ultimate source of energy for all metabolic processes is oxygen. Energy becomes available for metabolic work through chemical reactions in the mitochondria that oxidize food materials.* Since the body cannot store as large a supply of oxygen as it can food materials, metabolically active cells depend upon a constant supply of oxygen brought to them by the respiratory and cardiovascular systems. However, muscle cells are unique with respect to the utilization of oxygen. *In muscle, oxygen serves as an indirect source of energy; the direct source of energy for muscle contraction is ATP.* A series of chemical reactions involving stored materials serves to replenish the supply of ATP as it is used for contraction.

Anaerobic Metabolism

Enough ATP is stored in each skeletal muscle to provide the chemical energy for performing only *two or three strong contractions of the muscle.* The chemical equation for that reaction is:

$$ATP \xrightarrow{\text{ATPase}} ADP + PO_4 + Energy$$

With addition of energy from the breakdown of another high-energy compound, phosphocreatine ($CrPO_4$) to creatine (Cr) and phosphate (PO_4), the by-products of the original reaction can be used to regenerate the supply of ATP, that is,

$$CrPO_4 \longrightarrow Cr + PO_4 + Energy$$
$$ADP + PO_4 + Energy \longrightarrow ATP$$

The relatively large reservoir of phosphocreatine can provide energy for muscle contractions over a period of *20 to 30 sec.* Regeneration of phosphocreatine is accomplished partly through the breakdown of glucose to lactic acid; the supply of glucose is replenished quickly by the breakdown of glycogen from storage depots in the muscle and the liver—a process called *glycolysis*.

Energy derived from this chain of reactions is capable of regenerating sufficient ATP to support vigorous muscle contractions for approximately 30 sec, and none of the reactions have required the expenditure of oxygen. Thus, these processes are called *anaerobic* (Gr. *a*, without, and *aero*, air) metabolism.

Aerobic Metabolism

Ultimately, all temporary reservoirs of chemical energy for muscle contraction are restored by oxidative metabolism of fats, carbohydrates, and proteins in the mitochondria of the muscle fiber. Carbohydrate, fat, and protein molecules are mobilized from storage sites in the body; enzymes split these large molecules into small units that can be oxidized in a series of chemical reactions called the *tricarboxylic acid cycle* (Krebs cycle). The end products of these reactions are carbon dioxide, water, and ATP for restoration and maintenance of energy stores.

Use of energy from anaerobic chemical reactions to power the contractile process for the first few minutes of strenuous physical exertion produces an *oxygen debt* that is repaid by continuing oxidative (aerobic) metabolism at a relatively high rate for several minutes after cessation of the exercise. The size of the oxygen debt constitutes a limiting factor for the continuation of exercise. The rate of buildup of the debt depends on the severity of the exercise. *Once the maximum oxygen debt has been attained, the rate of energy expenditure cannot exceed the rate of energy production through oxidative metabolism.* In addition to the rate at which chemical reactions proceed through the tricarboxylic acid cycle, other *factors that limit the steady-state performance of a person are the adequacy of operation of the respiratory and cardiovascular systems in supplying oxygen to the active cells and in removing the end products of metabolism.*

EFFICIENCY OF MUSCULAR WORK

The relative efficiency of the muscular system in performing mechanical work (that is, the mechanical work output per unit of energy put into the muscular system) has been calculated to be approximately 20 to 25 percent. This means that lifting a particular load a certain distance requires four to five times as much chemical energy as might be expected if all of the energy were directed at moving the load. This additional energy shows up as heat. When muscles are exercised vigorously, considerable heat is produced, and special physiologic mechanisms are set into motion to regulate body temperature. The reader is advised to consult a textbook on physiology for further information on the regulation of body temperature.

The rate at which energy is being expended in the body to sustain life (resting level), or to support physical activity, can be measured either by monitoring the rate of heat production or by monitoring the uptake of oxygen from the air being breathed. Expressed in terms of heat production, a typical *resting level of energy expenditure is*

TABLE 3-1. Relative Energy Cost in METS* During Various Activities

Self-Care Activities	METS	Locomotion	METS
Supine rest	1.0	Walk 2.0 mph	2.0
Sitting relaxed	1.0	Walk 2.5 mph	2.5
Standing relaxed	1.5	Walk 3.0 mph	3.0
Eating	1.5	Walk 3.5 mph	4.0
Dressing, undressing	2.0	Walk down stairs	4.5
Washing hands, face	2.0	Crutches and braces	6.5
Wheelchair propulsion	2.0	Walk upstairs, eight 9-inch steps	
Showering	3.5	11 steps/min	3.3
Using bedpan	4.0	22 steps/min	5.4
		33 steps/min	8.0

*Metabolic equivalents—multiples of the approximate resting energy expenditure.

approximately 1 Calorie per min* for a young adult weighing 70 kg (154 lb). This represents a total energy expenditure of approximately *1500 Calories per 24 hours to maintain the cellular processes of the body at rest* (resting metabolic rate). Walking at 5 km per hour (3.1 miles per hour) will increase the energy expenditure to about 5 Calories per min, and climbing a flight of stairs rapidly will increase it to about 8 Calories per min. Expressed in terms of oxygen consumption, the same person would use about 0.2 liters (L) of oxygen per min resting, 1 L per min walking at 5 km per hour, and 1.6 L per min climbing stairs. Measurements in trained athletes have yielded a maximum rate of oxygen consumption of approximately 6 L per min. In recent years, another term, the MET (multiples of resting metabolic rate), has become widely used to communicate the energy requirements for various activities. *One MET is arbitrarily defined as the resting oxygen consumption of the individual.* (A typical example is 3.5 ml of O_2 per kg of body weight per min.) The energy cost of any additional activity is then expressed as some multiple of the resting metabolic rate. For example, the energy cost of walking 5 km per hour would be expressed as 5 METS. The relative energy costs of various self-care activities are listed in Table 3-1, along with representative values for walking at different speeds.

The energy cost of any particular activity can be made to vary considerably depending upon the intensity with which the activity is pursued. Table 3-2 contains the range of energy costs (in METS) of other common activities (see also Passmore and Durnin, 1955).

---

*One Calorie, or large calorie (Cal), is the amount of heat required to raise the temperature of 1 kg (2.2 lb) of water 1°C. This is the unit commonly used to express the energy content of food that is eaten. One small calorie (cal) is the amount of heat required to raise the temperature of 1 gm of water 1°C (1 Calorie = 1000 calories). Many of those writing in newspapers and popular magazines erroneously use the lower-case spelling of the unit, but they nearly always mean the large calorie. The large calorie is sometimes called a kilocalorie.

TABLE 3-2. Approximate Range in Energy Cost (METS) of Common Activities

Activity	METS
Back packing	5–11
Bed exercise (arm movement, supine or sitting)	1–2
Bicycling (pleasure or to work)	3–8
Bowling	2–4
Cleaning windows	2–4
Conditioning exercises (calisthenics)	3–8
Crutch-walking*	2–8
Dancing (social and square)	3–7
Football, touch	6–10
Golf	
Using power cart	2–3
Walking (carrying bag or pulling cart)	4–7
Handball	8–12
Hiking, cross-country	3–7
Jogging, 5 mph	7–8
Making beds	2–4
Paddleball (or racquetball)	8–12
Pushing power mower	3–5
Propelling wheelchair	2–5
Stair climbing	4–8
Swimming	4–8
Table tennis	3–5
Tennis	4–9
Volleyball	3–6

*An important consideration for crutch-walking is the energy cost per meter walked.

MUSCLE FIBER TYPES

The problem of combining all the properties needed to perform the various functions of skeletal muscles was solved by incorporating three* different types of muscle fibers—each with different properties—into the muscle. The majority of skeletal muscles consist of a mixture of all three types, with the proportion of one type greater than another.

The first type of fiber is dark (like the meat on the leg of a chicken) and contains large numbers of mitochondria and a high concentration of myoglobin (muscle hemoglobin that stores oxygen). The second type of fiber is pale (like the breast of a chicken) and contains fewer mitochondria and only small amounts of myoglobin. Pale muscle fibers are larger in diameter than dark muscle fibers; they develop greater force of

---

*Some investigators have described more than three types (Burke, 1981), but for simplicity only the three main types of muscle fibers will be discussed here.

contraction and complete a single twitch in a significantly shorter time than dark muscle fibers, but they also fatigue more quickly. The third type of fiber is intermediate in color, numbers of mitochondria, size, and twitch characteristics. When samples of muscle are sectioned and stained with appropriate chemicals to reveal the presence of specific classes of enzymes, the mitochondria of dark muscle fibers are found to have a preponderance of oxidative enzymes (associated with aerobic metabolism). Pale muscle fibers are found to have a preponderance of glycolytic enzymes (associated with anaerobic metabolism) in their mitochondria. Thus, muscle fibers may be classified on the basis of appearance (anatomic and histologic) and functional (physiologic) characteristics (Table 3-3). For most purposes, the terms *slow-twitch* and *fast-twitch* muscle fibers are used to describe the two extremes. *Slow-twitch muscle fibers are fatigue resistant and fast-twitch muscle fibers have a tendency to fatigue rather quickly.*

Human trunk and limb muscles contain various proportions of the three types of muscle fibers. In addition, the few studies that have been reported (Gollnick et al, 1972; Johnson et al, 1973; Edgerton et al, 1975; Thorstensson, 1976) suggest a large variation from subject to subject regarding the proportions of fast-twitch and slow-twitch muscle fibers in a particular muscle. However, in spite of the subject-to-subject variation, the proportion of slow-twitch fibers is high in the human soleus muscle (as great as 85 percent of the fibers) and low in the orbicularis oculi (10 percent). The proportion of slow-twitch fibers in representative muscle groups has been ranked (in descending order) by Johnson and associates (1973) as follows: soleus, adductor pollicis, tibialis anterior, biceps femoris, peroneus longus, deltoid, gastrocnemius, biceps

TABLE 3-3. Characteristics of Skeletal Muscle Fibers Based on their Physical and Metabolic Properties*

Property	Muscle Fiber Type		
	Slow-Twitch	Intermediate	Fast-Twitch
Muscle fiber diameter	Small	Intermediate	Large
Color	Red	Red	White
Myoglobin content	High	High	Low
Mitochondria	Numerous	Numerous	Few
Oxidative enzymes	High	Intermediate	Low
Glycolytic enzymes	Low	Intermediate	High
Glycogen content	Low	Intermediate	High
Myosin ATPase activity	Low	High	High
Major source of ATP	Oxidative phosphorylation	Oxidative phosphorylation	Glycolysis
Speed of contraction	Slow	Intermediate	Fast
Rate of fatigue	Slow	Intermediate	Fast
Other names used	Type I	Type II B	Type II A
	SO	FOG	FG

*Adapted from Burke, RE and Edgerton, VR: *Motor unit properties and selective involvement in movement.* Exer Sport Sci Rev 3:31, 1975.

brachii, quadriceps, sternocleidomastoideus, triceps brachii, and orbicularis oculi. The degree to which a particular muscle exhibits physiologic characteristics of contracting slowly and tonically (sustained contraction) and of resisting fatigue can be expected to follow this same distribution. In reverse order, beginning with the orbicularis oculi muscle, they will exhibit physiologic characteristics of contracting briskly and phasically (brief contraction) and of fatiguing quickly.

THE MOTOR UNIT

In the anterior horns of the gray matter of the spinal cord are located the large motor cells that constitute the link to the final pathway of motor response (see Fig. 3-4, A, C). Such a cell body, together with its axon and all the muscle fibers it innervates, is named the *motor unit*. The number of muscle fibers innervated by a single motor nerve fiber varies from as few as 5 in some eye muscles, which have fine control, to as many as 1000 or more in a large muscle (such as the gastrocnemius), which does not require a high degree of control. The average number of muscle fibers per motor unit in a given muscle is determined by dividing the number of muscle fibers by the number of large motor axons innervating that particular muscle (innervation ratio). Table 3-4 lists the number of motor units and average number of muscle fibers per motor unit found in studies performed on human muscles (from the review prepared by Buchthal and Schmalbruch, 1980).

Muscle fibers excited by one axon are believed to occupy an average territory of 5 to 10 mm in diameter, allowing space for the fibers of 15 to 30 motor units within the

TABLE 3-4. Number of Motor Units and Average Number of Muscle Fibers per Motor Unit in Human Muscle

Muscle	No. of α-Motor Axons	No. of Muscle Fibers Per Muscle $\times 10^3$	No. of Muscle Fibers Average Per Motor Unit	No. of Muscle Spindles Per Muscle	No. of Muscle Spindles Per Motor Unit
Biceps brachii	774	580	750	320	0.41
Brachioradialis	330	130	390	65	0.20
Interosseus dorsalis 1	119	40.5	340	34	0.29
Lumbricalis 1	98	10.3	110	53	0.54
Opponens pollicis	133	79	595	44	0.33
Masseter	1020	1000	980	160	0.16
Temporalis	1150	1500	1300	217	0.19
Gastrocnemius medius	580	1000	1720	80	0.14
Tibialis anterior	445	270	610	284	0.64

From Buchthal, F and Schmalbruch, H: *Motor unit of mammalian muscle.* Physiol Rev 60:95, 1980, with permission.

same territory. Thus, fibers of many motor units intermingle in a given area of the cross section, the density of fibers being somewhat greater in the center of the motor unit than in the periphery. Most individual muscle fibers have no physical contact with other muscle fibers of the same motor unit (Kugelberg, 1981).

As the name "motor unit" implies, all the muscle fibers within a given motor unit contract or relax nearly simultaneously; that is, it is not possible for some of the muscle fibers of a motor unit to contract while others in the same motor unit relax. Also, if the muscle fibers of a motor unit are activated by the nerve sufficiently to contract, those fibers will contract maximally. This is known as the *all-or-none law*. The law, however, applies only to individual motor units, and physiologic mechanisms exist for the fine gradation of the force of contraction of the muscle as a whole.

GRADATION OF STRENGTH OF MUSCLE CONTRACTION

In general, *increased strength of contraction of a muscle, as a whole, occurs in three ways:* (1) *by initially activating motor neurons with the smallest innervation ratio, thereby activating few muscle fibers;* (2) *by increasing the number of motor units activated simultaneously (recruitment);* and (3) *by increasing the frequency of stimulation of individual motor units,* thereby increasing the percentage of time that each active muscle fiber is developing maximum tension. The fact that the smallest motor neurons are the first to be recruited and the largest motor neurons are recruited last is called the *size principle of recruitment* (Henneman, 1981). Since small motor neurons innervate slow-twitch muscle fibers, they participate in most functional activities. Only when contractions requiring great strength are attempted do the largest fast-twitch motor units become active.

NERVE FIBERS

Peripheral Neurons

Neurons come in all shapes and sizes depending on their placement in the nervous system (see Fig. 3-4) and the functions for which they are responsible. Figure 3-8 shows the characteristics of a sensory and a motor neuron. A typical neuron consists of a *cell body* (containing the nucleus), several short radiating processes *(dendrites),* and one long process (the *axon*) that terminates in twig-like branches and may have branches (collaterals) projecting along its course. The axon, together with its covering (sheath), forms the *nerve fiber.* The larger motor and sensory nerves are wrapped with a covering containing a white lipid substance called *myelin.* The myelin sheath is laid down so that it forms regular indentations along its length known as *nodes of Ranvier* (named after a French histologist, Louis Ranvier, 1835–1922).

A peripheral nerve trunk is composed of many nerve fibers bound together by supporting connective tissue (see Fig. 3-4, C). Functionally, three main classes of nerve

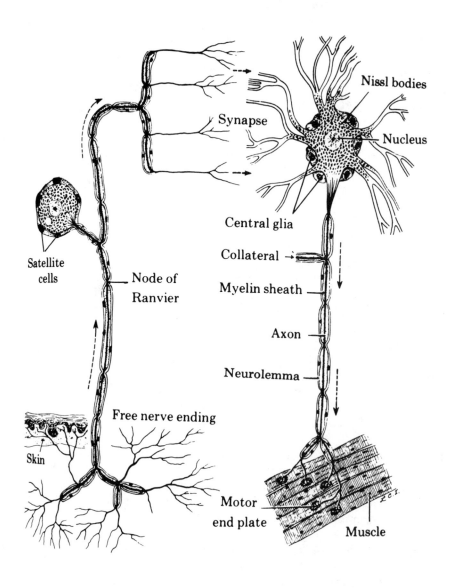

SENSORY NEURON   MOTOR NEURON

FIGURE 3-8. Diagrammatic representation of two types of neurons. The satellite cells and central glia are supporting cells that surround the nerve cell body. Synaptic connections between the terminal processes of the sensory neuron and the dendrites of the motor neuron are not shown. In the nervous system, such synaptic connections are numerous. (From King, BG and Showers, MJ: *Human Anatomy and Physiology*, ed 6. WB Saunders, Philadelphia, 1969, p 59 with permission.)

fibers are found in the peripheral nerve: (1) *Motor fibers* conduct nerve impulses from the spinal cord to skeletal muscle fibers for the control of voluntary muscular activity. Their cell bodies are located in the gray matter of the spinal cord and brain stem. These are also called *efferent* (L. *ex*, out, plus *ferre*, to carry) nerve fibers. (2) *Sensory fibers* carry impulses arising from various receptors in the skin, muscles, and special sense organs to the central nervous system where the impulses are interpreted. The cell bodies lie in special ganglia located along the roots of origin of the sensory nerves. These are also called *afferent* (L. *ad*, to, plus *ferre*, to carry) nerve fibers. (3) *Autonomic fibers* (efferent in function) are concerned with the control of smooth muscle and glandular activities. Discussion of the autonomic nervous system is beyond the scope of this book.

CLASSIFICATION OF NERVE FIBERS ON THE BASIS OF AXON DIAMETER

When histologists and anatomists began studying the characteristics of neurons supplying various motor and sensory structures in the body, they classified neurons on the basis of the diameter of their axons. The largest fibers were labeled type A and the smallest type C; those of intermediate diameter thus became type B. The A and B fibers are all myelinated, whereas the C fibers are unmyelinated. It later became convenient to subdivide the type A category on the basis of fiber diameter into subcategories called alpha (α), beta (β), gamma (γ), and delta (δ). The speed at which a nerve impulse travels along the length of an axon is related to the diameter of the axon. *Larger axons conduct impulses at a faster velocity. Adding a myelin sheath causes the axon to conduct an impulse even faster.* The largest myelinated axons (type A, alpha, with a diameter of 20 μm) conduct an impulse at a maximum velocity of approximately 120 m per sec. The longest motor axons are those extending from the lumbar segments of the spinal cord to muscles in the foot—a distance of approximately 1 m. Thus, a minimum of 8 msec (0.008 sec) would be needed for a nerve impulse to travel the length of the largest motor axon. The largest sensory axons are also of the A, alpha, type. Consequently, a similar amount of time would be needed for a sensory impulse to travel from a receptor in the foot to the spinal cord. However, the *average* velocity of conduction of the large motor and sensory fibers in a peripheral nerve is in the range of 50 to 70 m per sec. Therefore, one can expect it to take at least 28 msec for a nerve impulse to travel the 2-m reflex arc from sensory receptor in the foot to motor cell in the spinal cord and back to a muscle in the foot. To this must be added the time needed (1) to generate the action potential in the sensory receptor (1 to 5 msec); (2) to transmit the signal across the synapse between sensory ending and motor cell (0.5 msec); (3) to transmit the signal throughout the sarcotubule system (1 to 5 msec); (4) to activate the contractile apparatus (1 to 2 msec); and (5) to produce shortening of the muscle (10 to 300 msec). The smallest nerve fibers (0.5 μm in diameter) convey nerve impulses from sensory endings in the skin that appear to produce sensations of pain when stimulated. These impulses are conducted at a velocity of approximately 0.5 m per sec.

CLASSIFICATION OF NERVE FIBERS ON THE BASIS OF SENSORY FIBER ORIGIN

A second classification, applied by sensory physiologists to afferent fibers, is based on a division of fibers into four groups on the basis of the type of sensory receptor from which they are conducting impulses. The first group (group I) is subdivided into subgroups Ia and Ib. *Group Ia fibers carry impulses from a particular type of sensory receptor located in muscles, called the muscle spindle primary receptor.* The structure and function of the muscle spindle will be described below. *Group Ib fibers carry impulses from sensory receptors located in tendons which attach muscle fibers to bone.* These are called *Golgi tendon organs* and will also be described later. The diameters of group Ia and Ib fibers are approximately the same, and they fall into the type A, alpha, category of the other classification. *Group II fibers* are equivalent to type A, beta, in size and carry impulses from the *secondary receptors in the muscle spindle.*

Central Neurons

Nerve fibers are also present in the central nervous system, that is, the spinal cord and brain (see Fig. 3-4, A). Some of the neurons reside entirely within the spinal cord and transmit impulses from the end of a peripheral sensory neuron to the dendrites or cell body of another neuron nearby. Such neurons are called *interneurons*, or internuncial neurons. Other neurons extend from a sensory receptor in the skin, muscle, tendon, or joint to the spinal cord. After entering the spinal cord, the sensory fiber may give off a branch that synapses with interneurons in the spinal cord, but the main fiber usually continues upward through the spinal cord to synapse on nerve cells in the brain. Such an uninterrupted sensory fiber is called a *first-order* sensory fiber. A sensory neuron that receives synaptic input from a peripheral sensory neuron and conducts action potentials from the spinal cord to sensory centers in the brain is called a *second-order* sensory fiber. Neurons that carry motor impulses from the brain to motor neurons in the spinal cord are called *upper motor neurons.* This separates them from the *lower motor neurons*, which conduct motor impulses from the spinal cord to activate muscle fibers.

NEURAL MODIFICATION OF EXCITABILITY

Most neurons discharge nerve impulses intermittently, that is, they exhibit a resting level of firing. The frequency of discharge is then modified by the influence of other neurons. All neurons send signals to other neurons by releasing small amounts of chemicals called *neurotransmitters* at the synapse, the junction between nerves (see Fig. 3-4, D). *A quantity of transmitter is released each time a nerve impulse arrives at the synapse.* The process is essentially the same as that which occurs in transmission at the myoneural junction (see Fig. 3-4, C). But *some of these neurotransmitters facili-*

tate a neuron (depolarize the postsynaptic membrane), thus tending to make it fire one or more nerve impulses; whereas *others inhibit the neuron (hyperpolarize the postsynaptic membrane),* thus tending to keep it inactive. These neurotransmitters are called *facilitatory* (excitatory) and *inhibitory* transmitters, respectively. Any given neuron synthesizes and releases either a facilitatory or inhibitory substance, not both, at its presynaptic terminals, and is therefore known as either a facilitatory or inhibitory neuron. Both facilitatory and inhibitory stimuli are constantly being transmitted from motor centers in lower parts of the brain to interneurons throughout the spinal cord. Similarly, motor neurons receive synaptic connections from thousands of neurons. Whether a given motor neuron becomes more active or less active depends on the *net* effect of all the facilitatory and inhibitory stimuli that arrive at the motor neuron at any given instant. An inactive motor neuron can be stimulated to discharge nerve impulses by: (1) increasing the facilitatory stimuli, while the inhibitory stimuli remain constant; (2) decreasing the inhibitory stimuli, while the facilitatory stimuli remain constant; or (3) a combination of increasing the facilitatory and decreasing the inhibitory stimuli. The last mechanism is probably the most common.

JOINT, TENDON, AND MUSCLE RECEPTORS

Specialized receptors are present in skeletal muscles, tendons, and joint structures. These receptors detect changes in tension and position of the structures in which they are situated, and a pattern of nerve impulses is generated in the receptor to convey this information to other parts of the nervous system. As a result, moment-to-moment changes in muscle length, force of muscle contraction, joint angle (position), speed of joint motion, and degree of joint compression or distraction are relayed to centers in the spinal cord and brain where the information is integrated with that coming from other sensory organs, such as those in the retina of the eye and the vestibular apparatus of the ear. The integrated sensory signals are used by the motor control centers in the brain to automatically adjust the location, type, number, and frequency of motor unit activation so that the appropriate muscle tension is developed to perform the desired movements.

Joint Receptors

Several different types of sensory receptors are found in the joint capsule and ligaments about the joints. Figure 3-9 shows the major anatomic features of those most commonly present. Most of these receptors emit several action potentials per second as a "resting" output. The receptor is stimulated by being deformed. Depending on the location and magnitude of deforming forces acting on the joint and the location of the receptor, certain receptors will be stimulated and discharge a high-frequency burst of nerve impulses when the joint is moved. They typically adapt slightly after the movement ceases (frequency of impulses decreases) and then transmit a steady train of nerve impulses thereafter. Further movement of the joint may cause one set of recep-

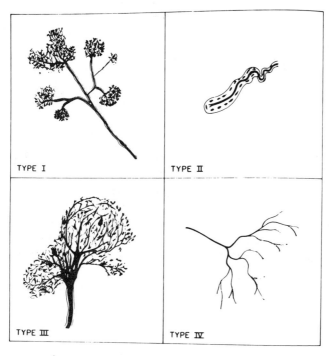

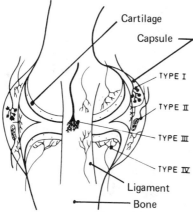

FIGURE 3-9. *Top,* semischematic illustration of the four joint receptors usually distinguished. *Bottom,* a diagram of the knee joint, showing the distribution of the various receptor types in the capsule and ligaments of the joint. The menisci are free from nerve fibers except at their attachment to the fibrous capsule. (From Brodal, A: *Neurological Anatomy,* ed 3. Oxford University Press, New York, 1981, p 56, with permission.)

tors to stop discharging impulses and another set to become active (Fig. 3-10). Thus, *the information from these joint receptors continually apprises the nervous system of the momentary angulation of the joint and of the rate of movement of the joint.*

Golgi Tendon Organs

Golgi tendon organs lie within muscle tendons near the point of attachment of the muscle fiber to the tendon (Fig. 3-11). An average of 10 to 15 muscle fibers is usually connected in direct line (series) with each Golgi tendon organ, and the receptor is stimulated by the tension produced by this small bundle of muscle fibers. Nerve impulses discharged by the tendon organ are transmitted over large, rapidly conducting afferent axons (group Ib fibers) to the spinal cord and cerebellum. Arrival of these nerve impulses at the spinal cord excites inhibitory interneurons which, in turn, *inhibit the motor neurons (A, alpha, neurons) of the contracting muscle,* thus limiting the force developed to that which can be tolerated by the tissues being stressed. Slips of tendon, however, can be *torn free from natural points of attachment by the abrupt application of a forceful contraction,* or by abrupt passive stretch of the tissues.

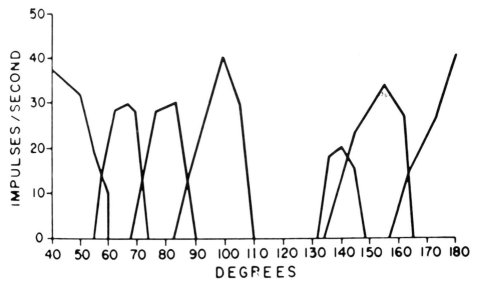

FIGURE 3-10. Discharge frequency of joint receptors during movement of the joint. Graphs of impulse frequencies for eight single nerve fibers innervating slowly adapting receptors in the capsule of the knee joint of the cat. The adapted impulse frequency is plotted against position of the joint in degrees. The figure is not representative for the distribution of endings that are successively activated during full movement, since, in general, activation of endings occurs more often immediately before or at full flexion or full extension than in the intermediate positions of the joint. The sensitive ranges (15 to 30 degrees) are representative of the behavior of most endings. (From Skoglund, S: *Anatomical and physiological studies of knee joint innervation in the cat.* Acta Physiol Scand 36[Suppl 124]:1, 1956, with permission.)

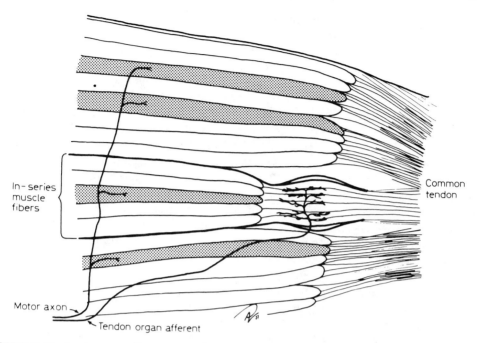

FIGURE 3-11. A schema to illustrate the anatomic relations among muscle fibers, a motor unit (stippled), and a Golgi tendon organ. Physiologic data indicate that a tendon organ is selectively sensitive to the forces produced by the in-series muscle fibers. A motor unit that activates a given tendon organ typically contributes only one fiber in series with the receptor. (From Houk, JC, Crago, PE, and Rymer, WZ: *Functional properties of the Golgi tendon organs*. In Desmedt, JE (ed): *Progress in Clinical Neurophysiology*, Vol 8. Karger, Basel, 1980, p 35, with permission.)

Therefore, to avoid injury, a muscle should be activated or stretched moderately at first, *gradually increasing* the force exerted on the points of attachment.

Muscle Spindle

The *muscle spindle* is a small but complex organ with multiple functions. Hundreds of studies have been conducted during the past 50 years to gain a better understanding of the structure and functions of this organ (Taylor and Prochazka, 1981). Although a great deal is now known, many questions about muscle spindle operation remain unanswered. The description presented here is a simplified version that disregards the finer distinctions regarding structure and functions reported in recent years (Matthews, 1981).

The lengths of human muscle spindles vary from 0.5 to 13 mm, but the usual length is 2 to 4 mm. They are fusiform in shape, that is, they are widest in the center and taper toward each end. Spindles are present in nearly all muscles, but are most numerous in the muscles of the arms and legs (see Table 3-3). They are especially abundant in the small muscles of the hand and foot. *The muscle spindle has both afferent and efferent innervation.* It functions as a *stretch receptor,* sending sensory impulses over afferent axons that inform other neurons in the spinal cord and brain of the length of the muscle spindle and of the rate at which it is being stretched. The muscle spindle also contains contractile fibers that are controlled by nerve impulses reaching them via small-diameter motor axons (efferent, type A, gamma) from the spinal cord. The *degree of shortening of the contractile portions of the muscle spindle regulates the sensitivity of the stretch receptor portion of muscle spindle.*

The muscle spindle is composed of a central nuclear bag containing the specialized stretch receptors and sets of 3 to 10 small muscle fibers, called intrafusal fibers, attached to each end of the bag (Fig. 3-12). The *intrafusal* (L. *intra,* within, plus *fusus,* spindle) *muscle fibers* are controlled by small-diameter motor nerve fibers from the spinal cord, called *gamma motor neurons* because of the size of their axons, or called *fusimotor neurons* because they supply motor impulses to the intrafusal muscle fibers. Thus, the middle, noncontractile part of the muscle spindle can be stretched by two different mechanisms. First, when the whole muscle is stretched, the spindle is also stretched. Secondly, when the contractile portions at each end of the muscle spindle are activated by impulses arriving over gamma motor nerves, the contractile portions shorten, thereby stretching the central portion of the spindle. In either case, stretch of the nuclear bag portion of the muscle spindle activates one or both of two sensory receptors residing there, called primary and secondary stretch receptors (see Fig. 3-12). Activation increases the frequency of nerve impulses emitted from these receptors. Afferent nerves from the *primary receptor* (group Ia) make synaptic connection with the motor neurons (A, alpha) controlling *extrafusal* (L. *extra,* outside of or in addition, plus *fusus,* spindle; in this case, referring to regular muscle fibers) *muscle fibers in the same muscle.* Abrupt stretch of a muscle, therefore, initiates a burst of impulses from the primary stretch receptor in the muscle fiber, which travels to the spinal cord and excites activity in motor units of the same muscle. Shortening of the muscle as a whole relieves stretch on the muscle spindles contained in the muscle, thereby removing the stimulus from the stretch receptors. Figure 3-13 illustrates the neural and muscular structures that participate in the stretch reflex. An abrupt stretch is applied by striking the patellar tendon with a hammer specifically designed to test the reflex response. The presence of a reflex contraction in the stretched muscle 100 to 200 msec after tapping the tendon reveals that the circuit is intact. In addition, the briskness and relative amplitude of the reflex contraction reflect the general level of excitability of alpha motor neurons innervating the stretched muscle.

The stretch reflex circuit is believed to operate in the automatic (reflex) regulation of muscle length when the desired length has been established by voluntary contraction of the muscle. Figure 3-14 shows a highly schematic representation of the initial condition (Fig. 3-14, A), followed by generation of additional sensory impulses when the joint is extended and the muscle spindle is stretched momentarily by the increased load in the hand (Fig. 3-14, B), and then reflexly returned to the original joint position by development of increased tension in the extrafusal muscle fibers (Fig. 3-14, C).

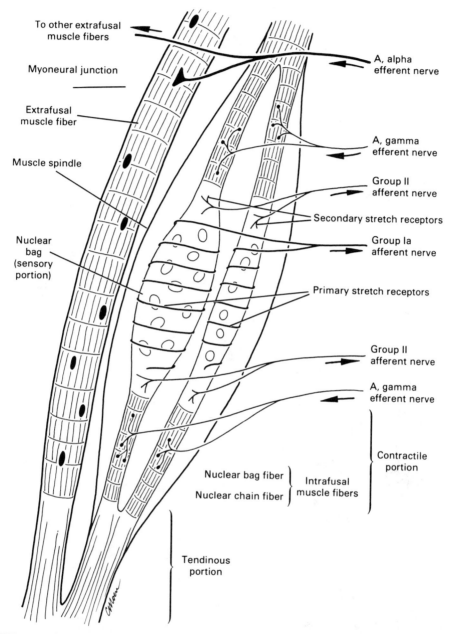

FIGURE 3-12. The muscle spindle. Diagram shows the anatomic relationships among the major anatomic components of a muscle spindle. Although most muscle spindles contain 3 to 10 intrafusal fibers, only 2 are shown here for simplicity. One regular (extrafusal) muscle fiber is also shown alongside the muscle spindle.

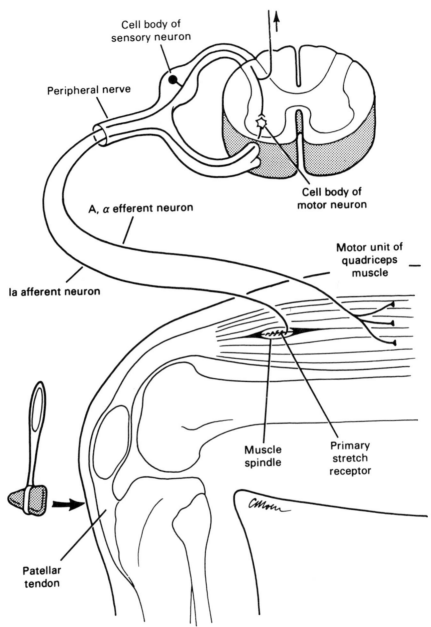

FIGURE 3-13. The stretch reflex. The four fundamental parts of the simple stretch reflex arc are (1) a receptor in the muscle that generates nerve impulses in proportion to the degree of deformation; (2) an afferent neuron that conducts the burst of sensory impulses from the receptor to the spinal cord; (3) an efferent neuron that conducts motor impulses from the spinal cord to extrafusal muscle fibers; and (4) an effector, the muscle, to respond to motor impulses. Note that the same sensory signals are transmitted to other parts of the central nervous system as well.

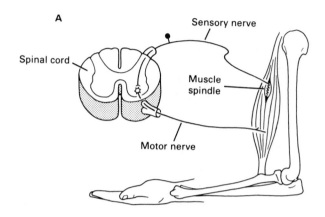

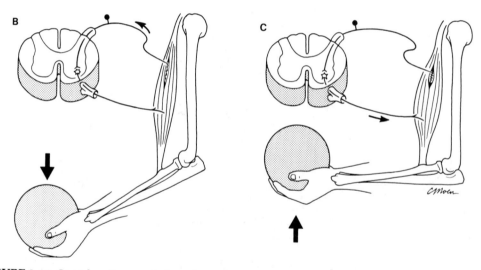

FIGURE 3-14. Stretch reflex regulation of muscle length. A muscle is under the influence of the stretch reflex when it is engaged in a steady contraction of a voluntary nature, as when a person's elbow is flexed steadily against a load (A). A sudden unexpected increase in the load (B) stretches the muscle, causing the sensory ending on the muscle spindle to send nerve impulses to the spinal cord (upward arrow), where they impinge on a motor nerve cell at a synapse and excite it. As a result motor impulses are sent back down to the muscle (downward arrow), where they cause it to contract (C). More complicated nervous pathways than the one shown may also be involved in the stretch reflex. Any real muscle is, of course, supplied with many motor nerve fibers and spindles. In addition the synaptic connections to even a single motor nerve cell are multiple. (Adapted from Merton, PA: *How we control the contraction of our muscles.* Scientific American 228:30, 1972.)

PRIMARY SENSORY ENDING

The primary sensory ending detects not only the relative amount of stretch but also the velocity of the stretch. As previously described, arrival of impulses from the primary receptor excites alpha motor neurons in the spinal cord, innervating muscle fibers in the stretched muscle. In addition, these *impulses excite interneurons which, in turn, inhibit alpha motor neurons supplying muscles that perform an action opposite to that performed by the stretched muscle* when it contracts (Fig. 3-15). Such inhibition promotes relaxation of the opposing muscle so that it can be elongated easily while the contracting muscle shortens.

SECONDARY SENSORY ENDINGS

The *secondary sensory endings* appear to detect the *amount of stretch.* Signals from secondary receptors are transmitted over smaller-diameter afferent neurons (called group II fibers), which synapse principally with interneurons and elicit more delayed and more variable patterns of muscle reflexes than obtained from the output of primary receptors.

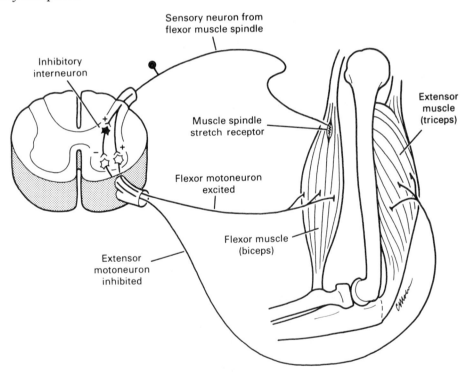

FIGURE 3-15. Reciprocal inhibition of motor neurons to the opposing muscle. Impulses from the stretched muscle excite motor units in the same muscle (facilitatory synaptic influence designated with a plus sign) and inhibit, through an interneuron, motor units in the opposing muscle (inhibitory synaptic influence designated with a minus sign).

SUMMARY OF MUSCLE SPINDLE FUNCTIONS

In essence, the muscle spindle functions as a *comparator*, comparing the length of the spindle with the length of the skeletal muscle fibers that surround it (see Fig. 3-14). If the length of the surrounding extrafusal muscle fibers is less than that of the spindle, the frequency of nerve impulses discharged from the receptors is reduced. When the central portion of the spindle is stretched because of gamma efferent activity, its sensory receptors discharge more nerve impulses, which reflexly excite alpha motor neurons to activate extrafusal muscle fibers. This mechanism is particularly important in the regulation of postural muscle tone.

Figure 3-16 summarizes the patterns of sensory receptor discharge recorded from nerves supplying the primary (Ia) and secondary (II) stretch receptors of the muscle spindle and the Golgi tendon organ (Ib) under various conditions. The major distinctions are that: (1) *the primary stretch receptor signals both the velocity of stretch and the length of the muscle spindle;* (2) *the secondary stretch receptor signals the length of the muscle spindle;* and (3) *the tendon organ detects the amount of tension being exerted by the muscle fibers.* In these roles, the primary stretch receptor is exhibiting qualities of both *phasic* (Gr. *phasis*, an appearance, a distinct stage) and *tonic* (Gr. *tonikos*, continuous tension) activity, while the secondary receptor and tendon organ are displaying tonic activity. A phasic receptor signals the rate of change of an event, while a tonic receptor signals the final result of the change. For example, the pattern of discharge from a purely phasic receptor during graded amounts of stretch is shown in Figure 3-17, B, and that from a purely tonic receptor is shown in Figure 3-17, C.

SEGMENTAL AND SUPRASEGMENTAL COMPONENTS OF MOTOR CONTROL

The earlier portions of this chapter have described the basic physiologic mechanisms responsible for the development of graded amounts of tension in motor units contained within a single muscle. To perform skilled motor activities requires a highly integrated set of motor commands to activate and inhibit appropriate muscles in the proper sequence. A complete description of what is known about the neural control of motor activities is beyond the scope of this book; however, a brief overview of several major mechanisms by which the excitability of motor neurons can be altered may be useful. In this context, the term *segmental* refers to the neural activity in circuits residing in particular neural segments of the spinal cord. The term *suprasegmental* refers to the influence of impulses from the brain on the excitability of neurons within the spinal cord.

Motor Centers

First, no movement can be performed effectively unless a *posture appropriate to the action is assumed* by suitable arrangement of the limbs and the body as a whole. Thus,

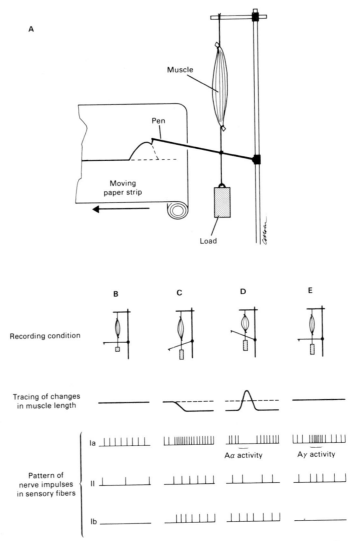

FIGURE 3-16. Discharge patterns of muscle spindle primary receptor (in group Ia sensory nerve fiber), secondary receptor (in group II fiber), and Golgi tendon organ (in group Ib fiber) under resting conditions (A), during stretch (B), during transient *contraction of the extrafusal muscle fibers* produced by activation via alpha motor fibers (C), and during *contraction of the intrafusal fibers* produced by activation via the gamma motor fibers (D).

the control of posture is one of the most important functions of the central nervous system. The structures chiefly responsible for the control of posture and movement, called motor centers, are located in several different parts of the brain. In considering the motor functions of the nervous system, keep in mind that the motor centers can function appropriately only if they receive an uninterrupted stream of afferent (sen-

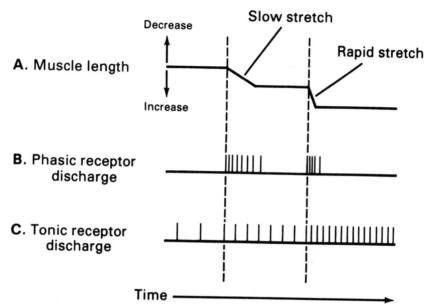

FIGURE 3-17. Discharge patterns of purely phasic and tonic receptors. The phasic receptor responds to the change in a condition, with the frequency of discharge proportional to the rate of change. The tonic receptor signals the existing status of the condition, such as muscle length.

sory) information about the status of all parts of the body and of the environment. To emphasize the role of the sense organs in the control of posture and movement, the term *sensorimotor system* is often used to connote the *combined afferent and efferent processes required to produce coordinated movement.* Movement is the end product of a number of control systems that interact extensively. The question of how voluntary movements are initiated is still unanswered (results of very recent studies indicate that the intent to begin a motion is associated with increased neural activity in the supplementary motor area of the cortex), but neurobiologists have established a considerable array of facts regarding the structure and operation of major circuits that execute the "orders" to perform functional activities.

Within the various regions of the brain and spinal cord, aggregations of anatomically and functionally related neurons are distinguished and set off from one another as separate *nuclei* or *ganglia. Tract* is the term used for a bundle of nerve fibers (axons) that joins the different regions of the brain and spinal cord. Because many of the nerve fibers are covered with a sheath of white insulating material, called myelin, the tracts appear white in unstained histologic sections. On the other hand, regions in which nerve cell bodies (which are not covered with myelin) are concentrated appear gray in color. In the spinal cord, the central region containing nerve cell bodies (gray matter) is completely surrounded by tracts of myelinated axons (white matter), some of which carry ascending impulses and others conduct descending impulses (see Fig. 3-4). In the cerebrum, the situation is reversed. Here, the cortex appears gray because the cell bodies of the cortical neurons lie in the surface layers; the tissue below is white because it consists of myelinated axons connecting cortical cells with other regions of the central nervous system.

The nerve fibers that descend from the motor cortex collectively form a bundle of fibers called the *corticospinal tract* (Fig. 3-18). As the name implies, most of the axons extend from a cell body in the motor cortex of the brain to the spinal cord where synaptic contact is made with motor neurons in the anterior horn of the spinal cord gray matter. The corticospinal tract is also called the *pyramidal* tract because many of the large motor cells are triangular in shape and have the appearance of small pyramids when a section of cortex is viewed under a microscope. Most of the corticospinal axons cross to the opposite side in the brain stem, as illustrated in Figure 3-18, proceeding downward in the lateral corticospinal tract of the spinal cord. Thus, the crossing fibers from the right and left motor cortex also form a pyramid in the brain stem. (The diagrammatic nature of Fig. 3-18 does not show the pyramid.) At the spinal segmental level, the axons of the pyramidal tract end predominately on interneurons. The organization of the pyramidal tract suggests that it is designed for precise control of individual muscle groups. Other cortical neurons, in the same motor areas that give rise to the long corticospinal axons, have short axons that synapse with second-order motor neurons lying in the basal ganglia or brain stem as illustrated in Figure 3-19. Their postsynaptic fibers (e.g., the reticulospinal and vestibulospinal tracts) do not enter the pyramids. For this reason, they and all other tracts descending into the brain stem that synapse there and then continue into the spinal cord are frequently termed, collectively, the *extrapyramidal* system. This distinction is a purely anatomic one. At one time, neurophysiologists supposed that voluntary motor control was effected through the pyramidal tracts and that automatic (involuntary) motor control was effected through the extrapyramidal system. Later studies cast doubt on the extent to which this distinction holds true. Currently, the question is still unresolved (Schwindt, 1981).

A schematic diagram of the spinal and supraspinal motor centers and their most important connections appears in Figure 3-20. The arrows connecting the various centers depicted in Figure 3-20 show the main direction of information flow underlying muscular activity. On the right in the illustration is an indication of the role each of these centers plays in producing movement. Each center is a site of processing and redirecting incoming signals. A conspicuous aspect of the diagram is the key position of the motor cortex. This is connected to the motor centers in the spinal cord, both indirectly by way of the brain stem and directly by way of the corticospinal tract. In addition, collateral branches leave the corticospinal tract, some passing to the brain stem and others acting on other high-level motor centers, the cerebellum and the basal ganglia. The brain stem consists of the midbrain, pons, and medulla oblongata (Fig. 3-21) and functions as a prespinal integrating system of great complexity. *Centers in the brain stem are chiefly responsible for automatic (reflex) control of the posture and spatial orientation of the body.* To accomplish this, they monitor and evaluate the afferent signals of many receptors throughout the body.

The most important sensory receptors for monitoring the orientation of the head with respect to the gravitational field are the receptors in the organs of equilibrium (the vestibular organs located in each inner ear) and the stretch and joint receptors of

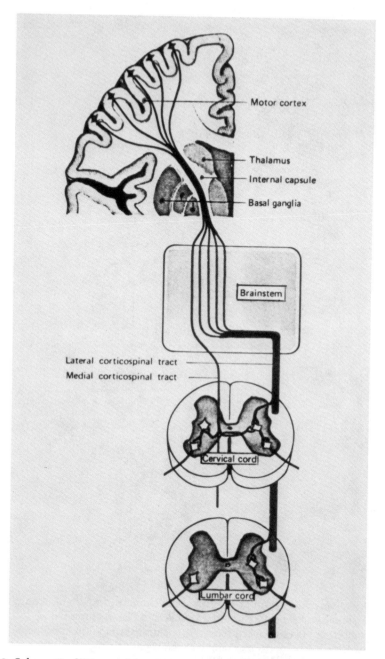

FIGURE 3-18. Schematic diagram of the course of the corticospinal tract from the motor cortex to the spinal cord. The collaterals to the basal ganglia, the cerebellum, and the motor centers of the brain stem have been omitted for simplicity (see Figs. 3-19, 3-20). For further description, see text. (From Schmidt, RF (ed): *Fundamentals of Neurophysiology*, ed 2. Springer-Verlag, New York, 1978, p 179, with permission.)

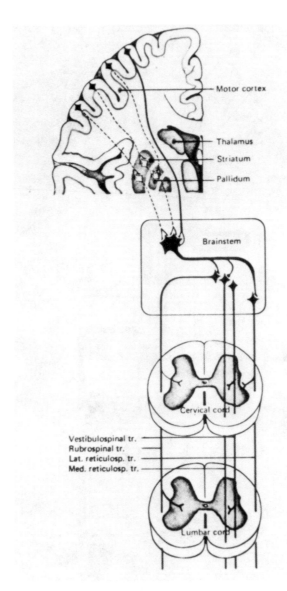

FIGURE 3-19. Schematic diagram of the courses of the most important extrapyramidal tracts from the supraspinal motor centers into the spinal cord. The neuron with a thick axon in the brain stem symbolizes the crossing of most of the extrapyramidal motor fibers to the opposite side at that level, and does not imply convergence. The pathways from motor cortex to basal nuclei are partly collaterals of the corticospinal tract and partly separate efferents. The details of connectivity among the brain stem structures involved in motor activity are extremely complicated; the representation here is greatly simplified. (From Schmidt, RF (ed): *Fundamentals of Neurophysiology*, ed 2. Springer-Verlag, New York, 1978, p 181, with permission.)

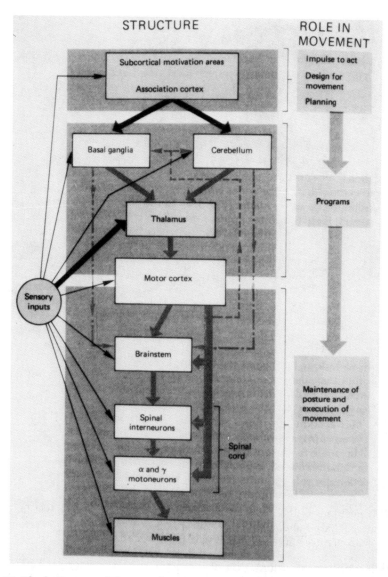

FIGURE 3-20. Block diagram of the spinal and supraspinal motor centers and their most important connections. For the sake of simplicity, all sensory inputs are summarized at the far left. The right-hand column indicates the chief role played by the structures in the middle of the diagram during the performance of movements. Note that the motor cortex is assigned to the transition between program and execution. (From Schmidt, RF (ed): *Fundamentals of Neurophysiology*, ed 2. Springer-Verlag, New York, 1978, p 176, with permission.)

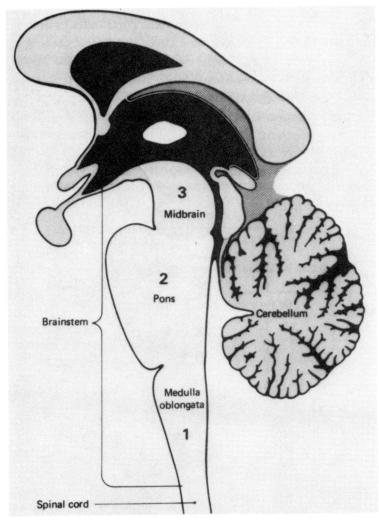

FIGURE 3-21. Positions of the main subdivisions of the brain stem. See text for explanation. (From Schmidt, RF (ed): *Fundamentals of Neurophysiology*, ed 2. Springer-Verlag, New York, 1978, p 187, with permission.)

the neck that monitor the orientation of the trunk with respect to the head. Information in the form of patterns of nerve impulses from these sources enables the brain stem motor centers to provide a continuous regulatory output, so that the upright body posture is adopted and maintained *entirely without the need for voluntary control.* Note, however, that voluntary motor commands can be superimposed upon the involuntary motor commands to achieve any particular posture or movement. The basal ganglia participate in the conversion of the plans for movement arising in the supplementary motor cortex into programs for movement. These centers are particularly significant with respect to the initiation and execution of slow movements. The basal ganglia are immediately adjacent to the thalamus, which is one of the most important sensory relay centers in the brain. Interconnected with all levels and functioning as an overall coordinator of activities is the cerebellum—a highly organized center with an extensive cortex of its own. The *cerebellum (see Fig. 3-21) appears to be chiefly concerned with programming rapid movements, correcting the course of such movements, and correlating posture and movement.* Thus, the cerebellum and basal ganglia serve different but related functions in the programming of cortically initiated movement patterns.

Sensory-Motor Integration

All the various suprasegmental motor pathways ultimately converge on a series of simple circuits that link each muscle with the spinal cord. The basic circuit includes the following parts: the *cell bodies of the motor neurons* in the spinal cord, their *efferent axons* extending out into the ventral roots; the *neuromuscular junctions,* the *muscle fibers* innervated by the axons; the *sensory receptors* with their *afferent axons* entering the spinal cord through the dorsal roots and their *synaptic terminations* in the spinal cord (see Fig. 3-4). The sensory neurons carrying impulses from a given muscle are connected with the motor neurons that transmit impulses back to the muscle, thus forming a closed loop that regulates the activity of each motor unit in the muscle (Fig. 3-22). This is the basic segmental component for control of the motor system. No movement (reflex or voluntary) can occur except through the operation of this circuit. Some of the sensory fibers from the muscle establish a direct connection with the motor neurons, whereas others do so indirectly through interneurons. These segmental circuits automatically regulate the length and tension of the muscles in accordance with various requirements. They are responsive peripherally to mechanical input (such as stretching of the muscle) and centrally to neural input from various motor centers. Mechanical deformation of the muscle spindle stimulates the stretch receptors, provoking action potentials that travel to the spinal cord to elicit a reflex response of the muscle (see Figs. 3-13, 3-14).

The sensory impulses from muscles are not restricted to influence only their own motor neurons. *This afferent input also spreads out through collateral branches of primary sensory neurons and through interneuron circuits to reach the motor neurons of all closely related muscles and, to a decreasing extent, those of more distant muscles.* Stretch or contraction of one muscle affects its own motor neurons most strongly, those of the muscle performing an opposite action somewhat less (where the effect is to *inhibit* any action; see Fig. 3-15), and those of other muscles which may assist in the motion still less (where the effect is to *facilitate* action). Thus, every primary loop is part of a larger feedback network serving a group of muscles. Transmission in local segmental circuits involves very little delay and ensures rapid responses. While this immediate response is occurring, the *same sensory signals are being transmitted to higher centers by way of collaterals, projection tracts, and secondary relays to widely separated parts of the nervous system* for more elaborate analysis of their information content. This permits integration of information about the status of the body and the

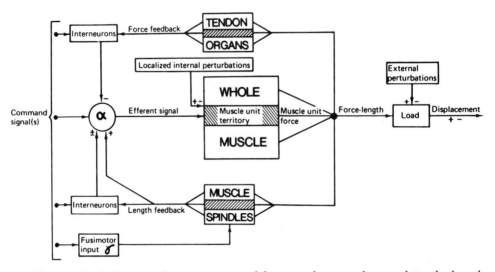

FIGURE 3-22. Block diagram of a current view of the control system that regulates the length of a particular muscle and the force of contraction while performing a motor act. According to this model, the relative amount and strength of muscle contraction are regulated by two feedback pathways, one from the muscle spindle stretch receptors signaling muscle length and velocity of motion, and the other from the Golgi tendon receptors signaling muscle force. The supra-segmental motor centers supply command signals that activate both alpha (α) and gamma (γ, fusimotor) motor neurons as well as interneurons. The degree of further activation is dependent upon how much the muscle actually shortens in relation to the amount of shortening intended. The influence of any additional forces acting internally or externally that may perturb (disturb) the intended motion is sensed, and corrective motor signals are generated. (From Binder, MD and Stuart, DC: *Motor unit-muscle receptors interactions: Design features of the neuromuscular control system.* In Desmedt, JE (ed): *Progress in Clinical Neurophysiology*, Vol 8. Karger, Basel, 1980, p 74, with permission.)

environment from all types of receptors in tendons, joints, and skin, as well as from visual, auditory, and vestibular receptors. After variable delays, suprasegmental mo-tor signals are relayed back to segmental levels to adjust posture and to perform motor activities. Thus "long loops," involving higher centers and more delay, help to regu-late the activity of the spinal circuits and of motor units that produce movement.

Kinesthesia and Proprioception

Under most conditions, a person can be consciously aware of the position of the vari-ous parts of the body relative to all other parts and whether a particular part is moving or still. This awareness has been given, among others, the names *kinesthesia* (Gr. *kinen*, to move, plus *aisthesis*, perception) and *position sense*. These two terms are usually treated as synonymous, and both are frequently used to cover all aspects of the awareness, whether static or dynamic. Strictly speaking, however, the term *position* sense should refer to the awareness of static position and the term kinesthesia to the awareness of joint motion. Kinesthetic signals are generated in various types of sensory receptors residing in muscles, tendons, and joints in response to bodily movements and tension on tendons. The impulses produced are transmitted predominately over group II afferent fibers to the spinal cord and to the cerebellum and sensory cortex, where they inform other sensory-motor centers of the exact locations of different parts of the body at each instant to assist in controlling posture and movement.

Proprioception (L. proprio, one's own, plus ceptive, to receive) is a more inclusive term than kinesthesia and refers to the use of sensory input from receptors in muscle spindles, tendons, and joints to discriminate joint position and joint movement, including direction, amplitude, and speed, as well as relative tension on tendons. Some neurophysiologists also include the vestibular sense organs in each ear as part of the proprioceptive system because the output of the vestibular sense organs provides conscious awareness of the orientation and movements of the head. Proprioceptive impulses are transmitted predominately over group I afferent fibers and are integrated in various sensory-motor centers to automatically regulate adjustments in contraction of postural muscles, thereby maintaining postural equilibrium. Also important for the maintenance of equilibrium are several types of somatosensory (Gr. soma, body, plus, L. sensorius, pertaining to sensation) inputs. For example, pressure sensations from the soles of the feet can provide information about the distribution of load between the two feet and whether the weight is more forward or backward on the feet. Visual images of the location of the body and body parts with respect to reference points in the immediate environment provide complementary information for the maintenance of equilibrium. Visual input may sometimes serve as the primary means of maintaining equilibrium when functioning of the proprioception system has been impaired.

MUSCLE TONE

Muscles of able-bodied subjects exhibit a firmness to palpation that is called muscle tone. This firmness is present in muscles at rest even in well-relaxed subjects; but it is lost if the motor nerve supplying the muscle is cut. Such an observation would lead one to conclude that muscle tone is produced by intermittent contraction of a small fraction of the muscle fibers comprising the muscle. However, very careful studies of relaxed muscles that exhibited at least a palpable amount of muscle tone have failed to detect any muscle action potentials to account for the tone (Clemmeson, 1951; Basmajian, 1952; Ralston and Libet, 1953). Thus, the tone of normally innervated, relaxed muscles appears to be the result of basic physical properties of muscle (elasticity, viscosity, and plasticity). On the other hand, the development of tension in particular muscles that are actively engaged in holding the different parts of the skeleton in their proper relationships to maintain a particular posture is called postural tone and is accompanied by recordable electric activity from the active motor units. The muscles used most often to maintain the body in an erect position, called antigravity muscles, are principally the flexor muscles of the upper extremities and the extensor muscles of the lower extremities. Motor centers in the cerebral cortex and basal ganglia, facilitatory and inhibitory centers in the midbrain and brain stem reticular formations, the cerebellum, and the vestibular apparatus (see Fig. 3-20) all supply nerve impulses that *influence the excitability of lower motor neurons* in the spinal cord segments supplying antigravity muscles. Postural tone of muscles is a reflex (i.e., involuntary) phenomenon, and afferent impulses (from sensory receptors) as well as efferent impulses (from gamma motor neurons) influence it. A normal amount of muscle tone ensures that the muscle is ready to resist any change in length, thereby helping to maintain posture, but that it is also ready to contract or relax promptly when appropriate control signals reach the motor neurons to produce coordinated movement. Tone may be influenced by disease or injury at various levels of the nervous system and thereby cause symptoms of insufficient muscle tone (hypotonia) or excessive muscle tone (hypertonia).

ENDURANCE AND FATIGUE

Endurance is the ability to perform the same act repeatedly over a period of time; loss of endurance may be an early sign of a cardiopulmonary or a neurologic problem. *Fatigue* is defined as a failure to maintain the required or expected force of muscle contraction. Any one of several physiologic mechanisms may be responsible for the state of neuromuscular fatigue present at a particular time (Edwards, 1981). For example, fatigue may be of peripheral origin in which there is impairment of excitation—contraction coupling, failure of muscle action potentials, or impaired transmission of nerve impulses across the myoneural junction. Or fatigue may be of central origin in which failure of neural drive results in reduction in the number of functioning motor units or reduction in the frequency of activation of each functioning motor unit.

The metabolic consequences of prolonged muscular activity that can lead to fatigue include depletion of the ATP supply for membrane functions (e.g., active transport of ions) and accumulation of the products of biochemical reactions, which slows the rate of subsequent reactions. Fatigue becomes important from a clinical standpoint when one or more groups of muscles become unable to continue with a given task that the individual desires to continue. When disease or injury has caused significant weakness of a muscle, its endurance can be expected to be limited. In general, repeated use of a muscle against moderate resistance improves its endurance, but excessive fatigue of an already weak muscle may damage the muscle and produce further weakness (Bennett and Knowlton, 1958; Hickok, 1961; Johnson and Braddom, 1971).

Clinical Considerations Regarding Motor Control

MUSCLE HYPOTONIA

Loss of transmission of motor impulses to muscles, caused by impaired functioning of either upper motor neurons or lower motor neurons, produces a reduction in muscle tone and a state of *flaccid* (L. *flaccidus*, weak, soft, lax) *paralysis*. If the lower motor neuron is intact, the muscle may still respond weakly to segmental reflexes; but without impulses from motor centers in the cortex, cerebellum, and brain stem, the muscle cannot participate in the maintenance of posture or the performance of motor activities. Loss of the lower motor neurons to a muscle produces profound flaccidity, loss of all reflex responses of the muscle, and progressive atrophy of muscle fibers.

MUSCLE ATROPHY

When a muscle is not used for long periods of time, the quantity of actin and myosin myofilaments in each muscle fiber decreases, leading to a reduction in diameter of individual fibers and loss of muscle strength. This process is called *disuse atrophy*, and it is particularly likely to occur when a person is on strict bed rest for more than two weeks or when a limb is immobilized in a sling or cast (Gutmann and Hnik, 1963; Browse, 1965). Atrophy of disuse can be delayed by intermittently contracting the muscle against resistance (Hislop, 1964).

Delivery of action potentials to muscle fibers in a motor unit is accompanied by delivery of trophic substances that prevent atrophy (Guth, 1968; Gutmann, 1976). Disease or injury of the lower motor neurons innervating a muscle removes the source of a continuous supply of trophic substances. The affected fibers undergo progressive *atrophy of denervation* until the muscle fibers are reinnervated by sprouts from nearby surviving motor axons or by axons regrowing from the proximal end of the cut nerve. If reinnervation has not been achieved within about two years, all of the contractile myofibrils will have been replaced by fibrous connective tissue and the "muscle" is no longer capable of developing active tension.

Recent studies have also shown that the muscle fibers and other non-neural tissues produce substances that the neuron needs for its continuing operation (Varon and Bunge, 1978). Such substances are called *neuronotrophins*, and they appear to enter the distal end of the axon where they are picked up and transported through the length of the axon to the nerve cell body. Thus, *materials are transported in both directions through the axon*—a process called *axoplasmic flow* (Grafstein and Forman, 1980). A continual supply of trophic substances is needed by both the muscle fiber and the nerve fiber to remain healthy. Use of the neuromuscular system serves as a stimulus for synthesis of the trophic substances, and lack of use leads to functional and structural deterioration.

PERIPHERAL NERVE INJURY

Peripheral nerves (see Figs. 3-4, 3-8) are frequently injured by laceration or pressure, resulting in paralysis of muscle fibers supplied by the motor axons and loss of sensation in skin areas and other structures supplied by the sensory axons. The median and ulnar nerves are susceptible to damage at the wrist where they may be severed by glass or knives. Nerves in the arm may also be damaged by pressure after a fracture of the humerus that may cause a radial nerve lesion, or the nerve may be trapped in the callus (L. *callus*, hard; in this case, an unorganized meshwork of calcium deposits) formation as the fracture heals. The sciatic nerve may be injured by wounds of the pelvis or thigh and quite commonly is damaged either completely or partially by dislocation of the hip. In rheumatoid arthritis, inflammation of the synovial sheaths of the flexor tendons as they pass under the flexor retinaculum (L. *retinaculum*, a rope or cable; in this case, a band of fibrous connective tissue at the wrist) may lead to compression of the median nerve in the carpal tunnel. Pressure from tourniquets and improperly applied plaster casts may also lead to interference in nerve conduction.

Deformities may be caused by the unopposed action of innervated muscles. For example, a claw hand deformity is prone to develop following lesion of the ulnar nerve. In this case, the strong pull of the long finger flexors and extensors is unopposed by the interossei muscles, and clawing occurs. Another common problem that develops is a consequence of lack of movement of paralyzed muscles. Without occassional movement, adhesions can form between tendons and the sheaths surrounding them, as well as between adjacent bundles of muscle fibers. Whenever the tissues crossing a joint remain in the same position for several weeks, they tend to adapt to the shortened position and to exhibit contracture. These complications can usually be prevented by maintaining full range of movement and increasing the flow of blood and lymph through the area by physical activity.

Loss of sensation is often a more serious problem for a patient than loss of muscle strength, for there is loss of awareness of where certain parts of the body are located and what they are doing (loss of proprioception). In addition, the insensitive part cannot feel when blood flow is occluded by external pressure or when the part is in contact with excessively hot or cold objects (loss of touch, pressure, pain, and temperature sensations). Thus the part is subject to traumatic injuries, ischemia (Gr. *ischein*, to suppress, plus *haima*, blood), burns, and subsequent infections.

MUSCLE HYPERTONIA AND SPASTICITY

Disease or injury of upper motor neurons supplying the lower motor neurons can often lead to a state of excessive muscle tone. The term *spasticity* (Gr. *spastikos*, pertaining to spasms) is used in clinical neurology to indicate the presence of most or all of the following clinical signs: (1) increased firmness of the muscle to palpation; (2) increased resistance of the muscle to passive elongation; (3) impairment of voluntary, as well as reflex, control of skeletal muscles (including sphincters of bladder and anus); (4) low threshold for muscle stretch reflexes and cutaneo-muscle reflexes; and (5) irradiation of any reflex response to involve muscles on the opposite side of the body and those innervated from higher and lower spinal segments.

Since spasticity is the end result of many pathologic conditions affecting the brain and spinal cord, it is of great clinical importance. The mechanisms responsible for producing spasticity are still poorly understood. Under normal circumstances, descending motor tracts from the brain stem—particularly the reticulospinal and vestibulospinal tracts (see Fig. 3-19)—deliver low-frequency trains of impulses to spinal motor neurons either directly or indirectly through interneurons. Thus, at any given instant, many local postsynaptic responses (subthreshold depolarizations) are occurring at widely scattered sites on the dendrites and cell body of the postsynaptic cell. Although these local postsynaptic depolarizations may not be dense enough to provoke complete depolarization and firing of the cell, they serve to maintain it in a slightly oscillating state of high excitability, ready to respond to more concentrated presynaptic input. The supply of facilitatory impulses is ordinarily balanced by a similar supply of "inhibitory impulses"* dispensed to lower motor neurons from inhibitory centers in the brain stem, cerebellum, and cerebral cortex. Inhibition of segmental circuits permits complete relaxation of muscles. The normal operation of inhibitory centers in conjunction with excitatory centers during the performance of motor activities causes the excitatory impulses to be channeled only to those motor units needed to produce the desired motions. Disease or injury of upper motor neurons conducting impulses from supraspinal centers that normally inhibit segmental circuits upsets the balance between facilitatory and inhibitory inputs to a portion of the lower motor neurons. Inadequate inhibition of excitatory impulses during attempted movement can cause overflow of excitatory impulses to muscles that should not have been activated, and contraction of those muscles may actually interfere with accomplishment of the desired movement.

The tone of any particular muscle fluctuates from moment to moment, depending on the balance of excitatory and inhibitory influences on the motor neuron pool supplying the muscle. "Pure" lesions of the motor cortex or of the lateral corticospinal tract (see Fig. 3-18) produce flaccid paralysis of upper motor neuron origin. However, removal of inhibitory influences ordinarily supplied from the reticulospinal region of the brain (located in the pons and medulla) produces severe spasticity. Following traumatic injury to the spinal cord, flaccid paralysis is present for several weeks. Then segmental reflexes below the site of spinal injury return and gradually become hyperactive. Muscles of the limbs, particularly the flexors of the arms and extensors of the legs (the antigravity muscles), often exhibit the greatest spasticity. Similar findings occur after brain lesions that injure tracts descending to the spinal cord (e.g., stroke). Even so, the characteristics of spasticity resulting from injury to the brain are frequently quite different from those seen in persons recovering from spinal cord injury.

If the neural damage has occurred at a high level in the central nervous system, then the tonic postural and spinal reflexes may be "released" from their normally inhibited state. The released reflexes may then exert effects upon the lower motor neurons and cause stereotyped patterns of increased muscle tone relevant to the reflexes released (Fiorentino, 1965; Brunnstrom, 1970). For example, when the patient's head is passively rotated to the side, postural tone increases in the extensor muscles of the arm on the "face" side and in the flexor muscles of the opposite arm (asymmetric tonic neck reflex). The hypertonicity will appear in opposite muscle groups when the face is turned to the opposite side. If, however, the head is flexed forward, an increase in tone will occur in the extensor muscles of both arms (tonic labyrinthine reflex). Thus, the pattern of spasticity can vary from moment to moment depending on many factors. One factor is the general position of the patient. Another is the nature of the stimulus being applied to the patient, and yet another is how much effort the patient is making to obtain a voluntary movement. Strong volitional efforts often facilitate the spastic patterning. This is possibly because the threshold of the appropriate motor

---

*The action potentials of inhibitory impulses are the same as those of facilitatory impulses, but the chemical transmitter released at the presynaptic ending of an inhibitory neuron produces hyperpolarization of the postsynaptic membrane rather than depolarization.

neuron pools is already low (because of insufficient inhibition) so that the arrival of even a few excitatory impulses over preserved corticospinal nerve fibers triggers the lower motor neurons into action.

If the central nervous system is damaged at a lower level so that only the spinal reflexes are released, then the spastic patterning may well be more related to flexion withdrawal. Withdrawal of a hand or foot is a natural reflex response to noxious (L. noxius, injurious) stimuli, but when inhibition is lacking, it can be the response to almost any stimulus: touching of bedclothes on the affected areas, vibration, noise, or sudden movement. Depending on where the stimulus is applied, there may be flexion or extension patterning, but flexion is more likely to be predominant. In addition, the presence of a bladder infection or skin ulcer can be the source of a continual supply of afferent impulses that facilitates the motor neuron pool and increases symptoms of spasticity.

CEREBRAL PALSY

Cerebral palsy (L. cerebrum, brain; palsy, paralysis) is not a single disorder, but a group of motor disorders caused by damage or maldevelopment (L. malum, ill or defective) of the brain that occurs prenatally (L. prae, before, plus L. natal, birth), perinatally, or postnatally. Although the lesion does not usually progress, the clinical picture of disordered movement and posture changes as the child gets older since the nervous system develops in the presence of the lesion.

In cerebral palsy, the neurologic lesion is often diffuse, causing impairment of many functions carried out by the brain, including speech and communication, vision, hearing, perception, emotions, and intellectual functions. The nonmotor handicaps may be caused by the original organic lesion, or they may be secondary to the motor handicap. Secondary handicap occurs when the child is unable to acquire normal learning experience because the child cannot move normally and explore the environment. The child cannot creep, crawl, or walk, or use the hands to discover the meaning of space and direction, textures, shape, or temperature. The child may not be able to look at, reach, or touch different parts of the face and body in order to learn body image and its spatial relationships. The paucity of normal everyday experiences disrupts normal perceptual and conceptual development. This and the child's poor motor development affect speech and language development. Without adequate control of muscles that position the head, the child cannot observe what makes a specific sound and cannot easily communicate with eye-to-eye contact with another person. Without head control, the child also misses perceptual information; the child cannot observe perceptual aspects such as the relationships of objects to self and to others that give meaning to words such as "near" and "far" or "up" and "down." Therefore, the contribution of the therapist to the motor development of the child with cerebral palsy has far-reaching effects on the child's total development.

STROKE

The region of the brain between the thalamus and basal ganglia, through which the bundles of corticospinal fibers pass, is called the internal capsule (see Fig. 3-18). Rupture or occlusion of an artery supplying nutrients to the region of the internal capsule on one side of the brain may so impair the function of axons passing through the area that they no longer conduct impulses (the phenomenon is often called a cerebral vascular accident or stroke). When this happens, not only the corticospinal tract but other motor tracts from cortex to brain stem (see Fig. 3-19) may be affected, producing paralysis of muscles whose spinal motor neurons were controlled by those upper motor neurons. After emerging from the internal capsule, 75 to 90 percent of the million or so fibers in the pyramidal tract cross to the opposite side in the brain stem (forming a prominent anatomic structure called the decussation of the pyramids). Thus, impairment of motor impulse conduction through an internal capsule produces paralysis of muscles on the side opposite the injury. Paralysis of muscles on one side of the body is called *hemiplegia*. Injury to other parts of the sensory-motor system produce other symptoms.

BASAL GANGLIA DYSFUNCTION

The best-known complex of symptoms resulting from disturbance of basal ganglion function is the Parkinson syndrome. Patients with this problem are conspicuous by the rigidity of their expressions, the absence of communicative gestures, the hesitant gait with small steps, and the trembling of their hands. A probable cause of the Parkinson syndrome is deterioration of the tract passing from the substantia nigra to the striatum, the transmitter for which (in the striatum) is dopamine. Symptoms can sometimes be successfully treated by the administration of L-dopa, the precursor of dopamine.

CEREBELLAR DYSFUNCTION

When the functions of the cerebellum are impaired, movements are performed in an uncoordinated manner. A person with impaired cerebellar function walks with a staggering gait and may be suspected of being intoxicated with alcohol. The motor problems include (1) general decrease in muscle tone (hypotonia); (2) inability to achieve properly timed and properly graded activation of muscles during attempted movement; (3) inability to produce a co-contraction of both flexor and extensor muscles to stabilize a joint; and (4) tremor (L. *tremere*, to shake) that appears during attempted movement and that increases in amplitude as the patient attempts finer control of the movement.

CHAPTER 4

INTERACTION OF MECHANICAL AND PHYSIOLOGIC FACTORS IN FUNCTION

The role of individual muscles, or a group of muscles, in producing movement or stabilizing body segments may be examined by palpating the muscle to judge when it is active or relaxed. Although palpation of muscles is an important clinical skill to be mastered, the method is of limited usefulness in advancing our knowledge of muscle function. Only one, or perhaps two, superficial muscles can be examined at one time, and there is no record for analyzing the timing or magnitude of muscle contraction. Since activation of a muscle fiber is associated with transient depolarization and repolarization of the muscle fiber membrane (see Fig. 3-5), recording electrodes placed on the skin overlying a muscle (or even introduced into the muscle) can be used to monitor the small changes in electric field produced by the conduction of muscle action potentials over groups of muscle fibers.

Einthoven (1901) used his newly developed string galvanometer to record the action potentials generated by cardiac muscle when the heart of an experimental animal contracted. The technique was further improved by Adrian and Bronk (1929) to study the activity of skeletal muscles. The development of amplifying and recording equipment during World War II made it possible to use improved methods for the study of muscular activity in living human subjects. The gathering of information by this means, with surface, needle, or indwelling wire electrodes, is called *electromyography* (L. *elektra*, lit, brilliant, pertaining to electricity; Gr. *myos*, muscle; and L. *graphicus*, to write). Each pair of electrodes is connected to a "channel" of the recording apparatus (Fig. 4-1). The use of multichannel instruments allows the contraction and relaxation patterns of several muscles to be recorded simultaneously during some particular movement or postural state of a joint. In this way, the sequence of activation and relaxation, as well as the relative amount of activity of particular muscles, can be studied as they perform various isolated or coordinated functions. Some of the earliest

119

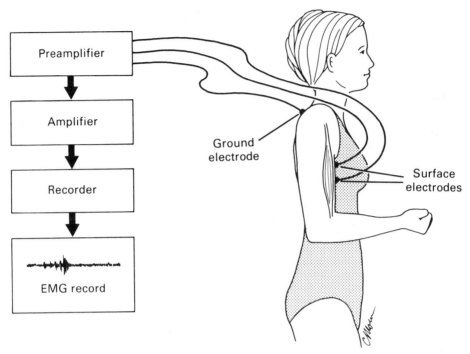

FIGURE 4-1. Electromyography. Electrodes are placed near the muscle to detect the changes in electrical potential associated with activation of muscle fibers. The electric activity "seen" by the electrodes is greatly amplified by electronic equipment and recorded for later analysis of the timing and relative amount of activity exhibited by the muscle(s) being monitored.

careful studies of kinesiology using electromyography were performed by Inman and coworkers (1944) in their analysis of motions of the shoulder. More recent reports of the use of electromyographic techniques for kinesiologic studies include those by Perry, Easterday, and Antonelli (1981) and by Devine, LeVeau, and Yack (1981). Basmajian (1978) and Ralston (1961) are excellent sources of information about instrumentation, pattern of electrical activity of major muscle groups in relation to function, and the uses and limitations of electromyographic methods.

TYPES OF MUSCLE CONTRACTION

Certain terms have been adopted to specify particular characteristics of the contraction of muscles and muscle groups. When a muscle contracts and produces force with *no change in the angle of the joint*, such contraction is said to be *isometric* (Gr. *isos*, equal, and *metron*, measure). For example, the subject is asked to flex the elbow, but the examiner resists the subject's effort and the movement is prevented. Isometric contraction is sometimes called a *static* or holding contraction.

The word *isotonic* is derived from the Greek *isos*, equal, and *tonus*, tension. The term was originally used by muscle physiologists to refer to the *contraction of a mus-*

cle detached from the body and lifting a load vertically against gravity (see Fig. 3-16, A). The connotation was that shortening of the muscle occurred and that the load on the muscle was constant throughout the excursion. When the load became great enough to exceed the ability of the muscle to lift it, the contraction became isometric. Truly *isotonic contractions seldom, if ever, occur when muscles are acting through the lever systems of the body.* Even so, the term is often used, although incorrectly, to refer to a contraction that causes a joint to move through some range of motion, as in flexing the elbow while holding a weight in the hand. Even though the weight remains the same throughout the movement, the tension requirements of the muscle change continuously with changing leverage (see Chapter 2). Furthermore, the rotary force exerted by the weight also changes with changing joint angles.

An *isokinetic* (Gr. *isos*, equal, and *kinetos*, moving) contraction occurs when the *rate of movement is constant.* In recent years, an electromechanical device (an isokinetic dynamometer*) has been developed that limits the rate of movement of a crank-arm or a pulley to some preset angular velocity regardless of the force exerted by the contracting muscles. In 1967, Hislop and Perrine described the concept and principles of isokinetic exercise. The axis of rotation of the crank-arm of the isokinetic device is aligned with the anatomic axis of the moving joint, and the device lever is matched to the skeletal lever (Fig. 4-2). A subject contracts the muscle group being exercised or evaluated, and the device controls the speed of body movement without permitting acceleration to occur. "During isokinetic exercise the resistance accommodates the external force at the skeletal lever so that the muscle maintains maximum output throughout the full range of motion" (Hislop and Perrine, 1967, p 116). Before this type of instrument was developed, an experienced therapist could apply a similar accommodating resistance throughout the range of motion by manually resisting the motion. Manually applied, accommodating resistance is still a valuable therapeutic technique. With practice, the therapist can continuously adjust the amount of resistance being offered so that the motion produced is approximately constant throughout the range, thereby approaching an isokinetic condition.

Contractions may also be classified as *concentric* or *eccentric* contractions, depending on whether the whole muscle shortens or lengthens, respectively, during the movement. For example, the *biceps muscle contracts concentrically to flex the elbow when lifting a glass of water to the mouth. The same muscle contracts eccentrically to slow the rate of descent of the glass when returning it to the table.*

CLASSIFICATION OF MUSCLES ACCORDING TO THEIR INTERACTION IN JOINT MOVEMENT

Anatomically, muscles are described by their *proximal attachments* (origin), *distal attachments* (insertion), and *actions* in producing specific joint motions. Although knowledge of the anatomic attachments and actions is essential to the study of kinesi-

---

*CYBEX, Lumex Corp, Ronkonkoma, NY.

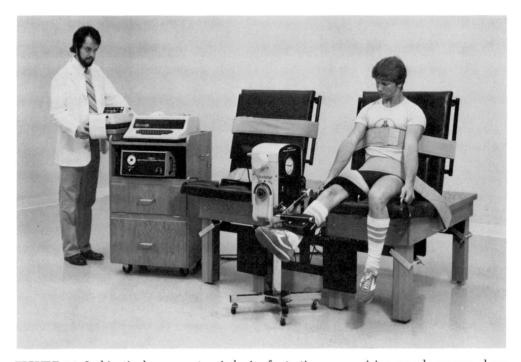

FIGURE 4-2. Isokinetic dynamometer. A device for testing or exercising muscle groups, showing the axis of the crank-arm aligned with the axis of the knee joint. One feature of the device is that the torque exerted by the muscles is recorded along with a record of the joint angle. Another feature is that the velocity of motion cannot exceed whatever value is preset into the device. Thus, the pattern of torque that can be generated throughout the range of motion can be recorded. (Courtesy of CYBEX, a Division of LUMEX, Inc., Ronkonkoma, NY.)

ology, it is important to recognize that these factors can be used to predict muscle function *only* under the limited circumstances where all of the following occur: (1) the proximal attachment is stabilized, (2) the distal attachment moves toward the proximal attachment (concentric contraction), (3) the distal segment moves against gravity or resistance, *and* (4) the muscle acts alone. These circumstances rarely occur in normal function because proximal attachments often move toward fixed distal attachments (closed kinematic chain), contractions are often eccentric or isometric, movement of the distal segment is often assisted by the force of gravity, and muscles seldom if ever act alone. They more often act conjointly. Even though a muscle or muscle group is named after a joint motion (i.e., flexor carpi ulnaris, flexor carpi radialis, or wrist flexors), the muscles *may* or *may not* be responsible for the motion. For example, when the hand is held with the palm facing the top of the table and the wrist is slowly flexed, the wrist flexors will be inactive, and the motion will be performed by an *eccentric contraction of the wrist extensors.* Thus, additional terminology is needed to classify muscles as they act in function.

Many different terms can be found in the literature to classify the function of muscles as they act in joint motion. These terms include agonist, prime mover, antagonist, synergist, true synergist, helping synergist, assistant mover, neutralizer, fixator, and stabilizer. Some of the words are synonyms, and some of the same words have different definitions. Although it is not difficult to determine if a muscle is or is not contracting (by palpation or electromyography), it is difficult to ascertain the *purpose* or reason for which a muscle is contracting. In order to reduce semantic debate, only three terms or their synonyms will be used in this text: agonist, antagonist, and synergist.

AGONIST

A muscle (or muscle group) which by its contraction is considered to be the principal muscle producing a joint motion or maintaining a posture is referred to as an *agonist* (Gr. *agon*, contest), or the *prime mover*. The agonist *always* contracts actively to produce a concentric, isometric, or eccentric contraction.

ANTAGONIST

The *antagonist* (Gr. *anti*, against) is a muscle (or muscle group) that possesses the opposite anatomic action of the agonist. Normally, the antagonist is a noncontracting muscle that neither assists nor resists the motion, but that *passively* elongates or shortens to permit the motion to occur. Thus, in the example of wrist flexion, when the palm is facing the table top, the wrist extensors are the agonists, and the wrist flexors the antagonists. The classification reverses when the dorsum of the hand is facing the table (forearm supinated) and the wrist is flexed against gravity. Here, the wrist flexors are the agonists, and the wrist extensors are the antagonists.

SYNERGIST

A muscle may be defined as a *synergist* (Gr. *syn*, with, together; and *ergon*, work) whenever it contracts at the same time as the agonist. The action of a synergist may be identical, or nearly identical, with that of the agonist—as when the brachioradialis acts with the brachialis during elbow flexion. A synergist may rule out an unwanted action of a prime mover, such as the pronator teres preventing the supination action of the biceps brachii during resisted elbow flexion, or the wrist extensors preventing wrist flexion when the long flexors of the fingers contract to close the hand. Synergists commonly act isometrically at joints far removed from the primary motion in order to *fixate*, or stabilize, proximal joints so that motion may occur at distal joints.

   Fixating functions are more frequently performed by muscles than the functions of agonists or antagonists. This important function is needed because when the agonist contracts, its force is distributed equally to both its distal and proximal attachments. Thus, *both* bones (segments) to which the muscle is attached could move. In order that the desired movement occur in one segment, the other segment must be fixed. This is accomplished by automatic muscle contractions to stabilize and prevent undesired motion of a segment. This important fixating action of muscles can be readily demonstrated as one closes the hand and grips forcefully. Even when the forearm is resting on a table, strong isometric contractions can be palpated in muscles of the forearm, arm, shoulder, scapula, and even the trunk.

The relationships of muscles as agonists, antagonists, and synergists are not absolute. They vary with the activity, position of the body, and the *direction of the resistance* that the muscle must overcome. These changing relationships are illustrated in the electromyographic records of the triceps brachii and the biceps-brachialis muscles during the motions of elbow flexion and extension (Fig. 4-3). When the seated subject flexes the elbow to lift a load in the hand, the flexors contract concentrically and are classified as the agonists. The antagonistic extensors are relatively relaxed and elongate to permit the motion of elbow flexion to occur. As the elbow is then extended to lower the load, the flexors perform an eccentric contraction and are still classified as agonists (Fig. 4-3, A). The extensors remain inactive and are still the antagonists. When, however, the subject is placed in the supine position with the shoulder in 90 degrees of flexion and performs the *same motions of elbow flexion and extension,* the agonist-antagonist relationships are reversed (Fig. 4-3, B). Here, the elbow extensors are the agonists for elbow extension (concentric contraction) and for elbow flexion (eccentric contraction), while the flexors are the antagonists for both motions.

An interesting switching of the agonistic-antagonistic classification in the same motions of elbow flexion and extension occurs when the subject is in the backlying position (Fig. 4-3, C). Here, the biceps-brachialis muscles are the agonists for the first part of elbow flexion, but as the elbow passes 90 degrees, the direction of the resistance force changes and the triceps becomes the agonist. The agonist for elbow extension in this position is the triceps to 90 degrees, but responsibility for controlling the remainder of the motion is assumed by the elbow flexors (eccentric contraction). Application of manual resistance throughout the motion of flexion and then extension (Fig. 4-3, D) further illustrates the principle that muscles act according to the resistance they meet rather than the motion of the joint.

Other examples of the varying relationships among these muscles are shown in Figure 4-4. In Figure 4-4, A, the biceps is acting as an agonist in the motion of supination (along with the supinator), and the triceps is acting as a synergist to prevent elbow flexion. The antagonists in this case would be the pronator muscles. In the movements of pronation and finger flexion to test grip strength (Fig. 4-4, B, C), the elbow extensors are acting as synergists to stabilize the elbow. The elbow flexors are relatively inactive even with a maximal grip effort.

FACTORS AFFECTING FUNCTIONAL STRENGTH OF A MUSCLE

Cross-sectional Area

Various investigators have shown a strong correlation between the cross-sectional area of an isolated animal muscle in the laboratory and the maximal force that the muscle can produce when excited with electrical stimuli. The physiologic cross section of a fusiform muscle (one that has all its fibers running parallel to the tendon of the muscle) is measured from a section cut through the thickest portion of the muscle at a right angle to its fibers, and with muscle being midway between complete elongation and complete shortening within the body. The *larger the physiologic cross section of a muscle, the more tension it can produce*. However, in the intact human being, the relationship between cross-sectional area and muscular strength is not quite as direct as in excised muscles of experimental animals. Cross-sectional area of a muscle is only roughly estimated by measuring the girth (circumference) of a limb. Girth measurements include not only muscle, but fat and bone as well. Also, these measurements do not take into account differences in the orientation of muscle fibers to the long axis of the muscle. The reason that large muscles are generally stronger is that the larger muscles have greater quantities of actin and myosin filaments and, therefore, greater numbers of cross-bridges that can be activated to produce muscular force during contraction.

Tables of physiologic cross sections of various muscles compiled by Fick (1911) are found in Appendix A. Cross sections vary a great deal in individuals, so that the figures in the tables must not be taken as absolute values. They are useful, however, in comparing the cross section of one muscle or muscle group with another, as an indication of the relative strength of each muscle or muscle group.

ABSOLUTE MUSCLE STRENGTH

The term *absolute muscle strength* is sometimes used to indicate the maximum tension a muscle is capable of producing per unit of physiologic cross section. Fick assumed the absolute muscle strength to be 10 kg per sq cm cross section, while von Recklinghausen (1920) reported the strength to be 3.6 kg per sq cm cross section. Haxton (1944) found the absolute muscle strength of the plantar flexors of the ankle to be 3.9 kg per sq cm cross section. Ramsey and Street (1940) determined the maximum tension of isolated muscle fibers in the frog and found that it varied from 2.5 to 4.4 kg per sq cm cross section, the average being 3.5 kg. Generally, 3 to 4 kg per sq cm (6.5 to 9 lb per sq cm) cross section is accepted as being reasonably correct. Theoretically, the quadriceps femoris muscle, which has a cross-sectional area of approximately 175 sq cm, should exert an absolute tension of 1100 to 1600 lb (500 to 700 kg). In the quadriceps problem (see Fig. 2-19), the muscle was calculated to produce a force of 380 lb with only a 30-lb weight on the foot. If the problem is recalculated using a weight of 80 lb, which is nearer to maximum resistance, the muscle force is more than 1000 lb.

Age and Sex

Most people recognize that males are generally stronger than females and each individual gains muscle strength from birth through adolescence, peaking at the age of 20 to 30 years and gradually declining with advancing age. For example, the grip strength of the dominant hand of males and females between ages 3 and 90 is plotted in Figure 4-5. The muscle strength of young boys is approximately the same as that of young girls up to the age of puberty. Thereafter, males exhibit a significantly greater

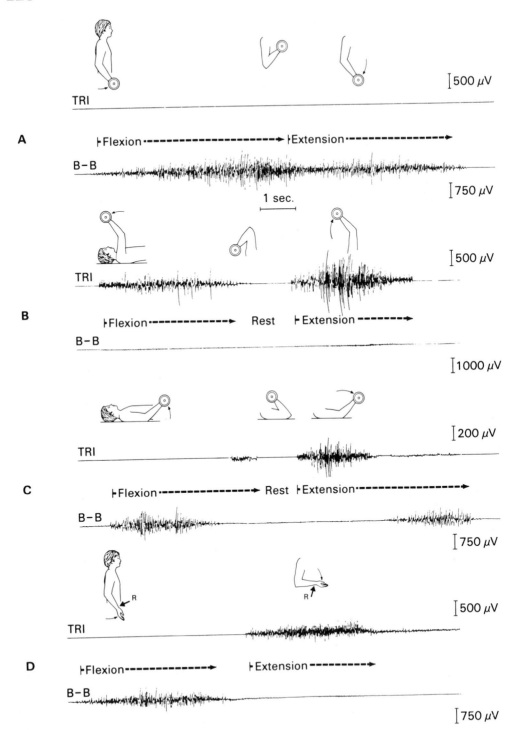

FIGURE 4-3. Electromyographic activity of the triceps brachii (TRI) and the biceps-brachialis (B-B) during the motions of elbow flexion and extension, with changes in the position of the body and the direction of the resistive force. (Range of motion of elbow flexion 0° to 120° and extension 120° to 0°.) (A) Subject sitting, shoulder in anatomic position and 10-lb weight in hand.

Flexion:	Agonist = B-B (concentric contraction)
	Antagonist = TRI
Extension:	Agonist = B-B (eccentric contraction)
	Antagonist = TRI

(B) Subject backlying, shoulder flexed to 90° and 10-lb weight in hand.

Flexion:	Agonist = TRI (eccentric contraction)
	Antagonist = B-B
Extension:	Agonist = TRI (concentric contraction)
	Antagonist = B-B

(C) Subject backlying, shoulder in anatomic position and 10-lb weight held in hand.

Flexion:	Agonist 0° to 90° = B-B (concentric contraction)
	90° to 120° = TRI (eccentric contraction)
Extension:	Agonist 120° to 90° = TRI (concentric contraction)
	90° to 0° = B-B (eccentric contraction)

(D) Subject sitting, shoulder in anatomic position with manual resistance to elbow flexion and then to elbow extension. (Slight to moderate resistance was applied at the distal forearm.)

Flexion:	Agonist = B-B (concentric contraction)
	Antagonist = TRI
Extension:	Agonist = TRI (concentric contraction)
	Antagonist = B-B

Note the decreased frequency and amplitude of electromyographic activity during eccentric contractions as compared with responses during concentric contractions of the same muscle, even though the resistance force and the velocity of motion were approximately the same.

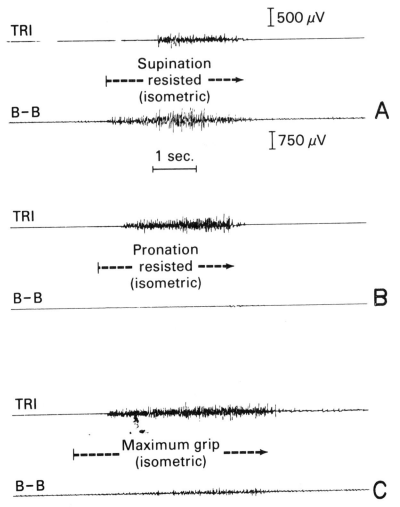

FIGURE 4-4. Synergistic actions of the triceps brachii (TRI) and biceps-brachialis (B-B) muscles. Electromyograph records with the subject sitting, elbow flexed to 90 degrees and forearm and hand supported. (A) Manual resistance to supination (isometric contraction and moderate resistance). (B) Manual resistance to pronation (isometric contraction and moderate resistance). (C) Maximal isometric grip strength using a hand dynamometer (force recorded = 117 lb or 53 kg).

grip strength than females, with the greatest differences occurring during middle age (between ages 30 and 50). The greater strength of males appears to be related primarily to the greater muscle mass they develop after puberty. Up to about age 16, the ratio of lean body mass to whole body mass is similar in males and females, as indicated by studies of creatinine excretion and potassium counts. But after puberty, the muscle mass of males becomes as much as 50 percent greater than that of females, and the ratio of lean body mass to whole body mass also becomes greater. On the other hand, muscle strength per cross-sectional area of muscle appears to be similar in males and

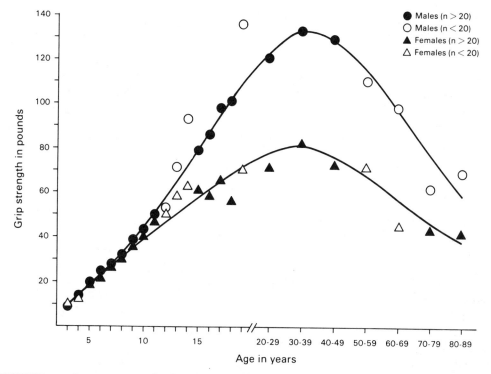

FIGURE 4-5. Average strength of grip of dominant hand in able-bodied male and female subjects between 3 and 90 years of age. N = 531 males and 537 females. Data for subjects 20 years of age and older were grouped by decades. Sample sizes greater or less than 20 are indicated by symbols in the legend.

females, as does the proportion of fast-twitch and slow-twitch muscle fibers in particular muscles (Komi and Karlsson, 1979).

Although muscular strength can be shown to be related to age and sex when considering the population as a whole, many exceptions to the general rule can be found because of the large variation in the rate at which biologic maturation occurs and the large variation in the amount of care that individuals take in keeping themselves in condition through proper diet and exercise.

Length-Tension Relations of Muscle

LENGTH-TENSION DIAGRAM (BLIX'S CURVE)

If a muscle is detached from its connections in the body and made to contract isometrically at different lengths, information on the muscle's ability to produce tension force at various points of its excursion can be obtained. By plotting the tension produced against the length of the muscle, the so-called length-tension diagram is constructed.

Blix, a Swedish physiologist, was one of the first scientists to carry out an extensive investigation of length-tension relations of muscle (1892–1895). The length-tension diagram, therefore, is often referred to as Blix's curve. Blix's experiments were undertaken on isolated frog muscle, and maximum contractions at different lengths were induced by electrical stimulation. Ramsey and Street (1940) further elucidated the principles governing length-tension relations by investigations on isolated fibers of frog muscle. Length-tension studies have also been undertaken on human muscle in patients with arm amputations with cineplastic tunnels,* which offer a unique opportunity for investigations of this kind (Bethe, 1916; Schlesinger, 1920; Inman and Ralston, 1968).

"Resting Length" or "Natural Length" of a Muscle

When a muscle or muscle fiber is *unstimulated and no external forces are acting on it, the muscle or muscle fiber is said to be at resting length* (RL). At this length, no tension is registered in the muscle, and this is the length to which the muscle tends to return when stimulation ceases, provided no external forces act upon it. The resting length of a muscle that has been detached from its connections with bones is comparatively easy to determine, whereas that of a muscle attached to skeletal parts *cannot* be determined.

The resting length of a muscle has also been defined as that *length at which the muscle can produce maximum tension* (Ramsey and Street, 1940). Since the maximum tension is produced when the muscle has been stretched approximately 10 percent beyond the "resting length" when no external forces are acting upon it, the two definitions are not consistent with one another, and the reader needs to be aware of which definition is being used in any particular situation.

Passive Tension Curve

If, starting from resting length (no external forces), an unstimulated muscle fiber is slowly elongated by an outside force, tension is produced in the fiber and rises first very slowly, then more rapidly (Fig. 4-6). Since the fiber is not stimulated, that is, the contractile elements are inactive, this is a passive tension for which the sarcolemma (see Fig. 3-1), not the actin and myosin filaments, is responsible (Ramsey and Street, 1940). This curve is known as the passive tension curve, or the passive stretch curve. Tearing of the structural components occurred at about 200 percent of resting length in the experiments of Ramsey and Street.

LENGTH-TENSION DIAGRAM FOR STIMULATED MUSCLE FIBER

The diagram in Figure 4-7 shows the result of an investigation of isometric contractions of a fiber at lengths shorter and longer than resting length. The muscle fibers

---

*Cineplasty (G. *kineo*, I move, and *plasticos*, forming), a surgical procedure in patients with arm amputations to construct a tunnel transversely through a muscle belly into which an ivory or stainless steel pin is inserted. With the pin "harnessed," the contraction of the muscle can activate the terminal device (artificial hand, or hook).

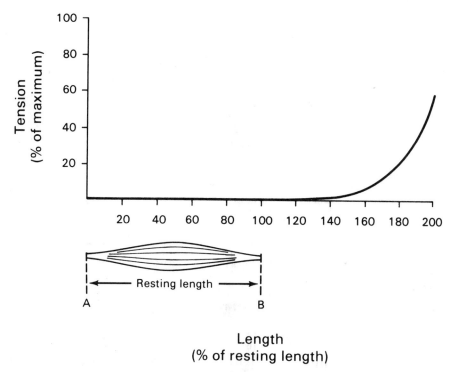

FIGURE 4-6. Passive tension curve of unstimulated muscle fiber, including fully elongated state of fiber. Length is expressed in percent of resting length; tension, in percent of maximum active tension. Muscle fiber A–B at resting length has been drawn in. (Adapted from Ramsey, RW and Street, SF: *Isometric length-tension diagram of isolated skeletal muscle fibers of frog.* J Cell Comp Physiol 15:11, 1940.)

used in the study described here were obtained from the semitendinosus muscle of frogs. The fiber was first stimulated at resting length, and the tension recorded. It was then slowly elongated by small increments and tetanized (stimulated at high frequency to obtain maximal tension) at each new length until it had been elongated to about 160 percent of resting length. The same procedure was then repeated at lengths less than resting length. The fiber at these lengths (prior to stimulation) was not taut but hung in a loop that had to be taken up by muscle contraction before the fiber could produce tension between the ends of the muscle.

The experiment was carried out between the points (1) where the fiber had too much slack for the active tension to be expressed through the ends of the muscle fiber (approximately 45 percent of resting length) and (2) where the overlap of actin and myosin filaments was reduced (see Fig. 3-3, E), thereby preventing coupling of the full number of cross-bridges. The upswing of the tension curve beyond 170 percent of resting length in Figure 4-7 was caused by the rise in passive tension on the fiber. The tearing point of the fiber occurred at about 200 percent of resting length.

In the living subject, the joints do not permit extreme shortening or lengthening of a muscle so that the muscle operates within a relatively small portion of the curve and

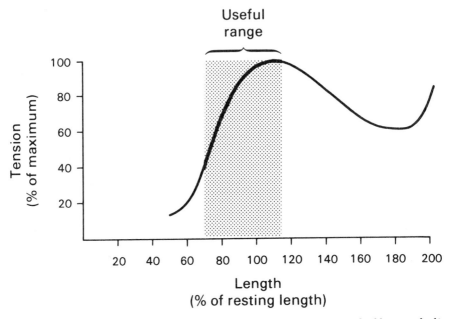

FIGURE 4-7. Length-tension diagram for isometrically stimulated muscle fiber, including extreme shortened and stretched states of fiber. (Adapted from Ramsey, RW and Street, SF: *Isometric length-tension diagram of isolated muscle fibers of frog.* J Cell Comp Physiol 15:11, 1940.)

well within safety limits. The *physiologically utilized portion of the length-tension curve* has been determined for the gastrocnemius muscle of the frog (Beck, 1921). This portion proved to be about 75 percent to 105 percent of the length at which maximum tension was produced—a range that corresponds to the ascending portion and the top of the curve in Figure 4-7. Individuals who have had muscles or tendons altered in length through surgical procedures or by limitation of joint motion may find that the tension that can be produced is near the limit of the useful range and therefore cannot produce as strong a contraction as before.

EXCURSION OF MUSCLES

The paired agonist-antagonist relationship of muscles in the lever system requires that each muscle have the ability to accommodate and change length both passively and actively to permit motion. Morrison (1970), for example, measured changes of 3 to 4 inches (8 to 10 cm) in the length of the quadriceps and hamstring muscles during normal walking. The *functional excursion* of a muscle is defined as that distance which the muscle is capable of shortening after it has been elongated as far as the joint(s) over which it passes allows. Weber (1851) determined the excursions of a large number of muscles and found that some could shorten to 34 percent of the longest length, and others could shorten to 89 percent, with a mean value of 50 percent. The highest excursions were for those muscles that cross more than one joint, such as the hamstrings. Kaplan (1965) and Boyes (1970) provide specific measurements of the excursion distances for each muscle of the hand and wrist. For example, Boyes (1970) measured an excursion of 3 inches (8 cm) for the flexor digitorum profundus muscle when the middle finger and wrist were moved from full wrist and finger flexion to full extension of these joints.

PASSIVE INSUFFICIENCY

When muscles become elongated over two or more joints simultaneously, they may reach the state of *passive insufficiency* and not allow further motion by the agonist. This antagonistic limitation of motion can be demonstrated with hip flexion in the able-bodied subject. The hip can be flexed to 115 to 125 degrees when the knee is also flexed, but when the knee is kept in extension, hip flexion is limited to 60 to 80 degrees because of passive insufficiency of the hamstrings muscles, which are now stretched over the hip and knee. Certain pathologic conditions may cause muscles and tendons to lose their normal range of excursions. These conditions include muscle tightness, spasticity, shortening from trauma or surgery, and adhesion of tendons to their sheaths. Thus, even though the agonist may contract strongly, motion may be severely limited by the lack of excursion of the antagonist. This restriction is commonly seen in patients with cerebrovascular accidents (hemiplegia) who have spasticity of the finger flexors. Even though these patients may have voluntary control of their finger extensors, they are unable to open the hand because of limitation in lengthening of the finger flexors.

TENDON ACTION OF MUSCLE

Passive tension may produce movements of joints when the muscle is elongated over two or more joints. This effect is called the tendon or *tenodesis* (Gr. *tenon*, tendon + *desis*, a binding together) action of muscle. In able-bodied subjects, the effect can be seen if the *relaxed* hand is alternately flexed and extended at the wrist. When the wrist is flexed, the relaxed fingers extend because the passive tension of the extensor digitorum, which has been elongated over the wrist and fingers. When the wrist is extended, the fingers flex because of the tension of the flexor digitorum profundus and superficialis muscles.

This tenodesis action is sometimes used functionally by quadriplegic patients with spinal cord transection resulting in a C6 level* of motor functions and who have the ability to contract wrist extensor muscles but have paralysis of muscles of the fingers.

---

*The designation of the level of a spinal cord injury is based on the *lowest* normally functioning nerve root segment of the spinal cord. If a patient has complete interruption of upper motor neuron connections to lower motor neurons in the seventh cervical segment and below, the patient is classified as having a C6 level (complete) of motor function. The level of sensory function may also be classified. Incomplete spinal cord injury results in partial preservation of voluntary control of a few muscles or partial preservation of sensation (or both) in regions of the body supplied by nerve roots originating in spinal cord segments below the injury.

When the wrist is permitted to flex, the fingers extend by passive insufficiency of the extensors and the hand can be placed over an object. As the wrist is voluntarily extended, the passive tension of the finger flexors produces increasing force on the object so that it may be picked up and held. If selective shortening of the long finger flexors has been permitted to occur (or the patient has spasticity in this muscle group), several pounds of grasping force can be generated.

ACTIVE INSUFFICIENCY

Active insufficiency refers to the weak contractile tension of the *agonist* when its attachments are close together. Here the muscle is on a slack and attempting to contract on the lower portion of its length-tension curve (see Fig. 4-7). This relative weakness can be demonstrated in able-bodied subjects by testing isometric strength of the hamstring muscles with the knee flexed and the hip extended as compared with the greater strength exhibited by these same muscles when the hip is flexed (Figs. 4-8, 4-17). The body is designed so that such weak positions are avoided in normal activities requiring great force. A large number of muscles, for example, cross more than one

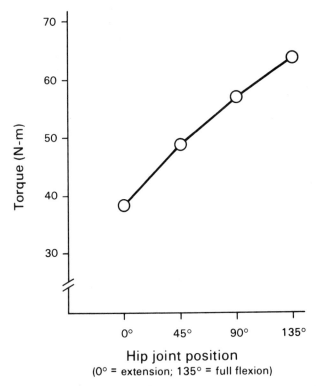

FIGURE 4-8. Length-tension changes in the hamstring muscles. Maximum isometric torque was measured at 30 degrees of knee flexion in four positions of hip flexion. 135° = full flexion; 0° = extension. (Plotted from data published by Lunnen et al, 1981.)

joint (multijoint muscles). Favorable length-tension relationships are maintained by movement combinations whereby the muscle is stretched over one joint while producing motion at another joint. Maximum isometric grip strength, for example, is greatest when the wrist is in a position of slight extension, which places the long finger flexors on a stretch (Fig. 4-9). The grip is markedly weakened when the wrist is maintained in flexion and the finger flexors are attempting to contract from a shortened position. The totally ineffectual grip produced when the wrist is held in full flexion is due to the combination of *active insufficiency* of the long finger *flexors* and *passive insufficiency* of the long finger *extensors*.

LEVERAGE AND LENGTH-TENSION INTERACTIONS

Another unique manner in which the body avoids the weakness of active insufficiency is by changes in the mechanical leverage in the range of joint motion. In the example of the biceps brachii muscle (see Fig. 2-32), the length-tension factor would be most favorable when the elbow was in a position of extension, but the maximum tension that can be produced during contraction of the muscle would decrease as the elbow approached and passed 90 degrees of flexion. To compensate for this loss in active

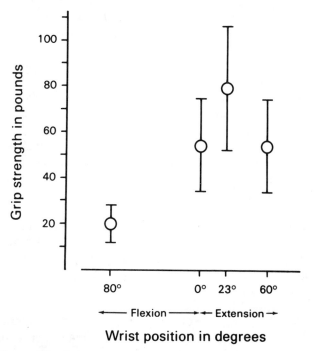

FIGURE 4-9. Maximum isometric grip strength in four positions of the wrist (mean and standard deviation). The wrist was maintained in 80 degrees of wrist flexion, a neutral position, and 60 degrees of extension while gripping; 23 degrees represents the mean position when subjects gripped without wrist restraint. N = 10 able-bodied adult subjects.

muscle tension, the leverage of the muscle (force arm distance) increases to a maximum at 90 degrees. In this instance, the torque that the muscle can produce actually increases, even though the muscle tension may decrease. The patella serves a similar purpose in the quadriceps muscle group. Not only does the patella increase the force arm distance, and consequently the torque of the muscle group, but this distance *increases* as the length-tension factor becomes less favorable. Kaufer (1971) measured a 49 percent increase in the force arm distance of the quadriceps from 120 degrees of knee flexion to complete extension (force arm changed from 3.9 cm to 5.8 cm). In the absence of the patella, both the initial force arm distance and the amount of increase with extension were less (force arm changed from 3.5 cm to 4 cm).

Isometric Torque Curves

The maximum isometric strength that a muscle group is able to produce can be measured indirectly by having the subject make a maximal effort against a fixed resistance on the bony lever. The force produced is recorded in pounds, kilograms, or Newtons by a force transducer (scale, dynamometer, tensiometer, or electronic strain gauge). The recorded force is then multiplied by the distance between the point of attachment of the resistance (force transducer) and the axis of the joint to find the resistance torque ($\tau = F \times \perp d$). This value is the same as the muscle torque since at equilibrium the sum of the torques is zero ($\Sigma\tau = 0$; $\tau_m = 0$ or $\tau_m = \tau_r$). If the measurement is repeated for the muscle group at different joint angles, an *isometric torque* curve can be plotted (Figs. 4-10 to 4-17).

Early investigators (Bethe and Franke, 1919; Williams and Stutzman, 1959; May, 1968) used this principle to study the magnitudes of muscle forces and the characteristic strength patterns of individual muscle groups. Although the results of those studies were often labeled as "torque curves," it should be noted that the measurements were expressed in units of force (kilograms or pounds). Since the resistance force varies inversely with the lever arm distance (whereas torque remains the same regardless of the lever arm length), the values obtained from one subject cannot be compared with those of other subjects unless the lever arm distance used in all tests was the same. Nevertheless, these studies have made a valuable contribution to the understanding of the characteristics of muscle strength. Since the lever arm length is constant in these tests, the *shapes* of the curves for force are parallel to those of torque.

Inspection of the curves shows that the torque of the muscle group changes markedly within its range of motion (40 to 80 percent from the lowest torque to the highest). Thus, maximum muscle strength depends on joint position. Most antagonistic pairs show equal force at some point in the range of motion (Williams and Stutzman, 1959). This relationship is illustrated in the curves for supination-pronation (Fig. 4-11), shoulder flexion-extension (Fig. 4-13), and hip abduction-adduction (Fig. 4-14). Comparisons or ratios of antagonistic muscle strength, then, require further definition as to the point(s) in the range of motion at which the measurements were made.

The curves also demonstrate the relative predominance of physiologic and mechanical factors. In most muscle groups, the length-tension factor is predominate, and the greatest torque occurs when the muscles are on a stretch before contracting (Figs. 4-10

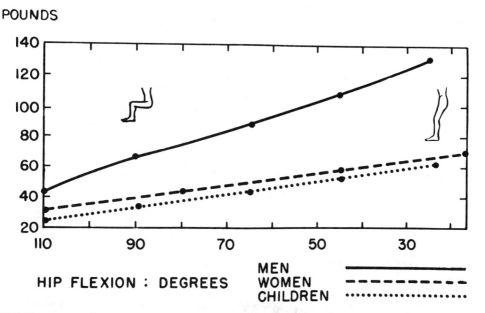

FIGURE 4-10. Hip flexion: comparison of men, women, and children. (From Williams, M and Stutzman, L: *Strength variation through the range of joint motion.* Phys Ther 39:145, 1959, with permission.)

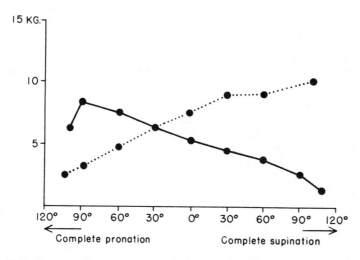

FIGURE 4-11. Torque curves for pronation and supination of right forearm, derived from determinations on four male subjects. Elbow at 90 degrees of flexion. Solid curve = supination. Dotted curve = pronation. Zero position = thumb upward. (Redrawn from Bethe and Franke, 1919.)

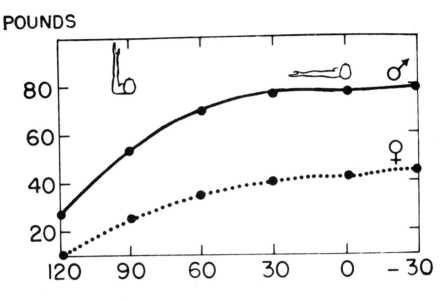

POUNDS

SHOULDER HORIZONTAL ADDUCTION : DEGREES

FIGURE 4-12. Shoulder horizontal adduction: comparison of college men and women. (From Williams and Stutzman, 1959, with permission.)

to 4-14). Pronation and supination of the forearm (Fig. 4-11) follow this principle, so that the maximum pronation torque occurs when the forearm is fully supinated and least when it is pronated. Conversely, supinator torque is greatest when the forearm is pronated. In other muscle groups, notably the elbow flexors (Fig. 4-15) and the knee extensors (Fig. 4-16), the mechanical factor predominates so that the peak torque occurs closer to the middle of the range of motion. The characteristic patterns of the relationship between joint angle and muscle strength can usually be related to functions that require great force such as maximum strength of the elbow flexors being available at a joint angle of 90 degrees, which is the position used in carrying heavy objects. Another example is the maximum strength of the knee extensors being available at a position of knee flexion that will provide great force to elevate the body in climbing stairs and rising from a chair. Pathologic conditions that produce changes in length-tension relationships or leverage of the muscle not only cause a decrease in muscle torque but may also alter where the peak torque occurs in the range of motion. Thus, some activities may be more difficult for patients to perform than would be indicated by the results of testing the strength of a particular muscle at a given angle of the joint.

Speed of Contraction

Speed means rate of motion. Velocity means rate of motion in a particular direction. The rate of shortening substantially affects the force a muscle can develop during

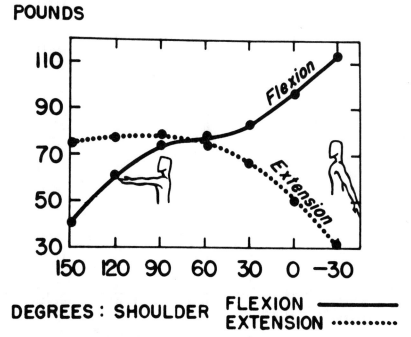

FIGURE 4-13. Comparison of agonist-antagonist muscle groups in college men. (From Williams and Stutzman, 1959, with permission.)

contraction. The relationship between the maximum force developed by an excised muscle and the speed of contraction is shown in Figure 4-18, A. When the load that the muscle is expected to lift is near zero, the speed of contraction is greatest (in this example, nearly 110 cm per sec). However, as the load on the muscle is increased in regular increments, the speed of contraction falls until a load is reached which cannot be lifted. At that point (200 N in this example), the speed of shortening is zero. The decrease in contractile force with increasing speed of shortening is explained on the basis of the number of links that can be formed per unit of time between the actin and myosin filaments (see Fig. 3-7). That is, the force development of the muscle is theoretically proportional to the number of links formed to pull the sliding filaments past one another. The more rapidly the actin and myosin filaments slide past each other, the smaller the number of links that can be formed between the filaments in a unit of time.

Lifting Versus Lowering a Load

Note that the *maximum force is developed when the muscle cannot move the load,* that is, the muscle is in a state of isometric contraction. Therefore, *maximum isometric strength at any joint angle is always greater than the strength of a dynamic, concentric contraction at the same angle.* However, this does not seem to be the case for eccentric (lengthening) contractions. *Maximum strength at a given joint angle is*

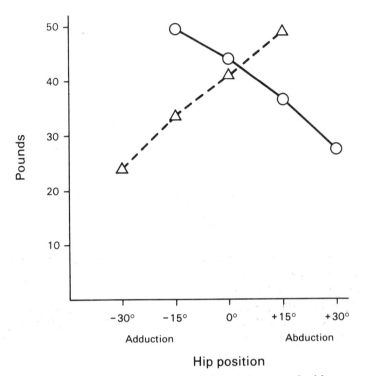

FIGURE 4-14. Maximum isometric contraction of the hip abductor and adductor muscles in 25 normal men. N = 50; age = 20–28 years. (Plotted from data published by May, 1968.)

greater when the muscle is lengthening (as it attempts to overcome too great a load) than when it is contracting concentrically or isometrically (Fig. 4-18, B). The greater strength of eccentric contractions is believed to be due to the excessive load stretching out the elastic components (which connect the contractile components to points of attachment) and all the energy of muscle contraction being directed toward drawing the points of attachment together. Since a lengthening contraction produces greater maximum force, a *greater load can be lowered than can be raised.* For the same *submaximal contraction*, fewer motor units are activated and less energy is expended to perform an eccentric contraction than a concentric contraction (see Fig. 4-3).

   Abbott, Bigland, and Ritchie (1952) devised an ingenious experiment to measure the relative difference in energy cost of performing *positive work* (such as that produced by lifting a load a certain distance by means of a concentric contraction) versus the cost of performing so-called *negative work* (lowering the load the same distance by means of an eccentric contraction). Two bicycle ergometers were placed back-to-back and coupled by a chain. When one cyclist pedaled in the conventional forward direction, the legs of the other cyclist were driven backward. When the first cyclist pedaled, the muscles shortened and performed positive work; the same muscles of the second cyclist were forcibly stretched as they resisted the motion and work was done on them. With practice, the cyclists learned to exert identical force and counterforce so that the pedaling speed remained constant during a given experiment. Experiments

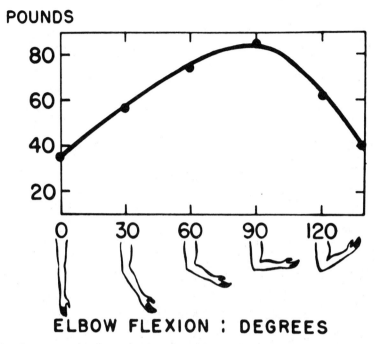

FIGURE 4-15. Isometric torque curve for elbow flexion in college men. (From Williams and Stutzman, 1959, with permission.)

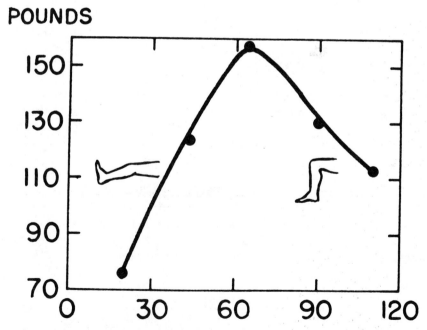

FIGURE 4-16. Maximum isometric knee extension in college men. (From Williams and Stutzman, 1959, with permission.)

POUNDS

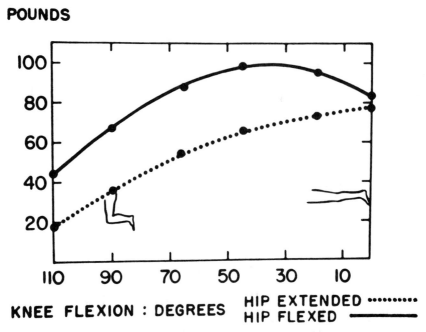

KNEE FLEXION : DEGREES   **HIP EXTENDED** ··········
                             HIP FLEXED ━━━━━━

FIGURE 4-17. Maximum isometric knee flexion: Effect of change of hip position on knee flexion force in college men. The difference between the two curves also illustrates the length-tension effect. (From Williams and Stutzman, 1959, with permission.)

were conducted at a variety of pedaling speeds and forces. Oxygen consumption was determined for each cyclist after steady-state conditions had been attained. The results of the experiments showed that the energy cost of forward pedaling was from 2.5 to 6 times greater than the cost of resisting (equal amounts of positive and negative work performed), depending on the rate at which the work was performed. The relative cost of resisting the motion *decreased* as the rate of motion increased. Thus, less energy is required to lower a given load quickly than to lower it slowly. Most of the energy is used to decelerate the load to prevent it from reaching the velocity it would attain in a free fall.

In a clinical setting, these principles can be applied in selecting activities appropriate to the functional status of a particular patient. Descending stairs at a modest rate costs only one fourth or one fifth of the energy needed to climb the same stairs. Thus, patients on cardiac or respiratory rehabilitation programs may be permitted to descend stairs before they are permitted to ascend them. Lowering a weight very quickly costs less energy than lowering it slowly; lifting a weight quickly can cost up to six times as much energy as lowering the same weight quickly.

Power of Muscular Contraction

The relationship between load and speed of contraction can be used to determine the load at which the maximum power is produced:

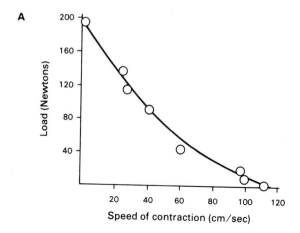

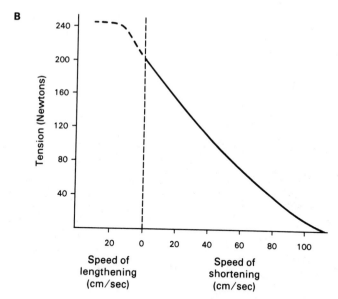

FIGURE 4-18. Speed of contraction versus load or tension. *(A)* The plotted values were obtained by recording directly from the tendon of the pectoralis major muscle in a subject whose arm had been amputated. Note that the speed of shortening decreased with increasing load. (Adapted from Ralston, HJ, et al: *Dynamic features of human isolated voluntary muscle in isometric and free contractions.* J Appl Physiol 1:526, 1949.) *(B)* Tension developed by the muscle when performing a maximum contraction in which the muscle lifted the load at a particular speed (shortening contraction) or lowered the load at a particular speed (lengthening contraction).

$$\text{Power} = \text{Force or Load} \times \text{Speed}$$

It represents the rate at which work is done:

$$\text{Load} \times \frac{\text{Distance}}{\text{Time}}$$

Plotting the relationship between power and load reveals that *power is greatest at approximately 30 percent of maximum load* (Fig. 4-19). Thus, packages weighing about 30 percent of one's maximal isometric strength would be optimal for the most rapid loading of a truck. Packages heavier or lighter than this would require a longer time to lift the same total weight of the product onto the truck. Of course, other factors such as fatigue and package shape would have to be considered, as well.

Isokinetic Torque Curve

The introduction of the isokinetic dynamometer (see Fig. 4-2) has permitted the recording of maximum muscle torques at different velocities of muscle shortening—*the isokinetic torque curve* (Fig. 4-20). Since the instrument records in torque (foot-pounds), the need to measure the lever arm distance is eliminated. Isokinetic torque curves provide a continuous record throughout the entire range of motion. The curves differ from plots of isometric contractions at different joint angles by always beginning and ending on the baseline (zero torque). At slow speeds of motion (10 to 30 degrees

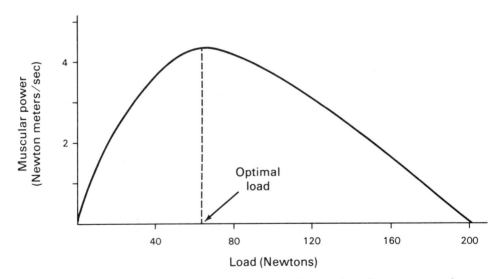

FIGURE 4-19. Relationship between load and power of muscular effort. Power is the rate at which mechanical work is accomplished. When the load is zero, no work is performed. Similarly, when the load exceeds the ability of the muscle to lift it, no work is performed and the power output is zero. The optimal load is the load at which power output is greatest.

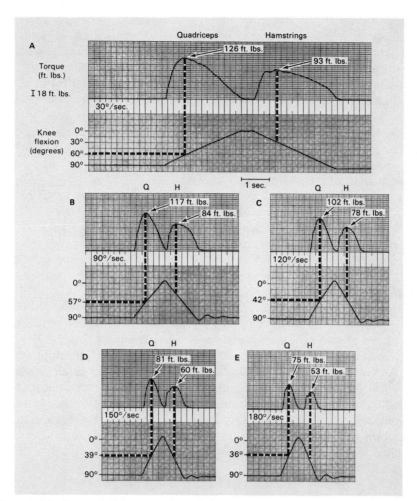

FIGURE 4-20. Maximum isokinetic torque of the quadriceps (Q) and hamstrings (H) muscle groups at different speeds of motion (A to E: 30, 90, 120, 150, and 180 degrees per sec, respectively). The upper tracing records torque and the lower tracing records knee joint position. The vertical dotted lines have been added to connect the point of peak torque with knee position. Subject was sitting with the back supported and the thigh stabilized.

per sec), the maximum isokinetic torque values are similar to isometric values. At faster speeds (30 to 210 degrees per sec), the physiologic velocity factor (see Fig. 4-18) becomes increasingly predominant, and the curves are altered. When the muscle is called upon to move the part rapidly, the amount of torque developed at each point in the range of motion decreases, and the time taken to reach peak torque increases. Thus, peak torques occur slightly later in the range of motion. This phenomenon is theoretically due to less time for the maximum number of cross-bridges between actin and myosin to be formed and less time for the elastic components of muscle to be stretched maximally. Fast, maximum isokinetic contractions permit the evaluation and training of muscles for their important dynamic characteristics such as the rapid explosive force, power, and endurance needed in running and other athletic activities.

Researchers (Moffroid and associates, 1969) studying isokinetics (see Fig. 4-20) have established norms and determined the reliability and validity of the device for measurements of torque, work, range of motion, and power. Moffroid and Whipple (1970) evaluated effects of training speeds on muscular endurance and on muscular force, thereby delineating further the principle that the amount of work done is not as important as the rate at which it is done. They found that:

1. Low-power (low speed, high load) exercise produces greater increases in muscular force only at slow speeds.
2. High-power (high speed, low load) exercise produces increases in muscular force at all speeds of contraction at and below the training speed.
3. High-power exercise increases muscular endurance at high speeds more than low-power exercise increases muscular endurance at slow speeds (Moffroid and Whipple, 1970, p 1699).

Through the use of the isokinetic dynamometer, Moffroid and Kusiak (1975) found new ways to "scrutinize . . . the . . . multifaceted measure of power." They examined muscle power more precisely than had been done previously. They defined five different kinds of power and proposed measures for assessment of power.

As a research measurement and exercise tool, isokinetics is an important addition to the field of kinesiology and rehabilitation. Only a brief description is presented here in order to acknowledge the inception of the concept and to provide some references for those who would pursue further study. The development of this more sophisticated measuring device has provided a more precise method of studying aspects of muscle performance, and its use emphasizes the importance of control and measurement of speed of movement.

CHAPTER 5
ELBOW AND FOREARM

The elbow is a structurally stable joint that contains two articulations within a single joint capsule: the ulno-humeral joint, which permits flexion and extension, and the proximal radio-ulnar joint, which permits pronation and supination. The two degrees of freedom serve hand placement by rotating the forearm and lengthening or shortening the distance of the hand to the shoulder. The elbow also is important in elevating the body as in pull-ups and push-ups.

BONES

Palpable Structures

EPICONDYLES

The epicondyles are bony prominences on the distal enlargements (condyles) of the humerus. Since they are readily identified, they serve as landmarks in this region. When the shoulder is externally rotated, the *medial epicondyle* lies close to the body; the *lateral epicondyle*, away from the body. But when the humerus is internally rotated, the medial epicondyle points to the rear; the lateral epicondyle, to the front. The medial epicondyle is known as the *flexor epicondyle* because it serves as the attachment for many flexor muscles of the wrist and digits. For similar reasons, the lateral epicondyle is referred to as the *extensor epicondyle*.

OLECRANON PROCESS

When the tip of the elbow is placed on the table with the forearm vertical, the prominent olecranon process of the ulna hits the table. This process is quite large, and by

147

following it distally, the *dorsal margin of the ulna* may be palpated all the way down to the *styloid process* of the ulna at the wrist. If the palpating fingers move medially from the olecranon process into the groove between it and the medial epicondyle, the ulnar nerve may be felt as a round cord. Friction across the nerve at this point or slightly more proximal produces a prickling sensation in the little finger; hence, the area where the ulnar nerve can be pressed against the bone is popularly known as the "funny bone."

HEAD OF RADIUS

The head of the radius is identified at a point just distal to the lateral epicondyle. When the elbow is fully extended, the circumference of the head of the radius may be felt rolling under the skin as pronation and supination are carried out. Once the head of the radius has been identified with the elbow extended, it should be easy to palpate when the elbow is flexed and the forearm is either supinated or pronated. (The location of the head of the radius with the forearm pronated is seen in Figures 5-5 and 5-9.)

Nonpalpable Structures

Bony structures that lie too deep to be palpated should be studied on the skeleton. Some of these are the *olecranon fossa*, the *trochlea*, and the *capitulum of the humerus*; the *trochlear notch* and the *coronoid process of the ulna*; the *neck of the radius*; and the *radial tuberosity*.

ELBOW JOINT (ARTICULATIO CUBITI)

Type of Joint

The elbow is a uniaxial joint of the hinge type (ginglymus) permitting flexion and extension by means of mixed gliding and rolling (one degree of freedom of motion). The trochlea of the humerus articulates with the trochlear notch of the ulna, while the capitulum of the humerus apposes the radius. The joint thus has ulnotrochlear and radiocapitular components that work in unison in flexion and extension. The strong structural stability of the joint is derived from both the bony configuration (corrugated) and the collateral ligaments.

Axis of Motion

The axis for flexion and extension of the elbow is represented by a line through the centers of the trochlea and the capitulum (Fig. 5-1, A). The approximate location of this axis in the living subject may be found by grasping the elbow from side to side slightly distal to the lateral and medial epicondyles of the humerus, which are easily palpated through the skin.

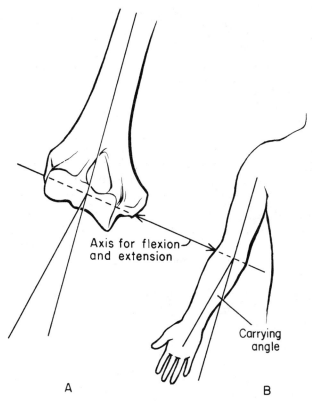

Axis for flexion
and extension

Carrying
angle

A   B

FIGURE 5-1. (A) Axis for flexion and extension of elbow courses through trochlea and capitulum (one degree of freedom of motion). (B) Carrying angle of elbow when forearm is supinated.

Carrying Angle

Since the trochlea extends more distally than the capitulum, the axis for flexion and extension of the elbow is not fully perpendicular to the shaft of the humerus; therefore, when the elbow is extended and the forearm supinated, the forearm deviates laterally in relation to the humerus, which accounts for the *carrying angle,* or cubital angle (Fig. 5-1, B). This angle varies somewhat in individuals, the angle usually being more pronounced in women than in men. Reports of studies in which the carrying angle was measured give mean values from 5 to 19 degrees, with mean differences between men and women of 0 to 6 degrees (Atkinson and Elftman, 1945; Steel and Tomlinson, 1958; Beals, 1976). The variations in these values can be attributed to the different methods of measurement. Excessive lateral angulation of the forearm with respect to the humerus is known as *cubitus valgus.*

The carrying angle has been suggested to serve the purpose of keeping objects carried in the hand away from the body. However, the natural and common way of carrying an object in the hand is with the forearm pronated, or partly pronated; in these positions in which the radius lies across the ulna, the carrying angle is obliterated.

Clearance is gained by abduction or internal rotation of the humerus at the shoulder, or both, or by lateral bending of the trunk.

RADIOULNAR ARTICULATION

Type of Joint

The connections between the radius and the ulna allow the radius to rotate in relation to the ulna so that in one position the two bones lie parallel (supination), and in another position the radius crosses over the ulna (pronation). The hand that is attached to the radius at the radiocarpal articulation follows the movement of the radius so that during supination the palm turns up, and during pronation the palm turns down. The movements of supination and pronation are made possible because there are two separate articulations between the radius and the ulna—one proximal, the other distal. The two joints acting together form a *uniaxial joint* (one degree of freedom) allowing pronation and supination only.

The elbow joint and the radioulnar joints thus both are uniaxial. In the elbow joint, the axis of motion is nearly transverse to the shaft of the bones, whereas in the radioulnar articulation, the axis of motion is almost parallel to the shafts of the participating bony segments.

Axis of Motion

The axis of motion of the radioulnar articulation is represented by a line through the center of the head of the radius proximally and through the center of the head of the ulna distally (Fig. 5-2). In order to locate the direction of this line in the living subject, the forearm is held supinated and the circumference of the head of the radius is identified as previously described. The head of the ulna is then palpated near the wrist on the side of the little finger. The location of the center of the heads of the two bones must then be visualized, and an imaginary line passing through these centers must be established.

Proximal Radioulnar Joint

The proximal radioulnar joint lies within the capsule of the elbow joint and may be described as a trochoid or pivot joint. The side of the head of the radius articulates with the radial notch of the ulna. The fibrous *annular ligament* forms a ring around the head of the radius. The annular ligament has firm fibrous connections with the ulna and is anchored to the neck of the radius by a broad ligament. The radial head thus rotates within a firm ring that permits transverse rotation while preventing movements in other directions.

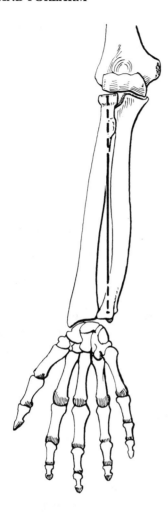

FIGURE 5-2. Axis for pronation and supination of forearm courses through head of radius proximally and head of ulna distally (one degree of freedom of motion). (Redrawn from Grant: *An Atlas of Anatomy.*)

Distal Radioulnar Joint

The articular surface of the radius (ulnar notch) is concave so that the radius (with wrist and hand) can pivot around the head of the ulna while staying in close proximity to it. An articular disk is interposed between the head of the ulna and the adjacent carpal bones.

Isolation of Pronation and Supination From Shoulder Rotation

When range of pronation-supination is observed or tested, the *elbow is held flexed and in contact with the side of the body.* This prevents the shoulder from participating. The entire range of pronation, starting from the fully supinated position, is less than 180 degrees. In turning the palm up and down, slight movements at the radiocarpal and intercarpal joints may also occur, particularly if the motion is performed passively, so that the range of motion as indicated by the palm is approximately 180 degrees.

If pronation and supination are carried out with the elbow extended, internal and external rotation of the shoulder occur simultaneously; and in that case, the palm can be turned through a much larger range.

GENERAL MUSCLE DISTRIBUTION IN ARM AND FOREARM

Two Muscle Groups Above the Elbow

By manipulating the soft tissue of the arm as seen in Figure 5-3, the biceps and the brachialis, flexors of the elbow, may be separated from the triceps, which extends the elbow. Anatomically, these muscle groups are separated both medially and laterally by intermuscular septa of the fascia. The biceps, originating above the shoulder joint and inserting below the elbow joint, has no direct connection with the humerus and can, therefore, be moved about more easily than muscles that take their origin on the humerus.

Three Muscle Groups in Forearm

GROUP ON RADIAL SIDE

The radial group of muscles is best manipulated when the elbow is flexed and the forearm is in midposition between pronation and supination. The group can then be partially separated from the other groups. In Figure 5-4, a pencil has been placed between the radial and the dorsoulnar group. The bulging shape of the radial group is seen in Figure 5-5 as the subject grasps around the adjacent dorsoulnar group. As may be judged from the illustrations (Figs. 5-4, 5-5), when the elbow is flexed, the muscle mass of the radial group lies on the flexor side of the axis of the elbow joint.

The radial group consists of three muscles: brachioradialis, extensor carpi radialis longus, and extensor carpi radialis brevis; the proximal attachments of all three occur in the region of the lateral epicondyle. They receive their innervation from the radial nerve and act in flexion of the elbow and (the latter two) in extension of the wrist. On the volar side of the forearm, this group lies close to the antecubital fossa where the tendon of the biceps is palpated.

GROUP ON DORSOULNAR SIDE

This group comprises muscles located on the dorsum of the forearm that are concerned with extension of wrist and digits and with supination of the forearm. They are

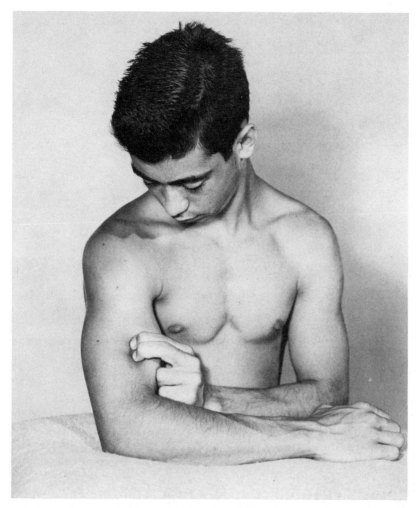

FIGURE 5-3. Grasp to separate biceps and brachialis from triceps.

innervated by the radial nerve. The subject in Figure 5-5 grasps around this group, which on palpation feels rather flat and which adheres more firmly to underlying structures than do the other groups. The approximate boundary between this group and the radial group is seen in Figure 5-4. The dorsal margin of the ulna separates it from the next group. Some of the muscles of this area have a close relation to those of the radial group, being partly covered by them.

GROUP ON VOLAR-ULNAR SIDE

Muscles on the volar-ulnar side of the forearm have their proximal attachments in the region of the medial (flexor) epicondyle of the humerus. Proximally, they are covered by the bicipital aponeurosis. Figure 5-6 illustrates how this group may be identified. The thumb is placed in the antecubital fossa and grasps around the pronator teres. The

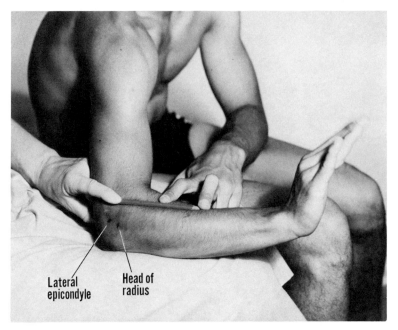

Lateral
epicondyle

Head of
radius

FIGURE 5-4. Separating radial group of forearm (brachioradialis, extensor carpi radialis longus, and extensor carpi radialis brevis) from the dorsoulnar group. Proximal cross-mark is lateral epicondyle; distal cross-mark, head of radius.

other digits are close to the dorsal margin of the ulna. Most of the muscles of this group are innervated by the median nerve and act in pronation of the forearm and in flexion of the wrist and digits.

MUSCLE DISTRIBUTION IN RELATION TO AXIS OF ELBOW JOINT

By grasping the elbow from side to side just distally to the epicondyles, the approximate axis of motion is located and a general idea of the muscle distribution relative to the axis is obtained. A muscle that passes anterior to this axis is a flexor or potential flexor, and one that passes posteriorly is an extensor or potential extensor.

Muscles Performing Flexion

The muscles that, according to Fick (1911, p 320), pass anterior to the axis of the elbow joint when this joint is flexed to a right angle are *brachialis, biceps, brachioradialis, pronator teres, extensor carpi radialis longus, extensor carpi radialis brevis, flexor carpi radialis,* and *palmaris longus.*

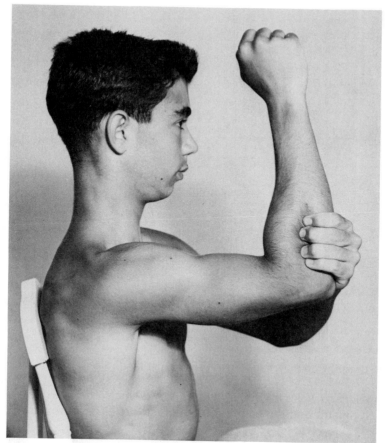

FIGURE 5-5. Grasp around dorsoulnar group, simultaneously showing area of palpation for supinator. The radial group is being pushed aside.

Which of the above muscles will be called upon to flex the elbow depends on the particular movement combination desired. The first four muscles are the principal flexors of the elbow, whereas the last four exert their action mainly at the wrist; the latter are likely to lie idle in elbow flexion unless wrist action is required simultaneously, as when an object grasped in the hand resists elbow flexion.

Briefly, the actions of the four principal elbow flexors are as follows:

Biceps brachii	—Flexor of elbow, supinator of forearm. (See Chapter 7 for biceps action at the shoulder.)
Brachialis	—Pure flexor of elbow.
Brachioradialis	—Flexor of elbow, has negligible action on forearm.
Pronator teres	—Flexor of elbow, pronator of forearm.

The elbow may be flexed with the forearm in pronation or supination, and in any desired position between pronation and supination. This is accomplished by activa-

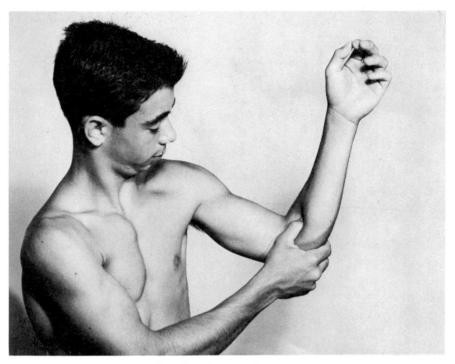

FIGURE 5-6. Grasping around volar-ulnar (pronator) group.

tion of the various muscles in proper proportions, taking advantage of the action of the biceps as a supinator and the action of the pronator teres as a pronator.

BICEPS BRACHII

The muscular portion of the biceps is located above the elbow. *Proximal attachment:* By two heads from above the glenohumeral joint. The *long head* is attached by a long tendon from the supraglenoid tubercle of the scapula. The tendon courses within the capsule of the glenohumeral joint and in the intertubercular groove of the humerus. The *short head* is attached, also by a long tendon, from the coracoid process of the scapula. The two heads have separate bellies in the proximal portion of the arm, and these fuse to form one belly in the middle of the arm. The muscle fibers belonging to the short head make up the medial portion of the common belly, whereas those of the long head make up the lateral portion. *Distal attachment:* Tuberosity of the radius and, in part, spreading out to form the bicipital aponeurosis (lacertus fibrosus). *Innervation:* Musculocutaneous nerve.

Inspection and palpation

The biceps brachii is one of the easiest muscles to identify; to the layman, "making a muscle" means tightening the biceps. The contour of the biceps in a muscular individual is seen in many of the photographs in this book. A maximum shortening of the muscle is effected by simultaneous flexion of the elbow and supination of the forearm (Fig. 5-7). With this movement combination, the muscular portion retracts considerably so that in the illustration the tendon appears to be quite long.

The tendon of the biceps is best identified in the "fold" of the elbow when the forearm is supinated. In a muscular subject, the tendon is rather broad, as shown by the examiner's grasp. The examiner's thumb indicates the location of that part of the tendon which dips into the antecubital fossa on its way to the tuberosity of the radius. The examiner's index finger is seen palpating the bicipital aponeurosis, which spreads out to cover the pronator teres and other muscles of this region.

The biceps and its tendon should next be palpated when the muscle is relaxed, as when the forearm rests on the table or in the lap. It is then possible to grasp around the muscle, lift it from underlying structures, and move it from side to side, a maneuver that is useful in separating it from the more deeply located brachialis muscle.

Finally, it should be observed that the biceps contracts strongly when a fist is made, as in squeezing an object in the hand, and that this contraction is automatic and cannot be inhibited by the will. The strength of the contraction is in direct proportion to the firmness of the grip. Note that the triceps contracts simultaneously (see Fig. 4-4, C).

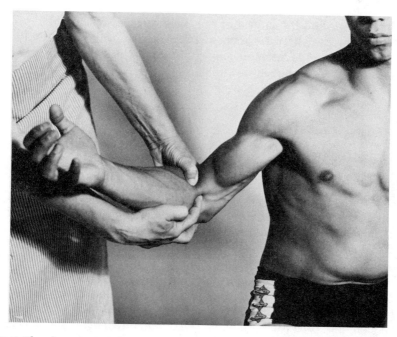

FIGURE 5-7. The characteristic contour of the biceps is brought out by flexion of the elbow and supination of the forearm. The examiner grasps around tendon of biceps in the "fold" of the elbow.

BRACHIALIS

The brachialis muscle has its *proximal attachment* halfway up the shaft of the humerus and is attached distally to the coronoid process of the ulna and adjacent areas of the ulna. *Innervation:* Musculocutaneous nerve.

Palpation

The muscular portion of the brachialis is located in the lower half of the arm, where it is largely covered by the biceps. The palpating fingers are placed laterally and medially to the biceps, an inch or two higher than the grasp seen in Figure 5-7. The subject's forearm should be pronated and resting in the lap or on a pillow, as seen in Figure 5-3, which secures relaxation of the biceps. If now the elbow is flexed with as little effort as possible, the contraction of the brachialis may be felt. Under the above conditions, the brachialis flexes the elbow with little or no participation by the biceps. Once the palpating fingers are properly placed, a quick flexion in small range may be performed, resulting in stronger contraction of the brachialis.

BRACHIORADIALIS

The most prominent and the largest of the three muscles of the radial group of the forearm, the brachioradialis varies considerably in size in individuals. *Proximal attachment:* To a ridge on the humerus above the lateral epicondyle. *Distal attachment:* Near the styloid process of the radius. *Innervation:* Radial nerve. Note that this muscle is a flexor of the elbow but as far as innervation is concerned it is associated with the extensors.

Inspection and Palpation

The brachioradialis is best observed and palpated when resistance is given to flexion of the elbow while the elbow angle is about 90 degrees and the forearm is in midposition between pronation and supination (Fig. 5-8). Figure 5-9 shows the contour of this muscle and its relation to the extensor carpi radialis longus and brevis. The muscle is superficial and can readily be palpated along most of its course. Above the elbow, it lies between the triceps and the brachialis. At and below the elbow, it forms the lateral border of the antecubital fossa. Its muscular part may be followed halfway down the forearm, but its point of *distal attachment* is less readily palpated because its tendon of attachment is flat and partially covered by tendons of muscles passing over the wrist to the hand and because these tendons are held down by ligamentous structures that cross obliquely from the ulnar to the radial side of the wrist. When the muscle contracts, its upper portion rises from the underlying structures so that its perpendicular distance to the elbow joint increases, which enhances its function.

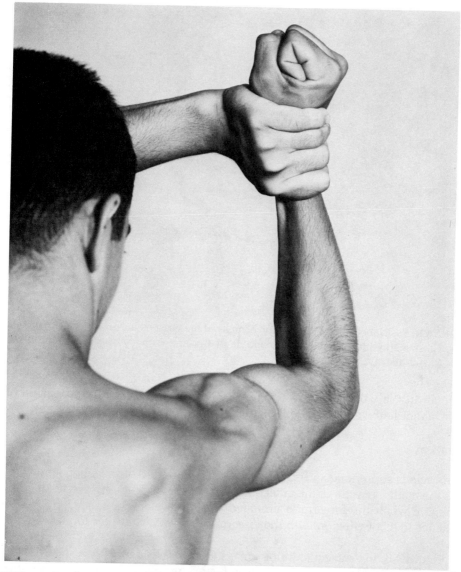

FIGURE 5-8. Brachioradialis is brought out by resistance to flexion of the elbow with the forearm in midposition between pronation and supination.

PRONATOR TERES

The bulk of the pronator teres muscle is located below the elbow. It courses rather close to the axis of the elbow joint so that it has comparatively poor leverage for elbow flexion. *Proximal attachment:* Medial epicondyle of humerus and a smaller portion from the coronoid process of the ulna. The muscle fibers cross obliquely from medial

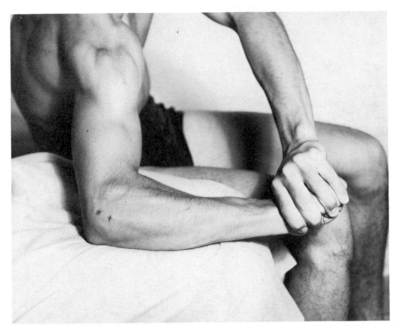

FIGURE 5-9. Resistance to wrist extension brings out the wrist extensors and also the brachiora-dialis. Cross-marks identify lateral epicondyle of the humerus (proximal mark) and head of radius (distal mark).

to lateral on the volar aspect of the forearm. *Distal attachment:* Lateral side of the radius, about halfway down the forearm. *Innervation:* Median nerve.

Palpation

The muscle is superficial and may be palpated in the fold of the elbow and below. It forms the medial margin of the antecubital fossa, and its fibers are easily identified in this region when the forearm is pronated while the elbow is flexed or semiflexed. Resistance to elbow flexion with the forearm pronated also makes for easy identification.

In Figure 5-6, the subject's thumb grasps around the edge of the pronator teres. If, from the position shown, the forearm is further pronated or resistance is given to pronation or flexion, the muscle hardens markedly.

The pronator teres lies close to the flexor carpi radialis, and both these muscles are covered by the bicipital aponeurosis. More distally, as it crosses over toward the radial side, the pronator teres is covered by the brachioradialis, and if the pronator teres is to be palpated close to its *distal attachment,* the brachioradialis must be relaxed. This is accomplished by resting the forearm in the lap or on the table. The forearm is then pronated, which activates the pronator while the brachioradialis remains essentially relaxed. The movement of pronation should be performed with little effort, or additional muscles in the region will become tense.

Muscles Performing Extension

The principal extensor of the elbow is the triceps brachii, with the small anconeus adding only insignificantly to the total strength of elbow extension.

TRICEPS BRACHII

The triceps brachii makes up the entire muscle mass on the posterior aspect of the arm. *Proximal attachment:* By three heads: the *long head*, the *medial head*, and the *lateral head*. The long head is attached to the infraglenoid tubercle of the scapula by a broad tendon that has a close relation to the capsule of the shoulder joint. The medial head is attached to the distal portion of the humerus and has a fleshy origin. The lateral head is attached to the lateral aspect of the humerus, a short distance below the glenohumeral joint. *Distal attachments:* The three heads join a sturdy broad tendon that attaches to the olecranon process of the ulna and that also sends an expansion spreading out over the anconeus muscle into the dorsal fascia of the forearm. *Innervation:* Radial (musculospiral) nerve.

Inspection and Palpation

The *long head* is identified in its proximal portion as it emerges from underneath the lowest fibers of the posterior deltoid (Figs. 5-10, 5-11). It may be followed distally halfway down the arm. The muscular portion of the *lateral head*, which is the strongest of the three heads, is palpated distal to the posterior deltoid. It is well recognizable in Figure 5-10. The long head and the lateral head join the common tendon of insertion from opposite sides, much like the two heads of the gastrocnemius approach the Achilles tendon. Note in the illustration the flat area between the lateral and the long heads. This is the broad superficial portion of the triceps tendon into which the two heads insert, partially from underneath and partially from the sides. The *medial head* is covered, in part, by the long head and is best palpated in its distal portion, near the medial epicondyle. For palpation of the medial head, it is suggested that the dorsum of the wrist be placed on the edge of a table and pressure be applied in a downward direction, the table supplying resistance to elbow extension. The medial head may then be felt contracting.

ANCONEUS

Proximal attachment: The region of the lateral epicondyle of the humerus. *Distal attachment:* The ulna, partly into the olecranon process, partly below this process. *Innervation:* Radial nerve.

Palpation

If one finger tip is placed on the lateral epicondyle and one on the olecranon process, the muscular portion of the anconeus is palpated distally at a point that forms a trian-

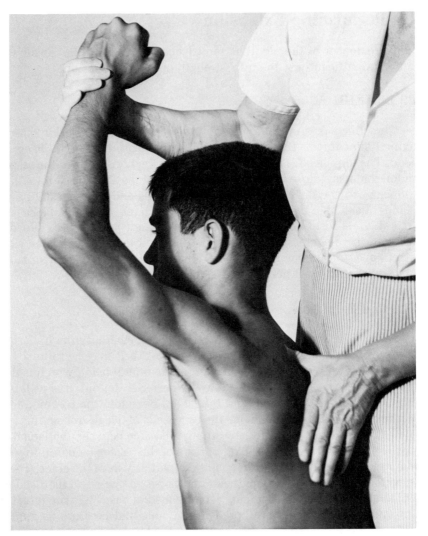

FIGURE 5-10. Triceps brachii and other muscles brought out by examiner's resistance to extension of elbow. Long head of triceps is responsible for contour at lower margin of arm. Note its relation to teres major and latissimus near the axilla. Lateral head appears separated from the deltoid by a groove. The flat area between the lateral and the long heads identifies the broad common tendon of attachment.

gle with the other two points. The anconeus may be identified in Figure 5-11, but should not be confused with the extensor carpi ulnaris that lies close to it. In the illustration, the two muscles appear almost as one; but by keeping in mind that the direction of the two muscles differs and that the anconeus lies more proximal and is very short, while the extensor carpi ulnaris runs down the forearm, each muscle may be identified.

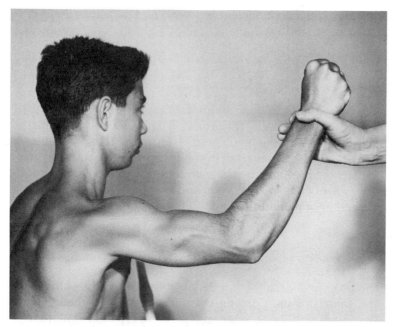

FIGURE 5-11. Triceps and anconeus. Elbow extension is resisted. The short, triangular-shaped anconeus lies close to the tip of the elbow and near the upper portion of extensor carpi ulnaris.

MUSCLE DISTRIBUTION IN RELATION TO AXIS OF PRONATION-SUPINATION

Muscles Performing Supination

In general, muscles capable of supination have their *proximal attachment* on the lateral (extensor) epicondyle of the humerus and adjacent structures, and cross the axis of pronation-supination posterior to the interosseous membrane, which unites the two bones of the forearm and which divides the forearm in posterior and anterior parts. The muscles are associated with the extensors of the wrist and the digits, in regard to anatomic position and innervation (radial nerve). The biceps brachii undertakes the task of supination in a different manner by exerting a pull on the tuberosity of the radius.

The muscles that, according to Fick (1911, p 348), are in a position that enables them to supinate the forearm are the *biceps brachii, supinator, brachioradialis* (extremely short range), *abductor pollicis longus, extensor pollicis brevis,* and *extensor indicis proprius.* The first two muscles are the most important supinators. The brachioradialis can be disregarded as a supinator. The last three are mechanically capable of aiding in supination but are primarily concerned with movements of the thumb and index finger and will be discussed in Chapter 6.

Location of the *proximal* and *distal* attachments and palpation of the biceps brachii have already been discussed.

SUPINATOR

The supinator is a deep muscle, located on the dorsal side of the interosseous membrane between the two bones of the forearm. It is covered by the anconeus, the extensor carpi radialis longus, and the brachioradialis. *Proximal attachments:* Lateral epicondyle of humerus and adjacent areas of the ulna. It is a fairly short and rather flat muscle, triangular in shape, which winds around the proximal portion of the radius close to the bone. *Distal attachments:* Volar and lateral surfaces of proximal part of the radius. *Innervation:* A branch of the radial nerve.

Palpation

The area where the supinator, although deeply located, may be palpated is shown in Figure 5-5. The fingertips are pushing the muscles of the radial group in a radial direction so that there will be no interference with palpation. The best position for palpation is perhaps to sit with the pronated forearm resting in the lap and to grasp the radial muscle group from the radial side, pulling it out of the way as much as possible. As the forearm is supinated through short range, the supinator may be felt under the palpating fingers.

Muscles Performing Pronation

All muscles capable of pronation are located in the forearm. In general, they arise from the region of the medial epicondyle of the humerus and/or adjacent areas of the ulna and cross the axis of pronation-supination on the anterior (palmar) side of the interosseous membrane. These muscles are closely related to the flexors of the wrist and digits in regard to both location and innervation (median nerve). One of the pronators, the pronator quadratus, is located more distally but, like the other pronators, crosses the axis of motion on the anterior side.

The muscles that, according to Fick (1911, p 351), are capable of pronating the forearm when the elbow is flexed at 90 degrees are the *pronator teres, flexor carpi radialis, palmaris longus, brachioradialis* (range of pronation is short, but longer than that of supination), *extensor carpi radialis longus,* and *pronator quadratus.*

The pronator teres and pronator quadratus are the most important pronators. The brachioradialis may be disregarded as a pronator because it is mainly concerned with flexion of the elbow. The other muscles are concerned with wrist movements and will be discussed in Chapter 6. The pronator teres has been discussed previously in this chapter.

PRONATOR QUADRATUS

This muscle crosses transversely over the ulna and the radius in the distal region of the forearm near the wrist. It is deeply situated on the palmar side, lying directly over the bones and the interosseous membrane, and is covered by the flexors of wrist and digits. *Attachments:* The distal one fourth of the ulna and radius on the volar surfaces. *Innervation:* A branch of the median nerve. *Palpation* is difficult or impossible, but the approximate length and direction of its fibers are indicated in Figure 5-12.

Selection of Muscles in Movement

In general, it may be stated that those muscles which best serve a particular purpose with the least amount of expenditure of energy are the ones selected by the nervous system to perform the task. For any movement combination, however, a perfect selection of muscles is achieved only by highly skilled individuals. Unskilled movements are wasteful of energy since muscles not necessarily needed for the movement contract along with those needed. As skill increases, the selection improves and gradation of contraction becomes more refined, resulting in smoother movements that are less fatiguing and, from the esthetic standpoint, are more pleasing to the eye.

The number of muscles involved in movements also is determined by the effort needed for a particular task. Thus, if great resistance is encountered, more muscles are recruited, not only at the joint or joints where the movements take place but also at joints far away from the scene of action. A typical example is that of making a fist, which involves primarily the flexors of the digits and the extensors of the wrist. When the effort increases, as in testing grip strength on a dynamometer, not only do the finger flexors and the wrist extensors increase their tension, but there is a successive recruitment of muscles at the elbow, the shoulder, and even the trunk until with greatest effort practically all muscles of the body appear to participate.

Many muscles act over more than one joint, and they are the ones usually selected for a task involving these joints. For example, the biceps brachii is a flexor of the elbow and a supinator of the forearm; when both these movements are wanted simultaneously, the biceps is the logical selection. This movement combination, of course, could also be performed by the brachioradialis and the supinator, as is indeed the case in musculocutaneous nerve injuries when the biceps and the brachialis are paralyzed. Ordinarily, for light tasks, the nervous system prefers to have one muscle do the job of two when such a muscle is available.

The brachialis, a one-joint muscle, is the perfect selection for flexion of the elbow if neither supination nor pronation is willed. For such motion, it would be wasteful to use the biceps since supination would have to be depressed by the pronators, and it would be equally wasteful to use the pronator teres, since pronation would have to be prevented by the supinators.

Often, it becomes economical to use a two-joint muscle to produce movement over one joint only, in which case synergic muscle action (or gravitational forces) stabilizes the other joint or moves that joint in the opposite direction. This latter arrangement

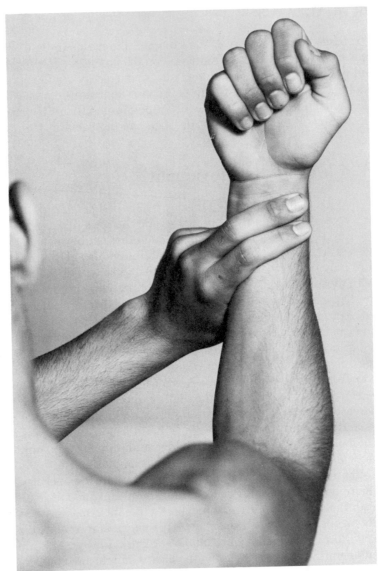

FIGURE 5-12. Demonstrating line of action of deeply situated pronator quadratus.

enables a muscle to do work in a relatively elongated state through a large range of motion, thus using a favorable portion of the length-tension diagram (see Chapter 4).

The foregoing discussion emphasizes that muscles may team up in many different ways and that synergism among muscles is always changing depending on requirements. Consequently, it can never be stated that two specific muscles are always synergists or antagonists; the muscles may be so labeled for specific movement combinations only.

The manner in which the individual muscles team up to flex the elbow has been the subject of much discussion and a considerable amount of dissension mainly because the variety of requirements and individual variations in skill have not been sufficiently appreciated. Recent electromyographic studies indicate that, as would be expected, there are considerable variations of muscle action among individuals, both in the selection of muscles and in the sequence of recruitment of the muscles.

BRACHIALIS

The brachialis is the least controversial of the flexors of the elbow. It is uninfluenced by the position of the forearm, being as effective when the forearm is pronated as when it is supinated. Studies by Basmajian and Latif (1957) show that the brachialis is always active as an elbow flexor with or without a load and whether the motion is rapid or slow.

BRACHIORADIALIS

This muscle is clearly a flexor of the elbow, but actions of supination and pronation have also been ascribed to it. Early anatomists called it the supinator longus. Fick states that, mechanically, it is capable of performing a limited range of pronation from the fully supinated position and a still more limited range of supination from the fully pronated position. Beevor (1903) considered the brachioradialis to be a pure flexor of the elbow. His observations have been substantiated by electromyographic studies (Basmajian and Latif, 1957) that showed that, with the elbow extended, no electric activity appeared in the muscle when the forearm was pronated from the fully supinated position or supinated from the fully pronated position, unless the motions were resisted. In that case, the brachioradialis may act for stabilization rather than for pronation and supination. Functionally, therefore, the brachioradialis may be considered a pure flexor of the elbow.

BICEPS BRACHII

An isolated, unopposed contraction of the biceps would produce simultaneous flexion of the elbow and supination of the forearm. Either of these actions can be suppressed by synergic action of other muscles.

Electromyographic studies cited above show that the biceps takes little or no part in slow flexion of the elbow when the forearm is pronated, even when a load of 2 lb, held loosely in the hand, is lifted or lowered. But when the forearm is supinated, the biceps acts in flexion of the elbow both with and without a load, in slow as well as in fast movements, and regardless of whether it acts in a shortening or lengthening capacity. With increasing speed and increasing load, however, the biceps acts also when the forearm is pronated.

COMPARISON OF ACTIONS OF THE BICEPS BRACHII
AND THE SUPINATOR

The biceps acts most effectively as a supinator when the elbow is flexed at an angle of about 90 degrees, a conclusion gained from observing the angle of approach of its tendon to the long axis of the radius. As the elbow extends, the effectiveness of the muscle as a supinator lessens; the effectiveness of the supinator muscle is not influenced by the elbow angle. Fick calculated that, at an angle of 90 degrees, the biceps is almost four times as effective as the supinator. When the elbow is extended, however, the effectiveness of the biceps is only twice that of the supinator.

Since the supinator's sole action is supination whereas the biceps is also a flexor of the elbow, it is logical to conclude that the supinator would be called upon to contract when supination without elbow flexion is willed, provided that the movement is performed slowly and without resistance. Clinically, this assumption may be confirmed as follows:

The subject is seated with the forearm resting in the lap. The palpating fingers are placed on the tendon of the biceps in the fold of the elbow. If supination is performed slowly and the forearm remains in the lap, the tendon of the biceps remains relaxed, and one may conclude that the movement is performed by the supinator. But, if a quick supination is performed, the biceps immediately springs into action and its tendon stands out markedly.

The above procedure is employed for isolated testing of the supinator, although in normal individuals no information about the *strength* of the supinator is obtained. The test is also useful in patients with radial nerve injuries to determine when regeneration of the nerve has progressed to the supinator. As long as the supinator is denervated, a slow supination of the forearm in the position described causes the biceps tendon to become prominent. When the supinator has been re-innervated, this is no longer the case.

The ability of the supinator to perform supination without the aid of the biceps has been verified by Basmajian and Latif (1957). In most subjects investigated, no electric activity was registered in either head of the biceps when the forearm was supinated while the elbow was in extension. But if resistance was applied to supination, the biceps became active also when the elbow was extended.

COMPARISON OF ACTIONS OF THE PRONATOR TERES
AND THE PRONATOR QUADRATUS

The pronator teres is the strongest of the pronators, and since it is superficial, its contraction can be ascertained by palpation. The role played by the pronator quadratus is difficult to assess since it cannot be palpated readily. Its cross section is almost two thirds of that of the pronator teres and compares favorably with that of the supinator. Its shortening distance, however, is small. One may assume that the pronator quadratus pronates the forearm unaided by other muscles if pronation is performed slowly without resistance and without active elbow flexion. These conditions are met if the subject lies prone with the forearm hanging vertically over the edge of the table and if little effort is used in pronation.

COMPARISON OF ACTION OF THE TRICEPS AND THE ANCONEUS

Both the triceps and the anconeus are extensors of the elbow, the triceps being by far the more powerful of the two. The triceps has a cross section about five times, and a shortening range about twice, that of the anconeus (see Table 3, Appendix A). The fascia over the triceps tendon continues over the anconeus, which has a close relation to the elbow joint and the proximal radioular joint. Both muscles, therefore, contribute to the protection of these joints.

Two-Joint Muscles of the Elbow and Shoulder

The two heads of the biceps and the long head of the triceps originate above the glenohumeral joint so that the lengths of these muscles are influenced by the position of the shoulder as well as that of the elbow joint.

BICEPS

The tendons of origin of both heads of the biceps are elongated when the shoulder is extended or hyperextended. Therefore, *elbow flexion combined with shoulder extension enhances the action of the biceps.* By means of this two-joint mechanism, the muscle maintains favorable tension while flexing the elbow through a large range. This combination—elbow flexion and shoulder hyperextension—is used in "pulling" activities and contributes materially to the strength of elbow flexion.

TRICEPS

The long head of the triceps, because of its attachment to the infraglenoid tuberosity of the scapula, is elongated when the shoulder is flexed. Therefore, *elbow extension combined with shoulder flexion enhances the activity of the triceps.* This two-joint mechanism is the reverse of the flexion combination and is used to advantage in "pushing" activities. The flexion and extension combinations are used alternately in scores of functional activities, such as sanding, polishing, pulling the beater of a loom, using a carpet sweeper, sawing wood, throwing a ball, and so forth. Examples of such two-joint mechanisms are numerous throughout the body.

BICEPS AND TRICEPS ACTING AS SYNERGISTS

In flexion and extension of the elbow, the biceps and triceps act antagonistically, but frequently they are called upon to contract simultaneously, such as when using a screwdriver. To force the screw in, the triceps extends or stabilizes the elbow in the position desired while the biceps supinates the forearm. This action can be confirmed by palpation. It should be noted that, when using a screwdriver, one tends to keep the elbow at an angle of approximately 90 degrees, at which angle the biceps has its highest efficiency for supination. In this activity then, the two muscles work together and thus act as synergists. Simultaneous contraction of the biceps and the triceps also occurs when a firm fist is made, in which case the two muscles act together to stabilize the elbow.

Pectoralis Major in Extension of the Elbow

When the hand is in contact with an object in front of the body, the pectoralis major, by exerting its pull on the humerus, contributes significantly to elbow extension. This is demonstrated when a heavy object is pushed away from the body and when push-ups are performed on horizontal bars or on the floor. The triceps and the pectoralis major then act in unison. In the quadriplegic patient who has innervation to the pectoralis major (C5 to C6) but not the triceps brachii (C7), the pectoralis major can produce some functional elbow extension. This can occur when the hand is fixed (closed chain) and the elbow is in 30 degrees or less of elbow flexion. Contraction of the pectoralis major extends the elbow and stabilizes it for light pushing activities.

Peripheral Nerve Injuries Affecting Muscles of the Elbow and Forearm

If the *radial nerve* is severed in the axilla, all the muscles supplied by this nerve will be paralyzed: the triceps, brachioradialis, supinator, wrist extensors, and long extensors of the digits. The nerve, however, may be injured distally to the branches supplying the triceps, as often occurs in fractures of the humerus, in which case the triceps is spared while the more distally innervated muscles are paralyzed.

In radial nerve injuries, in spite of the loss of the brachioradialis, elbow flexion is affected but little since the other flexors remain intact. Supination can be performed satisfactorily by the biceps without the supinator, but some strength in supination is lost.

A *musculocutaneous nerve injury* affects the biceps and the brachialis, causing a marked weakness of elbow flexion. Elbow flexion, however, can still be performed even against some resistance, since the brachioradialis and the pronator teres remain intact (Brunnstrom, 1946). With the loss of the biceps, supination is much weakened but can be carried out by the supinator alone; however, only a small amount of resistance can be overcome (Brunnstrom, 1946).

A *median nerve injury* affects elbow flexion very little, for although the pronator teres is paralyzed, the main flexors are intact. Pronation is severely affected since both the pronator teres and the pronator quadratus are innervated by the median nerve.

CHAPTER 6
WRIST AND HAND

The hand is a complex multipurpose organ. As a prehensile organ (L. *prehensus*, to seize), the hand can grasp with forces exceeding 100 lb (445 N or 45 kg) as well as hold and manipulate a delicate thread. In addition, the hand is used for pushing, striking blows, and even locomotion with crutches or wheelchairs. As a sense organ for touch, the hand is an extension of the brain to provide information to the visual system about the environment. The hand is also an important organ for expression and nonverbal communication.

Placement and stabilization of the hand are dependent on the shoulder, elbow, and wrist. With these multiple degrees of freedom, the palm or surface of the hand can be rotated in a full circle (360 degrees) and placed on any surface of the body with the exception of the ipsilateral arm and forearm.

BONES

Palpable Structures of the Wrist

HEAD OF THE ULNA

If the wrist is grasped from side to side at its narrowest portion, as seen in Figure 6-1, the bony eminence proximal to the examiner's index finger on the dorsum of the wrist is identified as the head of the ulna. In the pronated position of the forearm, this eminence is seen beneath the skin. If one fingertip is placed on the highest part of this bony eminence and the forearm is slowly supinated, this portion of the bone recedes and can no longer be palpated, because during supination the distal portion of the

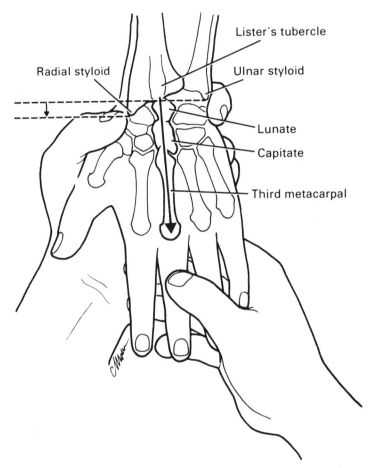

FIGURE 6-1. Bony landmarks on the dorsum of the wrist. The approximate location of the axis for radiocarpal flexion and extension is a line connecting the tips of the palpating thumb and forefinger of the proximal hand.

radius rotates around the head of the ulna, thus partially hiding the head of the ulna from palpation.

STYLOID PROCESS OF THE ULNA

The position of the examiner's index finger in Figure 6-1 indicates the approximate location of the styloid process. The tendon of the extensor carpi ulnaris, however, courses in this region and interferes with palpation. By sliding the index finger over this tendon in a palmar direction, the styloid process becomes more accessible for palpation. This process is smaller and feels sharper than the head of the ulna, and it may be palpated both in the pronated and in the supinated position of the forearm.

STYLOID PROCESS OF THE RADIUS

The position of the examiner's thumb in Figure 6-1 indicates the point where the styloid process of the radius may be palpated. This process extends somewhat more distally than the corresponding process of the ulna.

The styloid processes serve as attachments to the ulnar and radial carpal collateral ligaments, respectively.

GROOVES AND PROMINENCES ON DISTAL END OF RADIUS

On the dorsal aspect of the broad distal end of the radius are found a number of grooves for tendons passing to the hand, these grooves being separated by prominences. The *tubercle of the radius,* sometimes referred to as Lister's tubercle, may be palpated about level with the head of the ulna (see Fig. 6-1). The tendon of the extensor pollicis longus lies in a groove on the ulnar side of this tubercle and, on palpation, appears to be hooked around it. The tubercle serves as landmark for locating several other tendons in this region: the deeply situated tendon of the extensor carpi radialis brevis; the tendon of the extensor indicis proprius, which crosses over the tendon of the extensor carpi radialis brevis; and the tendon of the extensor digitorum communis to the index finger, which is superficial and visible under the skin. The deep tendons, however, are difficult to identify with certainty by palpation.

CAPITATE BONE (OS MAGNUM)

Occupying a central position at the wrist (in line with the middle finger), the capitate bone is best approached from the dorsum where a slight depression indicates its location (Fig. 6-2). The axis of motion for ulnar and radial abduction goes through this bone in a dorsal-palmar direction.

SCAPHOID (NAVICULAR) BONE

The scaphoid bone is palpated distal to the styloid process of the radius (see Fig. 6-2). Ulnar deviation of the wrist causes the bone to become prominent to the palpating fingers, while radial deviation causes the bone to recede. The scaphoid is the most commonly fractured of the carpal bones. The scaphoid bone and the *trapezium* (greater multangular) make up the floor of the "anatomic snuff box" (fovea radialis), the depression seen between the tendons of the thumb extensor muscles (extensor pollicis longus and brevis) when these muscles are tensed. It should be remembered that the scaphoid belongs to the proximal row and the trapezium to the distal row of carpal bones.

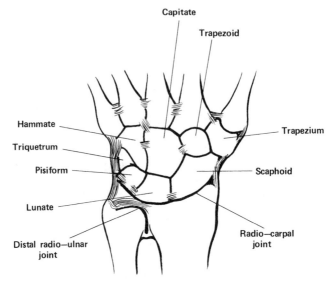

FIGURE 6-2. The proximal row of carpal bones contains the scaphoid, lunate, pisiform, and triquetrum. The distal row contains the trapezium, trapezoid, capitate, and hammate. The mid-carpal joint is formed by the articulating surfaces of these two rows.

TRAPEZIUM (GREATER MULTANGULAR)

The trapezium can be palpated proximally to the first carpometacarpal joint of the thumb (passively flex and extend the thumb) and distal to the identified scaphoid (see Fig. 6-2).

LUNATE BONE (SEMILUNAR)

The lunate is palpated distal to Lister's tubercle and proximal to the capitate (see Fig. 6-1). In normal subjects, the lunate becomes prominent to the palpating finger as the wrist is passively flexed and recedes as the wrist is passively extended. The lunate is the most frequently dislocated bone in the wrist (Hoppenfeld, 1976).

PISIFORM BONE

The pea-shaped bone palpated on the palmar side of the wrist near the ulnar border is the pisiform bone, which can be grasped and moved from side to side. It serves as the point of attachment for the tendon of the flexor carpi ulnaris.

OTHER CARPAL BONES

The trapezoid (lesser multangular), the triquetrum (triangular), and the hammate (unciform) bones seen in Figure 6-2 are more difficult to identify directly by palpation.

They can, however, be precisely palpated using their relationships to carpal bones and bony structures that are more easily palpated.

Palpable Structures of the Digits

FIVE METACARPALS

Each metacarpal has a *base* that articulates proximally with one or more carpal bones and with adjacent metacarpals (see Fig. 6-2), a *shaft* that is slightly curved, and a *head* that articulates with the base of a proximal phalanx. Each metacarpal can be palpated throughout its length on the dorsum of the hand. Note the *tubercle at the base of the fifth metacarpal,* which is located just distal to the examiner's index finger in Figure 6-1, and which serves as the distal attachment for the extensor carpi ulnaris. At the base of the second metacarpal bone (dorsally), an eminence may be felt that serves as the distal attachment for the extensor carpi radialis longus. The palmar surface of the base of the second metacarpal also presents a rough area which serves as the attachment for the flexor carpi radialis, but this lies in a position that is too deep for palpation. The head of each metacarpal bone presents a convex articular surface that becomes part of the metacarpophalangeal joint, and that may, in part, be palpated when the joint is flexed.

PHALANGES

The two phalanges of the thumb and the three phalanges of each of the other digits may be palpated without difficulty. To differentiate the phalanges of the thumb, the terms *proximal* and *distal* are used; for the other digits, *proximal, middle,* and *distal.* These terms are preferred to first and second, and to first, second, and third, respectively.

JOINTS

Radiocarpal Joint

TYPE OF JOINT

The radiocarpal joint is classified as a condyloid joint with two degrees of freedom of motion. The articular surface of the radius is *concave,* and the concave surface includes an articular disk located toward the ulnar side (see Fig. 6-2). The articular surfaces of the scaphoid and lunate are convex to correspond with the concavity of the radius. Note that neither the ulna nor the triquetrum has articulating surfaces for this joint and that both are separated from the distal radioulnar joint by an articular disk.

CAPSULE AND LIGAMENTS

The capsule of the radiocarpal joint is loose and allows extensive wrist movements. Motions of ulnar (adduction) and radial deviation (abduction) occur at the radiocarpal joint around an axis through the capitate bone. Note that ulnar deviation is approximately twice that of radial deviation. A portion of wrist flexion and extension occurs at the radiocarpal joint, and the remainder occurs at the midcarpal joint (between the proximal and distal rows of carpal bones). An elaborate ligamentous apparatus binds the osseous structures together and reinforces the capsule. The strong *ulnar collateral ligament* extends from the styloid process of the ulna proximally to the carpal bones distally (see Fig. 6-2). In its upper portion, it blends with the articular disk of the radiocarpal joint. One part of this ligament attaches to the pisiform bone and is in close relation to the tendon of the flexor carpi ulnaris muscle. The *radial collateral ligament* is attached to the styloid process of the radius proximally and to several of the carpal bones distally. It is in close relation to the tendons of the abductor pollicis longus and the extensor pollicis brevis muscles.

Midcarpal Joint

While the small motions between individual carpal bones are essential for normal hand function, the midcarpal joint (between the proximal and distal rows of metacarpals) has been identified as a major locus for flexion and extension motions.

Wrist Joint

Although the "wrist joint" has been simply classified as a condyloid joint, note that it is a complex of many joints and possesses multiple degrees of freedom. An important complexity is the changing axis of motion for wrist flexion and extension. The majority of the motion of wrist flexion occurs at the radiocarparpal joint (50 degrees), with less motion occurring at the midcarpal joint (35 degrees) (Kapandji, 1970a). Conversely, the major portion of wrist extension occurs at the midcarpal joint, with a lesser contribution at the radiocarpal joint. This movement of the axis of motion, illustrated in Figure 6-3, can be readily appreciated in the need to move the axis of the goniometer when evaluating motion of the wrist and is an important consideration in specific mobilization of wrists with limited motion.

Carpometacarpal Joints of Digits II to V

The trapezoid, capitate, and hammate bones of the distal row of carpal bones articulate with metacarpals II to V in a rather irregular fashion to form mortices (Gr. *murtazza*, joined or fixed in). While movements at these joints are small, motions of rotation and flexion-extension are important for hand functions and provide a large

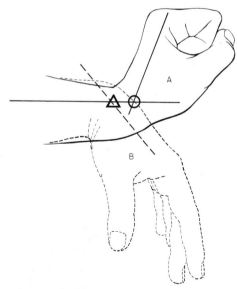

FIGURE 6-3. For maximum range of motion at wrist, the first should be closed in extension *(A)* and open in flexion *(B)*. The axis for extension (o) is distal to the axis for the flexion (Δ).

change in the shape of the transverse arch of the hand (Fig. 6-4). The third metacarpal (middle finger) is relatively stable, while the second, fourth, and fifth metacarpals provide increasing mobility. Thus, as the extended hand is opened, the span of the fingers increases to surround objects, and as the hand is closed in grasping, the fingers are approximated to increase the force of the grasp.

Carpometacarpal Joint of the Thumb

The base of the metacarpal bone of the thumb articulates with the trapezium, and this joint has a true saddle shape (see Fig. 1-8). The joint capsule is thick but loose, thus permitting great freedom of motion. The joint allows the thumb to move into *opposi-*

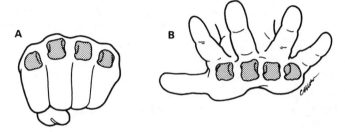

FIGURE 6-4. Transverse arch of the hand showing the position of the metacarpal heads *(A)* when making a fist, and *(B)* when opening the hand.

tion so that the palmar surface of the tip of the thumb is directed toward the palmar surface of the other digits. Anatomically, the term *opposition* refers to the carpometacarpal joint of the thumb only, but clinically, *opposition of the thumb* has come to mean the entire movement of bringing the palmar surface of the thumb in contact with one or more of the other digits. *Reposition* is the reverse of opposition.

The saddle joint of the thumb also permits movements of *abduction* and *adduction*, and these movements take place about an axis that is perpendicular to the axis of opposition and reposition.

Metacarpophalangeal Joints of Digits II to V

The metacarpophalangeal (MCP) joints of digits II to V are of the condyloid type, the rounded surfaces of the heads of the metacarpals articulating with the shallow concave surfaces on the bases of the proximal phalanges. The articular surfaces of the heads of the metacarpals extend more toward the palmar than toward the dorsal side to permit closing of the fist. When the MCP joints are in extension, abduction is relatively free, and the span of the fingers is wide. In 90 degrees of flexion, no abduction or adduction motion is possible. This is due to the flattened volar surface of the metacarpal heads and the tightening of the collateral ligaments. The MCP joints are thus stabilized mechanically to reinforce gripping.

At their bases, the metacarpal bones lie side by side, connected by firm joints, but they spread apart distally so that their heads do not contact each other. An extensive ligamentous apparatus, however, binds them together. The *deep transverse metacarpal* (transverse capitular) *ligament* on the palmar side of the metacarpal heads limits the distance by which the heads may be separated.

The metacarpal bones have different lengths, so that when a fist is made the knuckles do not form a straight line. The metacarpals belonging to the index and middle fingers are approximately the same length, while those of the ring and little fingers are shorter.

AXES OF MOTION

The axes for *flexion and extension* and for *abduction* and *adduction* both pass through the head of the metacarpal bone, the former being a transverse axis, the latter having a dorsal-palmar direction. The joint surfaces also allow a circumduction movement which can be performed actively. Passively, the accessory motions of distraction, rotation, dorsal-volar glide, and lateral glide are permitted and have the greatest motion when the MCP joint is in extension.

Metacarpophalangeal Joint of the Thumb

The MCP joint of the thumb is usually described as a hinge joint, but functionally, it possesses all the characteristics of the other MCP joints, even though range of motion is more limited. Two small sesamoid bones, interconnected by a ligament, are found on the palmar side of the joint. The tendon of the long flexor of the thumb passes in a groove between the sesamoid bones.

AXES OF MOTION

Movements permitted in this joint are flexion and extension and a small amount of abduction and adduction (see page 202). The axis for flexion-extension passes transversely, that for abduction-adduction in a dorsal-palmar direction through the head of the metacarpal bone. Both axes are oriented to the plane of the thumb. The relation to the plane of the palm varies in accordance with the position of the carpometacarpal joint.

Range of motion in flexion-extension is quite variable in individuals. In some subjects, flexion is less than 45 degrees; in others, as much as 90 degrees. Abduction-adduction of the metacarpophalangeal joint of the thumb is of smaller range than at the corresponding joints of the other digits. To observe the presence of this motion in the thumb, the metacarpal bone must be stabilized firmly, or the carpometacarpal joint will participate.

Interphalangeal Joints

Each of the digits II to V has two interphalangeal joints, while the thumb has only one. These joints are hinge joints, permitting flexion and extension only. Range of motion is larger at the proximal than at the distal joints of digits II to V. The interphalangeal joint of the thumb has a range of approximately 90 degrees.

MUSCLES OF THE WRIST AND HAND

The muscles listed below should be studied on the skeleton, on the cadaver, and in the living subject. For an understanding of the actions of these muscles, it is important to consider: (1) over which joint or joints each muscle passes; (2) the line of action of the muscle; (3) the distance of the muscle to the axis of motion of the joint at various positions of the joint; (4) the relative length of the muscle; and (5) the functional unit to which the muscle belongs.

MUSCLES ACTING ON THE WRIST AND DIGITS (AND ELBOW)

Muscles Acting on Wrist (and Elbow)
Extensor carpi radialis longus
Extensor carpi radialis brevis
Extensor carpi ulnaris
Flexor carpi radialis
Palmaris longus
Flexor carpi ulnaris

Muscles Acting on Wrist and Digits (Extrinsic muscles of the hand)
   Extensor digitorum
   Extensor indicis proprius
   Extensor digiti minimi proprius
   Extensor pollicis longus
   Extensor pollicis brevis
   Abductor pollicis longus
   Flexor digitorum superficialis
   Flexor digitorum profundus
   Flexor pollicis longus

Muscles Acting on Digits Only (Intrinsic muscles of the hand)
   Four lumbricals
   Three (four) palmar interossei*
   Four dorsal interossei
   Thenar muscles
      Opponens pollicis
      Abductor pollicis brevis
      Adductor pollicis
      Flexor pollicis brevis
   Hypothenar muscles
      Opponens digiti minimi
      Abductor digiti minimi
      Flexor digiti minimi brevis
   Palmaris brevis

The innervation of muscles acting on wrist and digits is as follows:

Radial Nerve
   Extensor carpi radialis longus
   Extensor carpi radialis brevis
   Extensor carpi ulnaris
   Extensor digitorum
   Extensor indicis proprius
   Extensor digiti minimi proprius
   Extensor pollicis longus
   Extensor pollicis brevis
   Abductor pollicis longus

---

*The deep portion of flexor pollicis brevis is sometimes described as the first palmar interosseus. In that case, the palmar interossei are four in number.

Median Nerve
Flexor carpi radialis
Palmaris longus
Flexor digitorum superficialis
Radial half of flexor digitorum profundus
and the two radial lumbricals
Flexor pollicis longus
Superficial portion of flexor pollicis brevis
Opponens pollicis
Abductor pollicis brevis (may have ulnar
innervation; Belson, Smith, and Puentes,
1976)

Ulnar Nerve
Flexor carpi ulnaris
Ulnar half of flexor digitorum profundus
and the two ulnar lumbricals
All interossei muscles
All hypothenar muscles
Palmaris brevis
Deep portion of flexor pollicis brevis
Adductor pollicis

The muscles may be thought of in groups, innervated as follows: The *radial nerve* supplies all the extensors of wrist and digits with *proximal attachments* on the forearm and in the region of the lateral epicondyle. The *median nerve* supplies most of the flexors of the wrist and digits with *proximal attachments* on the forearm and in the region of the medial epicondyle. The *ulnar nerve* supplies most of the small muscles in the hand. Exceptions are "half-half" supply of flexor digitorum profundus and lumbricals (median and ulnar), ulnar nerve supply to flexor carpi ulnaris, and median nerve supply to thenar muscles.

WRIST MOVEMENTS

Movements of the hand in relation to the forearm (see Appendix B), without consideration of simultaneous finger movements, will be considered here. Synergic action of wrist and finger muscles will be discussed under Hand Function.

Nomenclature

Movements of the wrist are described as *flexion and extension* and as *radial and ulnar abduction*. By combining these motions, the complex movement of *circumduction* may be performed, during which the hand executes a circling movement. Orientation for radial and ulnar abduction is a line drawn longitudinally through the forearm and the middle finger (see Fig. 6-1).

Palpation of Muscles Acting in Extension of the Wrist

If the wrist is extended with the fist closed, the *tendon of the extensor carpi radialis longus* becomes prominent and is palpated as seen in Figure 6-5. The tendon lies on the radial side of the capitate bone but on the ulnar side of the tubercle of the radius, and courses toward the base of the metacarpal bone of the index finger, to which it is attached. The distal attachment of the *extensor carpi radialis brevis* is the base of the metacarpal bone of the middle finger. The tendon of the extensor of the index finger crosses over the extensor carpi radialis brevis, making identification of the muscle by palpation somewhat difficult. Its tendon can usually be felt rising if the thumb is moved in a palmar direction, in a plane perpendicular to the palm of the hand.

The muscular parts of the two wrist extensors, together with the brachioradialis, make up the radial muscle group at the elbow. By manipulating the muscle tissue, this group may be separated from the other extensors on the dorsum of the forearm and from the flexor group on the palmar side of the forearm. To locate the radial extensors of the wrist, the brachioradialis is first identified by resistance to elbow flexion with the forearm halfway between pronation and supination (see Fig. 5-8). The muscular

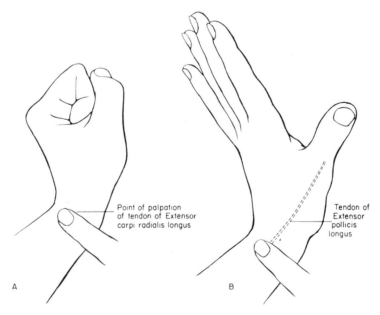

Point of palpation of tendon of Extensor carpi radialis longus

Tendon of Extensor pollicis longus

A

B

FIGURE 6-5. *(A)* Palpation of tendon of extensor carpi radialis longus when fist is closed. *(B)* When fingers are extended, extensor digitorum communis takes over task of extending wrist. Note that tendon of extensor pollicis longus also courses on extensor side of wrist, not far from the tendon of extensor carpi radialis longus.

portion of the extensor carpi radialis longus is then located close to the brachioradialis, toward the dorsal side of the forearm. It is a superficial muscle and may readily be identified when resistance is given to extension of the wrist (see Fig. 5-9). The extensor carpi radialis brevis is found somewhat more distally.

The *extensor digitorum* participates in extension of the wrist *only* when the fingers are simultaneously extended; in fact, the finger extensors then appear to take over the task of wrist extension altogether. To feel the shift from wrist extensors to finger extensors, the wrist should first be extended with the fist closed, and the prominent tendon of extensor carpi radialis longus palpated (see Fig. 6-5, A). While maintaining the wrist in this position, the fingers are extended (see Fig. 6-5, B). It will then be noted that the prominent tendon being palpated "disappears," a sign that the muscle "lets go" or diminishes its contraction. This shift is regulated entirely automatically. For a more detailed analysis of the relationships between the wrist extensors and the finger extensors, the reader is referred to Beevor's Croonian Lecture (1903).

The tendon of the *extensor carpi ulnaris* is palpated between the head of the ulna and a prominent tubercle on the base of the fifth metacarpal bone, the latter serving as its point of distal attachment. The tendon becomes prominent if the wrist is extended with the fist closed, and even more prominent if the wrist is simultaneously ulnarward abducted (Fig. 6-6). The tendon is also easily palpable when the thumb is extended and abducted as seen in Figure 6-25.

The muscular portion of the extensor carpi ulnaris is best palpated about 2 inches (5 cm) below the lateral epicondyle of the humerus, where it lies between the anconeus and the extensor digitorum (see Fig. 5-11). From this point on, it may be followed

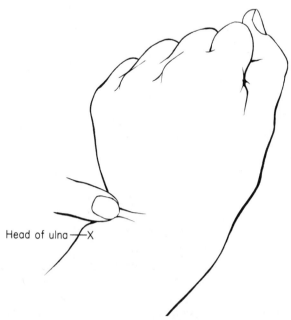

Head of ulna—X

FIGURE 6-6. Palpation of extensor carpi ulnaris in fist closure.

distally along the dorsal-ulnar aspect of the forearm in a direction toward the head of the ulna.

Palpation of Muscles Acting in Flexion of the Wrist

The three tendons of the wrist flexors become prominent if resistance is given to flexion of the wrist (Fig. 6-7). The most centrally located tendon is that of the *palmaris longus*; it varies in size in different individuals, or it may be missing altogether. Radial to it, the strong tendon of the *flexor carpi radialis* is identified. This tendon lies in a superficial position in the lower part of the forearm, is held down by the transverse carpal ligament at the wrist, and disappears into a groove in the trapezium bone. It cannot be followed to its distal attachment on the base of the second metacarpal bone. The tendon of the *flexor carpi ulnaris* lies close to the ulnar border of the forearm and may be palpated between the styloid process of the ulna and the pisiform bone, to which it is attached.

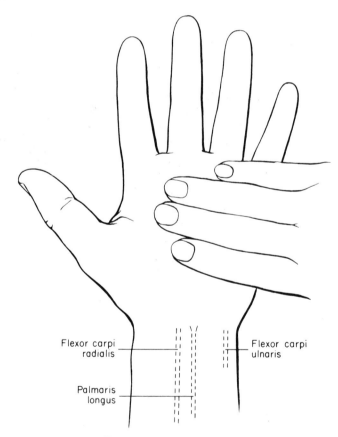

FIGURE 6-7. Resistance to wrist flexion applied in palm of hand brings out tendons of wrist flexors.

If the fist is tightly closed and wrist flexion is simultaneously resisted, one or more tendons of the *flexor digitorum superficialis* become prominent in the space between the palmaris longus and the flexor carpi ulnaris (Fig. 6-8). The tendon of the fourth finger appears to rise to the surface. In individuals lacking the palmaris longus, a more complete display of the tendons of the long finger flexors may be observed if flexion of the wrist is resisted and the subject then flexes one finger after the other, or flexes all fingers simultaneously (Fig. 6-9).

Muscles Acting in Radial and Ulnar Abduction of the Wrist

The palmaris longus and the extensor carpi radialis brevis have a central location at the wrist; the other wrist flexors and extensors are situated either toward the radial or

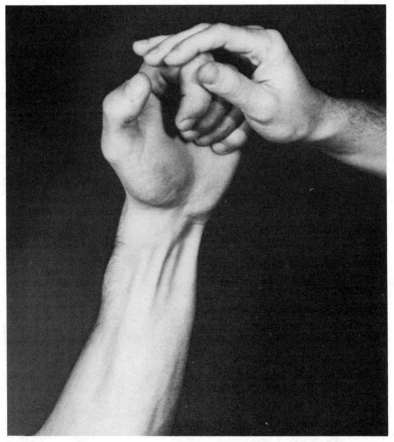

FIGURE 6-8. When a tight fist is made and wrist flexion is resisted, four tendons are visible: on the ulnar side of the wrist, the flexor carpi ulnaris; next, the flexor digitorum superficialis; then, the prominent palmaris longus; and on the radial side, the flexor carpi radialis.

toward the ulnar side of the wrist. They are therefore capable of producing movements from side to side as well as flexion and extension.

When the extensor carpi ulnaris and flexor carpi ulnaris combine their actions, ulnar abduction of the wrist results. The extensor carpi radialis longus and the flexor carpi radialis, aided by the abductor pollicis longus and the extensor pollicis brevis, produce radial abduction. The latter two muscles have a favorable line of action for performing radial abduction, and they do so regardless of the position of the thumb, whether flexed, extended, abducted, or adducted.

The wrist furnishes typical examples of how muscles may act either as synergists or antagonists. For instance, in flexion and extension of the wrist, the flexor carpi ulnaris and the extensor carpi ulnaris are antagonists, but in ulnar abduction of the wrist these two muscles act as synergists.

HAND FUNCTION

The function of the hand depends on the teamwork of many muscles, of those acting on the wrist as well as on the digits. The wrist muscles are an integral part of hand function, since they prevent undesired wrist movements and keep the finger muscles at a length that is favorable for producing tension. An extensive ligamentous apparatus, particularly well developed on the dorsum of the digits (here variably named *extensor sleeve, aponeurotic sleeve* or *extensor hood*), is admirably designed to enhance and regulate the function of the muscles moving the digits (see Fig. 6-17).

Many of the muscles participating in hand function are pluriarticular muscles, that is, they pass over several joints before reaching their point of insertion. A pluriarticular muscle, if contracting in an isolated fashion, tends to produce movements in all the joints over which it passes. Such movements, however, do not usually materialize,

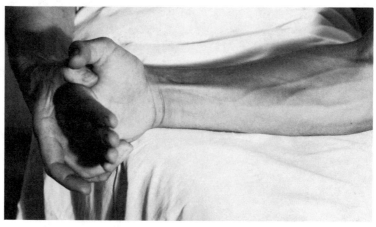

FIGURE 6-9. Absence of palmaris longus. The prominent tendon is that of the flexor carpi radialis. When this subject moves the digits, the play of the flexor tendons can be observed well. Ordinarily, the palmaris longus partially obstructs the view.

since synergic muscles spring into action to stabilize one or more joints where movements are undesirable.

In studying the function of the hand, close attention must be paid to the manner in which various muscles combine their actions as the hand is used for grasp and release and for various skilled movements. The muscles that make up such a "team," or movement synergy, are so strongly linked together neurophysiologically that the individual is unable voluntarily to omit a muscle from the combination to which it belongs (Beevor, 1903).

Closing the Fist

ROLE OF THE WRIST EXTENSORS IN GRASPING

When the fist closes, the fingers fold into the palm of the hand or close around an object by the action of the long finger flexors (profundus and superficialis), probably aided by some of the intrinsic muscles of the hand. Since these long finger flexors have proximal attachments in the forearm and their tendons pass on the flexor side of the wrist, these muscles, if unopposed, would cause the wrist to flex during grasp. Such action is prevented by the stabilizing action of the wrist extensors. The strength of contraction of the wrist extensors is in direct proportion to the effort of the grip—the harder the grip, the stronger the contraction of the wrist extensors.

If the wrist is allowed to flex during finger flexion, the grip is markedly weakened (see Fig. 4-9); in fact, it then becomes almost impossible to close the fist completely (Fig. 6-10). This difficulty arises partly because the finger extension apparatus may not permit further elongation (passive insufficiency), and partly because of the marked approximation of the proximal and distal attachments of the finger flexors,

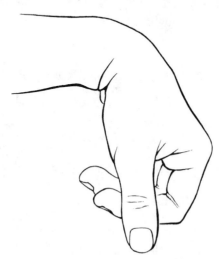

FIGURE 6-10. Weakness of grasp when wrist is fully flexed. In this position, it becomes difficult or impossible to close the fist completely.

which weakens their contraction so that they may attain a length at which they are unable to produce effective tension (active insufficiency).

PALPATION OF THE WRIST EXTENSORS IN GRASPING

For palpation of the *extensor carpi radialis longus*, the subject places the lightly closed fist on the table or in the lap, forearm pronated, and the examiner palpates on the radiodorsal aspect of the wrist, as explained previously. By having the subject alternately close the fist firmly and relax the grip, the rise and fall of the tendon of the extensor carpi radialis longus may be felt and its contracting muscle belly identified in the forearm close to the brachioradialis. To eliminate the possibility of palpating the wrong tendon, the tendon of the extensor pollicis longus should first be identified. This poses no difficulty because the tendon is visible under the skin when the thumb is held in extension.

The *extensor carpi radialis brevis* also participates in wrist fixation for grasp, but its tendon protrudes less than that of the extensor carpi radialis longus and is therefore somewhat more difficult to identify. Its tendon may be palpated on the dorsum of the wrist, in line with the third metacarpal bone, when the fist is firmly closed.

Another, perhaps even better, method of identifying the tendon of the extensor carpi radialis brevis is to have the subject place the lightly closed fist in the lap, ulnar side down, and then move the thumb in a horizontal plane and in a palmar direction. This thumb movement involves the action of the palmaris longus muscle, the tendon of which passes down the middle of the palmar aspect of the wrist. The extensor carpi radialis brevis, the tendon of which occupies a similar position on the dorsum of the wrist, is the logical muscle to use for wrist fixation so that wrist flexion by the palmaris longus is prevented.

The *extensor carpi ulnaris* also participates in wrist fixation for grasp. When a fist is made, its tendon and muscle belly may be palpated in the location previously described (see Fig. 6-6).

ROLE OF THE LONG FINGER FLEXORS IN GRASPING

Flexor digitorum superficialis and profundus serve the second to fifth digits for flexion at the interphalangeal joints. Since the tendons of these muscles pass on the palmar side of the wrist and of the metacarpophalangeal joints, they also tend to produce flexion of these joints. In using the hand for grasping, flexion of the metacarpophalangeal joints is necessary for proper shape of the hand, while flexion at the wrist is undesirable because it decreases the force exerted by the flexors by shortening them. Fortunately, wrist flexion is prevented by synergic contraction of the wrist extensors.

The superficialis, attaching to the base of the middle phalanx, flexes the proximal interphalangeal joint. The profundus tendon, after perforating the superficialis tendon, attaches to the base of the distal phalanx and acts as a flexor of the distal as well as the proximal interphalangeal joint. The profundus is the only muscle capable of flexing the distal joint.

PALPATION AND TESTING OF THE LONG FINGER FLEXORS

The *flexor digitorum superficialis* is located underneath the flexor carpi radialis and the palmaris longus, and the general direction of the muscle is from the flexor (medial) epicondyle to the center of the palmar side of the wrist. It is difficult or impossible to palpate the muscle at its proximal attachment since this is widespread and in part tendinous, or to distinguish the separate muscle bellies serving the four fingers. But, movement of the tendons of the superficialis may be observed in the forearm and at the wrist beneath the tendons of the flexor carpi radialis and palmaris longus, and particularly in the space between the tendons of the flexor carpi ulnaris and the palmaris longus. In this region, as previously mentioned, the tendon serving the fourth finger usually stands out prominently if a firm fist is made while the wrist is somewhat flexed. In subjects lacking the palmaris longus, observation is considerably easier.

Isolated action of the flexor digitorum superficialis is obtained if the proximal interphalangeal joint is flexed while the distal one remains inactive, a movement which is best performed with one finger at a time (Fig. 6-11, A). The coordination needed for this movement can be mastered by most individuals; if some difficulty arises, the examiner should stabilize the proximal phalanx.

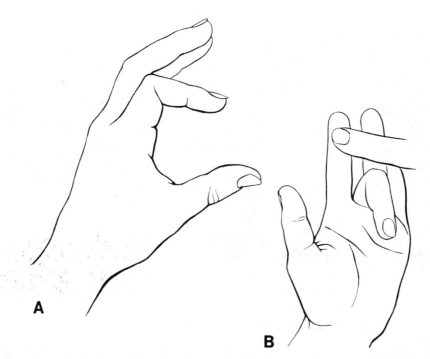

FIGURE 6-11. *(A)* Isolated action of the flexor digitorum superficialis of the index finger. *(B)* Method for testing individual flexor digitorum superficialis muscles by holding all other fingers in extension.

Another way in which the superficialis of one digit may be tested without participation by the profundus is for the examiner to maintain the other digits in full extension at all joints (Fig. 6-11, B). This inactivates the profundus so that the subject is unable to flex the distal joint.

The *flexor digitorum profundus* is deeply located, being covered by the superficialis, flexor carpi ulnaris, palmaris longus, flexor carpi radialis, and pronator teres. It is muscular only in the upper half of the forearm. The muscle bellies serving the individual fingers are not nearly as well separated as those of the superficialis.

In spite of the deep location of the profundus, its contracting muscle belly may be palpated, provided that tension is minimal in the more superficial muscles. To achieve relative relaxation of the overlying muscles, the subject is seated with the forearm supinated and resting in the lap while the wrist is extended by the weight of the hand (protruding over the lap). When the arm is in this position and the subject closes the fist fully but with moderate effort, the profundus may be felt rising under the examiner's fingers, which are placed in the region between the pronator teres and the flexor carpi ulnaris, about 2 inches (5 cm) below the medial epicondyle of the humerus.

In testing the profundus, one finger at a time is stabilized over the middle phalanx, as seen in Figure 6-12. During this test, it may be observed that the index finger is able to move well without drawing the other fingers into action, and the middle finger can be moved alone comparatively well, while isolated flexion of the fourth and the fifth fingers is difficult or impossible.

Ordinarily, a subject is unable to move the distal interphalangeal joint separately when no fixation of the middle phalanx is given. This is understandable, because the tendon of the profundus acts on the two interphalangeal joints simultaneously. Under normal circumstances, there is no extensor mechanism capable of extending the proximal joint separately. There are subjects, however, whose proximal interphalangeal joints allow hyperextension, and these persons will succeed in flexing the distal joints in an isolated fashion (Fig. 6-13). The middle band of the extensor mechanism then "locks" the proximal joint in hyperextension, preventing the profundus from flexing it. When the proximal joint is hyperextended, the lateral bands become slack and therefore can exert no action on the distal joint.

Differential action of the two long finger flexors in grasping has been revealed by electromyography. Studies by Long and Brown (1964) and reiterated by Long (1968) indicate that the flexor digitorum profundus is the most important muscle for *unresisted* flexion of the fingers. When each subject closed the hand until the fingertips

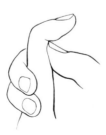

FIGURE 6-12. Testing flexor digitorum profundus of index finger.

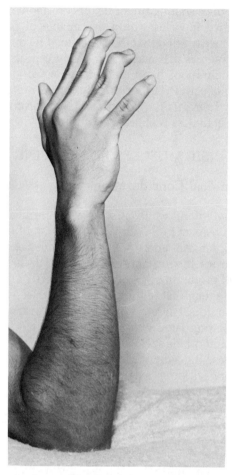

FIGURE 6-13. A subject who is capable of stabilizing the proximal interphalangeal joint in hyperextension can flex the distal joint in an isolated fashion by flexor digitorum profundus. Ordinarily, the profundus acts on both joints.

lightly touched the palm, this muscle showed consistent and strong electric activity. The flexor digitorum superficialis was found to be less consistent in its action, and its activity appeared to be related to the position of the wrist. When the wrist was extended, little or no activity was registered. Activity increased progressively as the wrist was flexed.

As previously stated, the neuromuscular system prefers to have one muscle do the job of two when such a muscle is available and when the tasks are light. Evidence that this rule applies to fist closure is now available. When the wrist is extended, length-tension relations of the flexor digitorum profundus are favorable for producing tensions, and sufficient tension is developed to close the fist. With progressive flexion of the wrist, however, length-tension relations of the profundus become less favorable, and the flexor digitorum superficialis is recruited to aid in fist closure.

The cross sections of the two long finger flexors are about equal in size (see Appendix A); therefore, the two muscles would be capable of producing approximately equal tension. It would be expected that the superficial flexor would contract strongly in forceful fist closure, such as that needed for firm grasping of tools. Close and Kidd (1969), in recording synchronous hand motion and action potentials in the muscles, did observe simultaneous activity in flexors digitorum profundus and superficialis. They graded the activity from medium to full, and they described the hand motions as pinch or grip or grasp, activities that seem to imply the need for added force.

ROLE OF THE INTRINSIC MUSCLES IN GRASPING

Anatomic and Mechanical Considerations

The location of the dorsal interosseous muscles would indicate that these muscles are essentially neutral with respect to flexion and extension of the metacarpophalangeal joints. But the palmar interossei and the lumbrical muscles course definitely on the palmar side of the axis for flexion and extension of these joints and are therefore mechanically capable of producing flexion. The leverage of the lumbrical muscles for flexion is more favorable than that of the palmar interossei—the former course on the palmar, the latter on the dorsal side of the transverse metacarpal ligament.

When a lumbrical is stimulated by a high-intensity electric current, the result is strong extension of the interphalangeal joints and flexion of the metacarpophalangeal joint to about 80 degrees. But when a low current is used (minimal to produce response), the interphalangeal joints extend but the metacarpophalangeal joint flexes very little or not at all (Backhouse and Catton, 1954). This suggests that the leverage of a lumbrical muscle for extension of the interphalangeal joints is far better than its leverage for flexion of the metacarpophalangeal joint. The high-current experiment also demonstrates that a lumbrical muscle when contracting maximally is capable of shortening effectively through a long range. Such long effective excursion is remarkable when one considers that, under the above experimental conditions, the proximal attachment of the lumbrical muscle must be poorly stabilized since the flexor digitorum profundus muscle is inactive.

Electromyographic Findings

When the fist is slowly and lightly closed, the lumbrical muscles have been found electrically silent (Backhouse and Catton, 1954; Long and Brown, 1964). Inactivity of the lumbrical muscles was also demonstrated when resistance was applied to simultaneous flexion of all three finger joints (Backhouse and Catton, 1954). The common conception that the lumbrical muscles actively aid the long finger flexors in closure of the hand must therefore be questioned. A different role for the lumbricals has been suggested by Landsmeer and Long (1965) and again by Long (1968), that these muscles may contribute to metacarpophalangeal flexion by their passive tension. Those investigators suggest that contraction of the flexor digitorum profundus exerts traction on the lumbrical muscles in a proximal direction and that, simultaneously, as the interphalangeal joints flex, these muscles are put on a stretch distally. It may well be that under these circumstances the passive tension curve could be used. This explanation, for the time being, however, must be looked upon as a hypothesis only. The electromyographic study of Close and Kidd (1969) does not support this theory for they observed simultaneous lumbrical and deep flexor activity during motions they describe as pinch and grasp. Perhaps the differences noted can be attributed in part to the total force requirement of the hand activity.

PALPATION OF THE INTRINSIC MUSCLES

The muscular portions of the lumbricals are located on the radial side of the tendons of the long finger flexors. In most hands, these tendons are best visible in the clawhand position, that is, when the metacarpophalangeal joints are hyperextended and the interphalangeal joints are flexed (Fig. 6-14). Identification of the lumbrical muscles by palpation is difficult since these muscles are small and covered with fascia and skin.

The palmar interossei are located deep in the palm of the hand beneath the lumbricals and between the metacarpal bones. They are even less accessible to palpation than the lumbricals. The dorsal interosseous muscles may be palpated from the dorsal side.

COORDINATED ACTION OF THE THREE FINGER JOINTS IN GRASPING

In normal hand closure, all three finger joints flex simultaneously, which enables the palm of the hand to make proper contact with an object grasped. As stated above, the

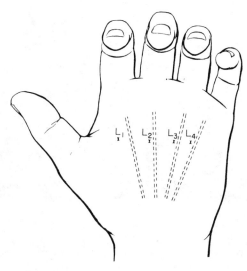

FIGURE 6-14. The muscular portions of the lumbricals are located on the radial side of the tendons of the long finger flexors.

flexor digitorum profundus is the principal muscle employed in light hand closure, apparently acting effectively over all three finger joints simultaneously. However, subjects with long-standing paralysis of the intrinsic muscles, even though the flexor digitorum profundus and superficialis are intact, have an ineffective grasp. Such a subject is still capable of making a fist, but the interphalangeal joints flex first and the metacarpophalangeal joints flex a fraction of a second later (Fig. 6-15). Without the intrinsic muscles, some difficulty arises when the subject attempts an activity that requires quick closure of the hand, as in catching a ball. Disturbance of the extrinsic-intrinsic muscle balance eventually results in a "claw" posture of the hand. Changes in capsules and ligaments and atrophy and loss of elastic properties of the intrinsic muscles are part of the picture.

Opening the Fist

ROLE OF THE WRIST FLEXORS IN EXTENSION OF THE FINGERS

The long extensor muscles of the fingers are attached in the forearm and pass over the wrist and then over the metacarpophalangeal joints. If these muscles were to contract in an isolated fashion, they would extend not only the joints of the fingers, but also the wrist. To prevent them from moving the wrist, the wrist flexors contract synergically, keeping the wrist in a neutral position or flexing it. The association between finger

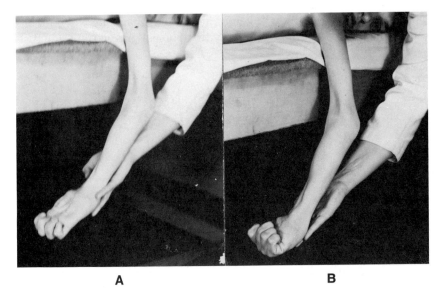

A B

FIGURE 6-15. Manner of closure of fist when intrinsic muscles of hand are paralyzed. The interphalangeal joints are first flexed by the long finger flexors (A). Then, in continued action, these muscles flex also the metacarpophalangeal joints, so that the fingers "roll" into the palm (B). Simultaneous flexion of all finger joints, such as needed in catching a ball, cannot be accomplished.

extensors and wrist flexors is strong, and it takes concentrated effort to interrupt the linkage.

If complete finger extension is alternated with grasp in rapid succession, it will be observed that the wrist as well as the fingers are in constant motion: flexion of the wrist accompanies finger extension; extension of the wrist occurs when the fist is closed. These combinations are automatic, and the less attention paid to the details of the performance, the more obvious they will be. Note that the wrist movements that take place are in a direction opposite to the finger motions, so that an alternate elongation of the finger extensors and the finger flexors over the wrist is obtained. Such elongation adds to the efficiency of these muscles in extending and flexing the fingers.

PALPATION OF THE WRIST FLEXORS IN EXTENSION OF THE FINGERS

When the fingers are extended, the tendons of the wrist flexors are palpated on the palmar side of the wrist: the flexor carpi radialis and the palmaris longus in the center, the flexor carpi ulnaris near the pisiform bone—all three muscles spring into action. With increased forcefulness of finger extension, increased tension can be felt in the wrist flexors.

EXTENSOR ASSEMBLY

The finger joints may be extended in many ways, such as extension of all finger joints simultaneously, extension of the interphalangeal joints with metacarpophalangeal joints flexed (Fig. 6-16), extension of the metacarpophalangeal joints while the interphalangeal joints are flexed (see Fig. 6-14), and in many in-between positions. For such variations of motion, the extensor digitorum is aided by the intrinsic muscles of the hand, the long finger flexors, and by muscles acting upon the wrist. The effect obtained when these muscles combine their actions in different manners is regulated in part by the dorsal aponeurosis (Fig. 6-17), particularly by its proximal portion, which forms the main part of the so-called *aponeurotic sleeve*.

The muscles that insert into the dorsal aponeurosis are the extensor digitorum, extensor indicis proprius, extensor digiti minimi proprius, lumbricals, and interossei.

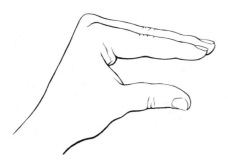

FIGURE 6-16. Flexion of metacarpophalangeal joints, extension of interphalangeal joints.

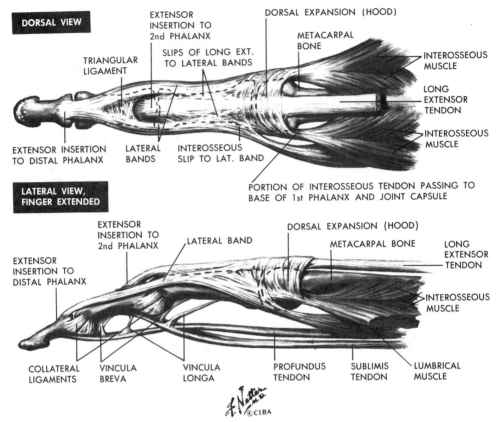

FIGURE 6-17. Dorsal and lateral views of anatomic structures of the extensor assembly of a finger (From *CIBA surgical anatomy of hand*. Clin Symp 21(3):34, 1969, with permission.)

The tendon of the *long extensor* of each finger passes on the dorsum of its respective metacarpophalangeal joint. Having passed this joint, the tendon not only gives off a "central deep ribbon" from its undersurface that acts to extend the joint (Bunnell, 1956), but is also bound to the capsule of the joint. The extensor tendon then continues distally and spreads into a broad aponeurosis that covers the dorsum and partially covers the sides of the proximal phalanx. Three more or less distinct tendon slips, incorporated in the dorsal aponeurosis, may be seen: the central one coursing dorsally to an attachment on the base of the middle phalanx and serving to extend the proximal interphalangeal joint; and the two lateral ones passing on the sides of the phalanx and forming the lateral bands.

The *four lumbrical muscles* pass on the flexor side of the metacarpophalangeal joints and join the dorsal aponeurosis on the radial side of each finger. By means of their attachment to the dorsal aponeurosis, the lumbricals are instrumental in extending the two interphalangeal joints.

The *interosseous muscles*, except for the dorsal components of the dorsal interossei, would be expected to flex the metacarpophalangeal joints and, by their attachment into the dorsal aponeurosis, to extend the two interphalangeal joints.

The tendons of the lumbricals and the interossei spread into the extensor aponeurosis by means of transverse and longitudinal fibers, the latter forming part of the lateral bands. Somewhat more distally, the lateral bands on each side of the finger divide as follows: The more central portions course dorsally, joining the central portion of the tendon of the extensor digitorum to extend the proximal interphalangeal joint; and the lateral portions bypass the proximal interphalangeal joint and then turn dorsally to extend the distal interphalangeal joint.

INTEGRATED ACTION OF EXTRINSIC AND INTRINSIC MUSCLES

Various theories have arisen with respect to interaction of intrinsic and extrinsic muscles in flexion and extension of the digits. Beevor (1903) observed that extension and hyperextension of the metacarpophalangeal joint are carried out by the extensor digitorum, but that this muscle has little or no effect on interphalangeal extension, an observation also made by Duchenne (1867). For extension of the interphalangeal joints, both Duchenne and Beevor held that intrinsic muscle action is required. Subjects with paralysis of the intrinsic muscles develop clawhand and are incapable of extending the interphalangeal joints. In these subjects, an effort to extend all three finger joints simultaneously only results in extreme hyperextension of the metacarpophalangeal joints while the interphalangeal joints remain flexed. Beevor further observed that in paralysis of the intrinsic muscles, if the metacarpophalangeal joints were kept passively flexed, the subjects could then use the extensor digitorum to extend the interphalangeal joints. He concluded that "it seems probable that in the clawhand the inability of the extensor digitorum to extend the terminal phalanges is due to its energy being expended on the first phalanges, which are not prevented from overextending by the interossei and lumbricales, as these are paralysed."

A widely accepted theory of the interaction of extrinsic and intrinsic muscles in the hand was formulated by Sterling Bunnell, whose extensive experience as a hand surgeon made him well qualified to discuss hand function (1938, 1942, 1956). He stressed in particular the movement of the aponeurotic hood (see Fig. 6-17) in coordinating the actions of the extrinsic and intrinsic muscles. When the hood is distal to the MCP axis, the intrinsic muscles have a line of pull to flex the MCP joint, and the interphalangeal joints are extended by action of the long extensor tendon. When the hood is pulled proximally by the long extensor tendon (see Fig. 6-17), the intrinsic muscles lose their leverage for MCP flexion, and their force is transmitted through the bands to produce interphalangeal extension. Bunnell described the mechanism "like the shifting of a gear" with the balance of power changing at about 45 degrees of flexion.

The theory that the extensor digitorum is instrumental in extending the interphalangeal joints when the metacarpophalangeal joints are flexed appears to be substantiated by observations on patients with paralysis of the intrinsic muscles. However, conclusions drawn from observations on pathologic cases cannot necessarily be applied to subjects with normal functioning of the neuromuscular system—this has been convincingly demonstrated by electromyography. The following is a brief review of some of the pertinent electromyographic findings reported by Backhouse and Catton (1954), Long and Brown (1964), Landsmeer and Long (1965), and Long (1968).

The lumbrical muscles do not assist the flexor digitorum profundus in closure of the fist as has been assumed in the past; they are consistently silent in this activity. In opening of the fist, synchronous activity is recorded in the extensor digitorum and the lumbricals, with the lumbricals exhibiting maximal activity. Contraction of the lumbrical muscles extends the interphalangeal joints but simultaneously might draw the tendons of the flexor digitorum profundus distally. The flexor digitorum profundus is electrically silent when the hand is opened, and therefore would offer poor fixation to the proximal attachments of the lumbricals. With the tendons of the flexor digitorum profundus drawn distally, digital extension is facilitated as the passive resistance of the profundus is overcome. That such passive resistance is present may be concluded from the semiflexed position of the fingers when the arm hangs relaxed at the side of the body. Earlier investigators (Poore, 1881; Sunderland, 1945; Kaplan, 1953) already suggested this function of the lumbrical muscles, but the theory was not universally accepted.

Anatomists have assumed that the interosseous muscles contribute to interphalangeal extension in opening the hand, but this has not been confirmed by electromyography. While the hand is being opened fully but without great force, the lumbrical muscles show high-level electric activity, and the interossei show little or no activity.

In performing metacarpophalangeal extension and interphalangeal flexion (see Fig. 6-14), high-level activity was registered in the extensor digitorum and the flexor digitorum profundus, whereas the flexor digitorum superficialis showed little or no activity. The lumbrical and interosseous muscles were essentially silent. Performance of the opposite motion—metacarpophalangeal flexion with interphalangeal extension (see Fig. 6-16)—was accompanied by high-level activity of the lumbricals and the interossei. Thus, these muscles appear to be primarily responsible for producing this motion. The electric activity in the extensor digitorum varied in individuals from zero to high level. These findings, in part, contradict Bunnell's theory of a gradual shift from intrinsic to extrinsic muscle action in extension of the interphalangeal joints when the metacarpophalangeal joints become more and more flexed. The variable response in extensor digitorum demonstrated by electromyography would indicate that some normal subjects, like those with paralysis of the intrinsic muscles, use the extensor digitorum, whereas others rely more or less exclusively on the intrinsic muscles. Possibly, the individual differences are related to the amount of effort employed by the subjects, in accordance with the general rule that the more effort that is employed, the more muscles that are recruited.

Abduction and Adduction of Digits II–V

NOMENCLATURE

Movements away from the midline of the hand are called *abduction*; movements toward the midline are called *adduction*. The *midline* is a line longitudinally through the center of the forearm and hand and through the middle finger; thus, when the fingers spread apart they are abducted, and when they lie close together they are adducted. The third finger, being in the midline, has radial abduction and ulnar abduction.

RELATION OF ABDUCTION AND ADDUCTION TO FLEXION AND EXTENSION

Abduction and adduction movements are free when the metacarpophalangeal joints are extended (collateral ligaments are loose); when these joints flex, the fingers automatically adduct, and the range of abduction becomes extremely limited or is absent (collateral ligaments tight). The natural tendency is to abduct the fingers as they extend; it may be said that *extension and abduction belong together*, as do *flexion and adduction*. If the fist is closed and opened in rapid succession, this pattern becomes obvious: the fingers abduct as they extend and adduct as they flex. In slower motions, and with some concentration, it is entirely possible to keep the fingers adducted as they extend. The extension-abduction combination appears to be part of a mass movement that is considerably easier to execute than other combinations.

MUSCLES ACTING IN ABDUCTION OF THE FINGERS

The four dorsal interossei are responsible for abduction of the second and fourth fingers, and for radial and ulnar abduction of the third finger. The fifth finger has its own abductor, the abductor digiti minimi, located on the ulnar border of the hand and being part of the hypothenar muscle group.

The dorsal interosseous muscles are located between the metacarpal bones, each muscle having double proximal attachments, that is, each is attached to two adjacent bones. The action of the dorsal interosseous muscles as abductors of the fingers may be concluded from knowing the location of their distal attachments:

First dorsal interosseus—radial side of base of index finger
Second dorsal interosseus—radial side of base of middle finger
Third dorsal interosseus—ulnar side of base of middle finger
Fourth dorsal interosseus—ulnar side of base of ring finger

Palpation

The muscular portion of the first interosseus is easily observed and palpated in the space between the metacarpal bones of the thumb and the index finger when resistance is applied to abduction of the index finger, by manual resistance or by using a rubber band, as seen in Figure 6-18. The second, third, and fourth dorsal interossei are more difficult to palpate in the narrow spaces between the metacarpal bones, but their attachments at the base of the proximal phalanges may be felt, although some practice is needed to do so. By applying a rubber band around the fingers in various combinations, the action of each of the finger abductors, including the abductor of the fifth finger, may be brought out.

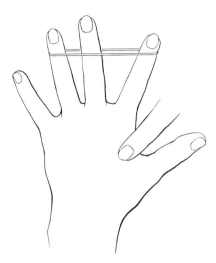

FIGURE 6-18. Palpation of muscular portion of first dorsal interosseus. Rubber band offers resistance to first and fourth dorsal interossei.

The *abductor digiti minimi* may be palpated on the ulnar border of the hand.

The *extensor digiti minimi*, with its proximal attachment above the wrist, has its distal attachment at the base of the proximal phalanx in such a manner that it is able both to extend and abduct the little finger. This muscle receives its innervation from the radial nerve. The ability of this muscle to abduct the little finger (in small range) is clearly seen in cases of ulnar nerve paralysis when the hypothenar muscle group is paralyzed. The little finger then tends to maintain a somewhat abducted position, and the subject is unable to adduct it.

MUSCLES ACTING IN ADDUCTION OF THE FINGERS

The palmar interossei are responsible for adduction of the index, ring and little fingers. These muscles, unlike the dorsal interossei, have only a single proximal attachment to the metacarpal bone of the digits that they serve. The palmar interossei may be tested by manual resistance to adduction of each finger separately, or by squeezing three small objects between the fingers (Fig. 6-19). If a piece of paper is slipped between two adjacent fingers and the subject is asked to hold on to it, one palmar and one dorsal interosseous muscle are tested simultaneously.

Some anatomists speak of the deep portion of the flexor pollicis brevis (innervated by the ulnar nerve), or of a division of the adductor pollicis, as the first palmar interosseous muscle. In that case, the index finger is served by the second, the ring finger by the third, and the little finger by the fourth palmar interosseus.

OPPOSITION OF THE LITTLE FINGER

The opponens digiti minimi, aided by the flexor digiti minimi and by the palmaris longus and brevis, is responsible for the motion referred to as opposition of the fifth finger. The movement is not nearly as well developed as opposition of the thumb. When both thumb and little finger move toward each other in opposition, ''cupping''

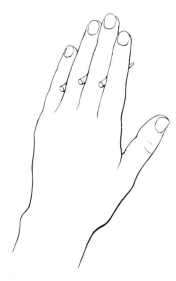

FIGURE 6-19. Testing the palmar interossei of the index finger, ring finger, and little finger.

of the hand results, that is, the hand narrows considerably from side to side (Fig. 6-20).

Thumb Movements

The marked mobility that the thumb possesses as compared with the other fingers is made possible *first*, because the saddle-shaped carpometacarpal joint of the thumb has two degrees of freedom of motion and the capsule is loose, permitting rotation and a third degree of freedom (Kapandji, 1970a); *second*, because the metacarpal bone of the thumb is not bound to the other metacarpals by ligaments, so that a wide separation between index and thumb can take place; *third*, because the movements that occur at

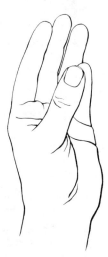

FIGURE 6-20. Opposition of thumb and little finger.

the metacarpophalangeal and interphalangeal joints of the thumb aid substantially to the versatility of thumb movements; and *fourth*, because the nine muscles that move the thumb can combine their actions in numerous ways in finely graduated movement combinations.

NOMENCLATURE

A considerable difference in terminology exists, which leads to potential confusion in the description of thumb movements, especially for those of the carpometacarpal joint. Movements at this joint have been variously labeled as flexion, extension, abduction, adduction, palmar abduction, opposition, reposition, and pronation, and as taking place either in the plane of the palm or in a plane perpendicular to the palm. To add to the confusion, movements are sometimes defined as related to the entire thumb rather than to movements of separate joints. Clinically, for example, *opposition of the thumb* means the ability to bring the palmar surface of the tip of the thumb in contact with the palmar surfaces of the other digits. Functionally, this is justifiable, but anatomically, each joint has to be dealt with separately.

The *carpometacarpal* joint of the thumb is a saddle joint (see Fig. 1-8) with two degrees of freedom of motion. If this conception is adhered to, movements at this joint may be defined as *opposition-reposition* and as *abduction-adduction* (which occurs in a plane perpendicular to the palm of the hand). The term *flexion-extension* is then reserved for the two distal thumb joints but is frequently used in reference to the carpometacarpal joint.

The axes of the *carpometacarpal joint* are determined by the shape of the "saddle" of the trapezium; the "rider" is the metacarpal bone. One axis passes longitudinally, the other transversely through the saddle, so that the "rider" may slide from side to side, or tip forward and backward in the "saddle."

The *metacarpophalangeal* joint of the thumb is more stable than the metacarpophalangeal joints of the other digits. Approximately 50 to 60 degrees of flexion can occur, whereas hyperextension and abduction-adduction are negligible.

The thumb contains only two phalanges and therefore has only one interphalangeal joint. Flexion is 90 degrees or less, and active extension is negligible. Passive hyperextension, as in pressing down on the thumb, may have a markedly larger range.

It is important to recognize that there is a wide range of terminology for thumb motions. In this text, the terminology used in *Gray's Anatomy* (Goss, 1973) and by Kendall and associates (1971) will be followed (Fig. 6-21).

MUSCLES ACTING ON THE CARPOMETACARPAL JOINT OF THE THUMB

All muscles that pass the carpometacarpal joint of the thumb have an influence on its movements. Those muscles that have their distal attachment on the metacarpal bone of the thumb (opponens pollicis, abductor pollicis longus) are primarily concerned with movement or stabilization of the joint; the muscles that have their distal attach-

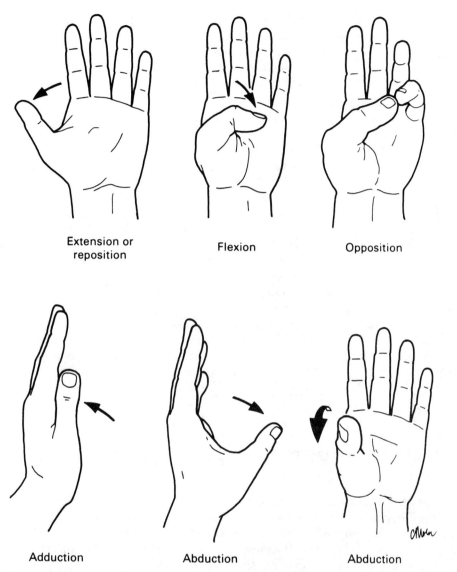

Extension or reposition   **Flexion**   **Opposition**

Adduction   **Abduction**   **Abduction**

FIGURE 6-21. Terminology used in this text for motions of the thumb. Extension and flexion occur in the plane of the palm, whereas abduction and adduction occur in a plane perpendicular to the palm. Opposition requires a rotation of the metacarpal at the carpometacarpal joint and contains elements of abduction and flexion.

ment on more distal segments act on one or both of the two distal thumb joints as well. To the latter group belong the abductor pollicis brevis, flexor pollicis brevis, adductor pollicis, extensor pollicis longus and brevis, and flexor pollicis longus.

Opposition is performed primarily by the *opponens pollicis* and the *abductor pollicis brevis*, both muscles having approximately the same line of action over the joint.

The abductor pollicis brevis is a superficial muscle, and it covers the opponens. The two muscles may be palpated in the radial portion of the thenar eminence. The *flexor pollicis brevis* may aid in maintaining opposition, once the joint has been positioned (Fig. 6-22); the muscle is palpated toward the ulnar side of the thenar eminence.

Reposition or extension is performed mainly by the *extensor pollicis longus* aided by the *extensor pollicis brevis* and *abductor pollicis longus*.

The tendon of the *extensor pollicis longus* may be palpated from the tubercle of the radius proximally to its distal attachment on the base of the distal phalanx. It forms the ulnar boundary of the anatomic "snuff box." The tendon of the *extensor pollicis brevis* is also visible under the skin, forming the radial border of the "snuff box" (Fig. 6-23). The tendon of the *abductor pollicis longus* lies partially covered by that of the extensor pollicis brevis. In the wrist region, where the two tendons emerge from their common compartment in the dorsal carpal ligament, the two tendons can usually be separated by palpation, but the abductor pollicis longus is not always visible.

Abduction is performed by the abductor pollicis longus, the extensor pollicis brevis, and the abductor pollicis brevis. The movement of *adduction* is executed mainly by the adductor pollicis and part of the flexor pollicis brevis (first palmar interosseus). Under certain circumstances (when the thumb is in a position of complete reposition) the extensor pollicis longus may also adduct.

It should be noted that a rider on a horse may slide from side to side in the saddle in various positions of forward and backward tipping of the saddle; similarly, abduction and adduction may be performed in various degrees of opposition and reposition. The muscles activated in abduction-adduction consequently vary in accordance with the amount of opposition present.

MUSCLES ACTING ON THE METACARPOPHALANGEAL JOINT OF THE THUMB

Flexion of the metacarpophalangeal joint of the thumb is performed by the *flexor pollicis brevis* and the *flexor pollicis longus*. Under certain conditions, the abductor pollicis brevis and the adductor pollicis also aid in flexing this joint. These two muscles pass on the flexor side of the joint, attaching into the base of the proximal phalanx of the thumb. They also send expansions to the extensor aponeurosis so that they may act in extension of the interphalangeal joint as well as in flexion of the metacarpophalangeal joint. Note the resemblance with the intrinsic muscles serving the other digits, which also may flex the metacarpophalangeal joint or extend the interphalangeal joints.

Extension of the metacarpophalangeal joint is performed by the extensor pollicis brevis and extensor pollicis longus.

Abduction and *adduction* of the metacarpophalangeal joint of the thumb are performed by the abductor pollicis brevis and the adductor pollicis, respectively, the latter movement being aided by the extensor pollicis longus as its tendon slides toward the ulnar side of the joint.

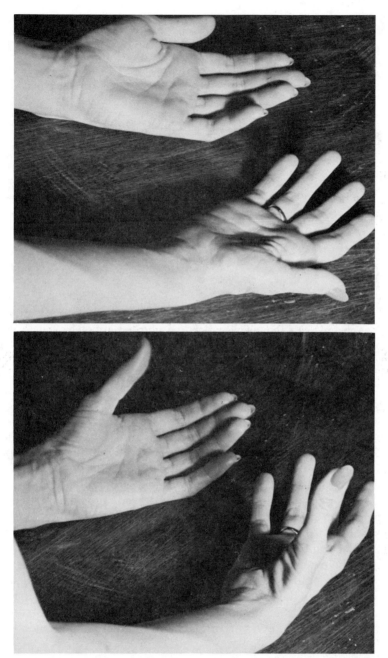

FIGURE 6-22. Partial paralysis after poliomyelitis of thenar muscles, particularly opponens pollicis. *(Top)* Subject is unable to initiate the opposition movement of the thumb. *(Bottom)* After thumb has been placed in opposition, subject is capable of maintaining position. It appears as if the flexor pollicis brevis were employed to do so. Note marked atrophy in the region of the opponens pollicis and abductor pollicis brevis.

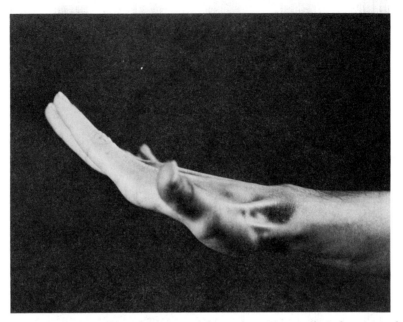

FIGURE 6-23. Anatomic snuff box between tendons of extensor pollicis longus and extensor pollicis brevis. Abductor pollicis longus tendon is visible adjacent to extensor pollicis brevis.

MUSCLES ACTING ON THE INTERPHALANGEAL JOINT OF THE THUMB

The *flexor pollicis longus* flexes the interphalangeal joint; the *extensor pollicis longus* extends it. Those thenar muscles that send expansions into the dorsal aponeurosis (abductor pollicis brevis, flexor pollicis brevis, and adductor pollicis) also aid in extension. These latter muscles may, unaided by the extensor pollicis longus, extend the interphalangeal joint. Such extension has been observed in patients with radial nerve injuries, when extensor pollicis longus and brevis are paralyzed. Strong and Perry (1966) investigated this observation by blocking the nerve to extrinsic muscles of the thumb in 11 subjects and noting the subsequent performance. They examined electromyographically the extensor pollicis longus, abductor pollicis brevis, flexor pollicis brevis, and adductor pollicis. Their results showed the abductor pollicis brevis to be the prime extensor when the extensors pollicis longus and brevis were inactive. They observed individual variations in the amount of interphalangeal joint extension, and they noted that this extension was accompanied by abduction and medial rotation of the thumb.

COORDINATED MOVEMENTS OF THE THREE THUMB JOINTS

When flexion and extension of the interphalangeal joint of the thumb are carried out without attention being paid to the manner of execution of the motion, the metacarpophalangeal and carpometacarpal joints become involved as well. The metacarpopha-langeal joint moves in the same direction as that of the interphalangeal joint; the carpometacarpal joint moves in the opposite direction. At the onset of the observa-tions, the hand should be relaxed so that the digits assume their natural positions. The carpometacarpal joint will then be in a midposition between opposition and reposi-tion. The interphalangeal and metacarpophalangeal joints will be slightly flexed. If in this position the interphalangeal joint is voluntarily and somewhat forcibly extended, the metacarpophalangeal joint will also extend. This is understandable since the ex-tensor pollicis longus passes on the extensor side of that joint. The carpometacarpal joint will move in the direction of opposition by the action of the thenar muscles, including the opponens pollicis. (The contraction of these muscles may be ascer-tained by inspection and palpation.) Conversely, flexion of the interphalangeal joint is accompanied by a reposition movement, effected by the extensor pollicis longus, ex-tensor pollicis brevis, and abductor pollicis longus; the tensing of the tendons of these muscles should be observed.

Interestingly enough, the functional relationship of the various muscles observed clinically in flexion and extension of the interphalangeal joint of the thumb is re-flected by electromyographic studies by Weathersby and associates (1963). In flexion of the interphalangeal joint (performed slowly and without resistance), these investi-gators recorded activity in the extensor pollicis longus, extensor pollicis brevis, and abductor pollicis longus, while the opponens pollicis was silent electromyographic-ally. In extension of the interphalangeal joint of the thumb, the opponens pollicis became active while the abductor pollicis longus and the extensor pollicis brevis were inactive.

The functional advantage of this arrangement is easily recognized. The movements of opposition and reposition performed in conjunction with extension and flexion of the interphalangeal joint, respectively, enable the extensor pollicis longus and the flexor pollicis longus to use a favorable portion of the length-tension diagram. A mechanism governing the closing and opening of the fist and serving the same pur-pose has been discussed previously.

SYNERGIC ACTION OF WRIST MUSCLES IN MOVEMENTS OF THUMB AND LITTLE FINGER

Synergic actions of the wrist muscles should be noted in the following movements:

1. When the little finger is abducted (by abductor digiti minimi), the flexor carpi ulnaris contracts to furnish counter-traction on the pisiform bone (Fig. 6-24). To prevent the flexor carpi ulnaris from abducting the wrist ulnarward, the abduc-tor pollicis longus contracts. Its tendon may be palpated as indicated in the illustration.

2. When the thumb is extended to the position seen in Figure 6-25, the tensed tendon of the extensor carpi ulnaris is palpated on the opposite side of the wrist. This muscle springs into action to prevent radial-abduction of the wrist by the abductor pollicis longus. The points of palpation of the tendons of both muscles

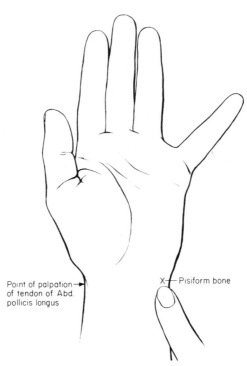

Point of palpation→ of tendon of Abd. pollicis longus

X—Pisiform bone

FIGURE 6-24. Palpation of flexor carpi ulnaris proximal to pisiform bone in abduction of little finger. Abductor pollicis longus contracts synergically.

are indicated. The tendon of the abductor pollicis longus lies close to, and is partially covered by, the tendon of the extensor pollicis brevis.

3. When the entire thumb is brought in a palmar direction (flexion) by the thenar muscles, the palmaris longus aids the movement by tensing the fascia of the palm. To prevent the palmaris longus from flexing the wrist, the extensor carpi radialis brevis contracts.

Peripheral Nerve Injuries Affecting Wrist and Hand

In *radial nerve paralysis*, the extensors of the wrist and the long extensors of the digits are paralyzed. A wrist-drop develops causing a hand position much like the one seen in Figure 6-3, B. The wrist cannot be actively extended nor can it be stabilized for effective grasp. In the drop-wrist position, the digits are partially extended, but such extension is due to tendon action, not to active contraction. The grasp becomes awkward and weak (see Fig. 6-10), but if the wrist is supported in extension by means of a splint (see Fig. 2-10, B), the strength of the grip is good because the flexor muscles are intact.

In *ulnar nerve paralysis*, the habitual position of the hand is a characteristic one (Fig. 6-26). The fourth and the fifth digits are the ones mostly affected since the flexor

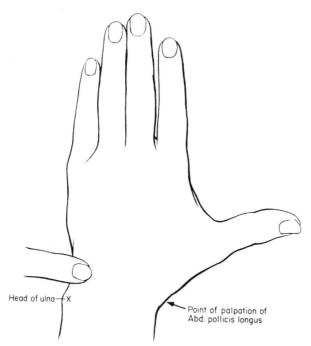

Head of ulna—X

Point of palpation of
Abd. pollicis longus

FIGURE 6-25. Palpation of extensor carpi ulnaris distal to the head of the ulna in extension of the thumb. Abductor pollicis longus may be palpated as indicated by the arrow.

digitorum profundus, the lumbricals, and the interossei belonging to these fingers are paralyzed and the hypothenar group is also out of function. The extensor digitorum tends to keep the metacarpophalangeal joints of digits IV and V hyperextended. If the examiner holds the metacarpophalangeal joints in a flexed position, however, the subject is capable of extending the interphalangeal joints by using the extensor digitorum. Although the abductor of the little finger is paralyzed, this finger is maintained somewhat abducted (by the extensor digiti minimi proprius), but it cannot be adducted because the action of the palmar interosseus cannot be taken over by any other muscle. Abduction and adduction movements of all digits served by the interosseous muscles are affected. Occasionally, however, there is some median nerve supply to the more radially located interossei, in which case some movements may be preserved.

A *median nerve paralysis* causes most of the flexors of the digits to lose action and therefore seriously affects the grasp. The digits on the radial side, having median nerve supply only, are affected to a greater extent than those on the ulnar side. Flexion and opposition of the thumb are lost, the thenar muscles atrophy, and the entire thumb is pulled in a dorsal direction by the extensor muscles so that it remains in the plane of the palm or is taken even further back toward the dorsum of the hand. The adductor is the only useful thenar muscle, and with the first dorsal interosseous muscle may enable the subject to hold a small object between the thumb and the index finger. Since the flexor digitorum superficialis and profundus, and also the lumbricals of the index and middle fingers, have median nerve supply, these two fingers lose

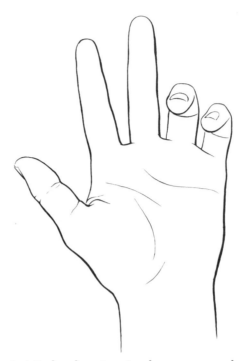

FIGURE 6-26. Characteristic hand posture in ulnar nerve paralysis. The fourth and the fifth fingers cannot be extended, since the long extensors of these digits, in the absence of the intrinsic muscles, cause hyperextension of the metacarpophalangeal joints but are incapable of extending the interphalangeal joints.

their ability to flex. The index finger tends to remain in an extended position while the middle finger, when the two ulnar fingers flex, may be drawn into some flexion. However, if the subject extends the wrist as far as possible, both index and middle finger may flex by tendon action, but this is not an active grasp.

Deficits in hand function are additionally influenced by sensory loss resulting from peripheral nerve injury. Hand rehabilitation programs have always included motor retraining; in recent years, these programs are emphasizing the importance of sensory retraining as well. The effect of sensory loss resulting from peripheral nerve injuries is to diminish power and precision of hand function (Wynn-Parry, 1981). Wynn-Parry divides re-education into stereognosis and localization of touch. He states that his experience has shown that patients can be trained to improve their sensory function remarkably and in too short a time to be explained by re-innervation.

Types of Prehension Patterns

The hand may be used in a multitude of postures and movements which in most cases involve both the thumb and the other digits. Napier (1956) describes two basic postures of the human hand, the "power grip" and the "precision grip." The power grip, used when full strength is needed, involves holding an object between the partially flexed fingers and the palm while the thumb applies counter pressure (Fig. 6-27, A). In the precision grip, the object is pinched between the flexor surfaces of one or more fingers and the opposing thumb (Fig. 6-27, B). It is used when accuracy and refinement of touch are needed. The thumb postures differ in the two grips. In power grip, the thumb is adducted, and it reinforces the pressure of the fingers. In precision grip, the thumb is abducted, and it is positioned to oppose the pulp of the fingers. Napier (1956) states that the nature of the task to be performed determines the working posture to be used and that these two postures incorporate the whole range of prehensile activity in the human hand.

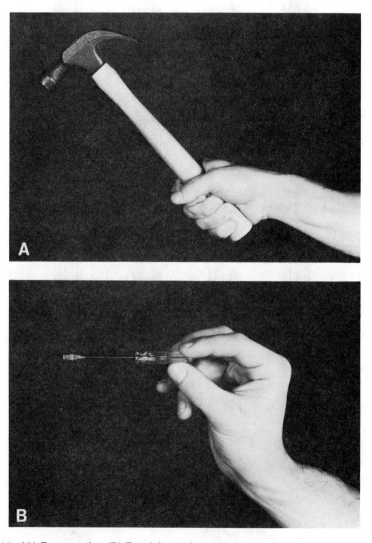

FIGURE 6-27. (A) Power grip. (B) Precision grip.

Other graphic terms have been used to describe hand prehension patterns. Their names imply that hand posture is conditioned by the shape of the object held. These terms should be noted, too, because they continue to be used in rehabilitation even though the terms power grip and precision grip are quite universally accepted.

Schlesinger (1919), in investigating designs for terminal devices for artificial arms, studied the versatility of the human hand in grasping and holding objects of various sizes and shapes. He distinguished among 12 different types of prehension; seven are described below:

HOOK GRASP. Digits II to V are used as a hook, as in carrying a brief case. The thumb is not necessarily active (Fig. 6-28).

CYLINDRIC GRASP. The entire palmar surface of the hand grasps around a cylindric object, such as a glass jar. The thumb closes in over the object (Fig. 6-29).

FIST GRASP. The fist closes over a comparatively narrow object, and the grip is secured by the thumb over the other digits, as in grasping a golf club or a hammer (see Fig. 6-27, A).

SPHERIC GRASP. The grasp is adjusted to a spheric object, such as a ball or an apple (Fig. 6-30).

TIP PREHENSION. The tip of the thumb is used against the tip of one or the other digits to pick up a small object, such as a bead, a pin, or a coin (Fig. 6-31).

PALMAR PREHENSION. The thumb opposes one or more of the other digits; contact is made by the palmar surfaces of the distal phalanges of the digits. This grip is used to pick up and hold small objects, such as an eraser or a pen. Larger objects may also be held in this manner by widening the grip (Fig. 6-32).

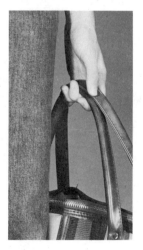

FIGURE 6-28. Hook grasp.

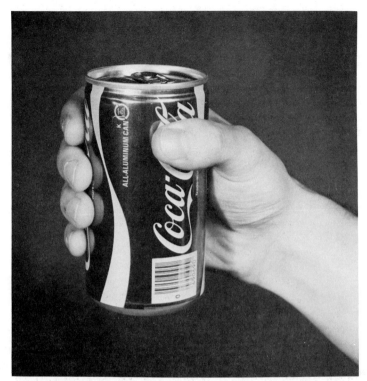

FIGURE 6-29. Cylindric grasp.

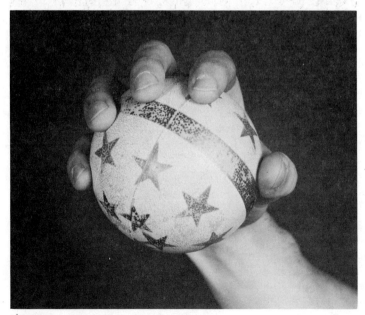

FIGURE 6-30. Spheric grasp.

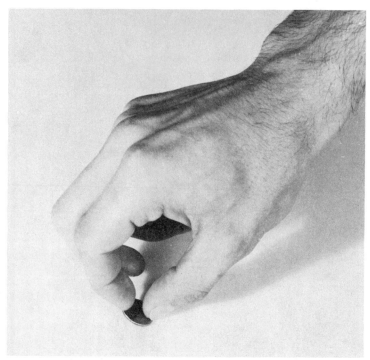

FIGURE 6-31. Tip prehension.

LATERAL PREHENSION. A thin object, such as a card or a key, is grasped between the thumb and the lateral side of the index finger (Fig. 6-33).

Schlesinger also points out that some of these prehension types may be compared to simple tools, such as a hook (hook grasp), pincers (tip prehension), and pliers (palmar prehension). Current terminology applies the mechanical analogue ''three-jaw chuck'' to the palmar prehension pattern of thumb pad opposing the index and middle digits.

Keller, Taylor, and Zahm, cited by Taylor and Schwartz (1955), investigated the frequency of three types of common prehension patterns in picking up objects and holding them for use. Their findings were as follows:

	Palmar	Tip	Lateral
Pick up	50%	17%	33%
Hold for use	88%	2%	10%

This study showed that palmar prehension is by far the most commonly used type for both picking up and holding small objects. An adaptation of this grasp was subsequently used in the design of terminal devices for artificial arms.

Palmar and tip prehension require that thumb and fingers be opposed to each other, and their frequent use in daily activities points to the importance of opposition of the thumb in the human hand.

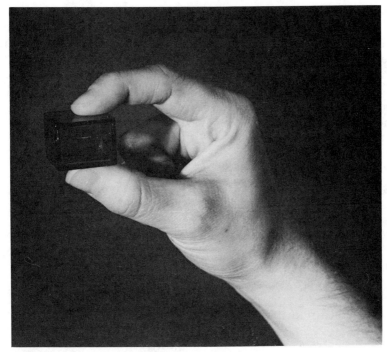

FIGURE 6-32. Palmar prehension.

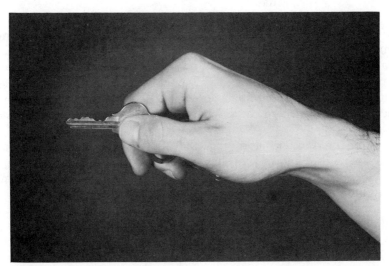

FIGURE 6-33. Lateral prehension.

Patients who have lost their ability to oppose the thumb but who are capable of adducting it, however, may use lateral prehension for grasping and holding small objects. Lateral prehension makes use of pressure of the thumb against the radial side of the index finger, which is held semiflexed. It is the prehension pattern of choice for patients with upper motor neuron lesions, in whom contact on the palmar surface of the fingers causes spasticity of the finger flexors, which is frequently the case. Such patients may be able to release an object held with lateral prehension, while an object which touches the palm of the hand may be very difficult to release.

Strength of Grip

Swanson, Matev, and deGroot (1970) studied normal grip and pinch strength to establish a baseline for evaluation of the disabled hand. Strength measurements were taken on 50 normal males and 50 females ranging in age from 17 to 60 years. Some of the mean values expressed in pounds are as follows:

	Age	Male	Female
Grip (major hand)	20	100	53
	20–30	107	54
	30–40	109	68
	40–50	108	52
	50–60	101	49
Chuck pinch (major hand)	17–60	17	11
Lateral pinch (major hand)	17–60	17	11

This study, in addition to providing some normal values useful for making comparisons, found only 4 to 9 percent decrease between the major and minor hands, which substantiates the 6 percent difference found by Toews (1964). This small differential does not necessarily hold true for individuals. Swanson and associates (1970) found 29 percent of the subjects had the same or greater grip strength in the minor hand. If a noticeable difference exists in the grip strength of the two hands, it is important to suspect pathology.

To determine forces of grip and pinch that should be provided in artificial hands, Keller and associates, cited in Klopsteg and Wilson (1968), measured the minimum prehension forces required in the manipulation of common objects and other activities of everyday life. They found, for example, that pulling on a sock required a 7.7-lb (≈ 3.4 kg) force, whereas manipulation of a screw cap like that found on a toothpaste tube required a 2.5-lb (≈ 1.1 kg) force, and holding a soup spoon a 1.6-lb ($\approx .72$ kg) force. It is estimated that adults with arm amputations, using prostheses, use 3 to 10 or 15 pounds (≈ 1 to 8 kg) prehension force in their activities (New York University, 1971).

Prehension forces available in the natural hand as shown by the Swanson and associates study (1970), or as calculated by using cross section of the deep and superficial finger flexors of 21.5 sq cm (Fick, 1911, p 396) and the 4 kg per sq cm factor giving an 85.8 kg total are considerably higher than forces required for most everyday activities.

Position of Function

Kinematic studies of daily living activities have provided information concerning the frequency of natural motions of wrist and forearm (Klopsteg, 1968). The most frequent angular positions of common use were 0 to 10 degrees of wrist extension, a neutral position (near 0 degrees) between radial and ulnar abduction and with the forearm held slightly pronated (30 to 40 degrees). Steindler (1955) speaks of the neutral or rest positions of 3 degrees of ulnar abduction, 12 degrees of wrist extension with the forearm held in a midposition between pronation and supination. These movement ranges serve as guides in rehabilitation management of the disabled hand. Further advice concerning optimum hand position is offered by Wynn-Parry (1981). When the hand must be immobilized for any reason, the wrist should be in 20 degrees of extension, the metacarpophalangeal joints in 45 degrees of flexion, the proximal interphalangeal joints in 30 degrees of flexion, the distal interphalangeal joints in 20 degrees of flexion, and the thumb in half abduction and half opposition with the interphalangeal joint flexed a few degrees. The forearm should be in a midposition between pronation and supination. Wynn-Parry states that a hand in which stiffness may develop will function better in this position than in any other.

CHAPTER 7

SHOULDER REGION

The shoulder region is a complex of twenty muscles, three bony articulations, and three soft tissue moving surfaces (functional joints) that permit the greatest mobility of any joint area found in the body (approximately 180 degrees of flexion, abduction, and rotation and 60 degrees of hyperextension; see Appendix B). The shoulder complex not only provides a wide range for hand placement but also carries out the important functions of stabilization for hand use, lifting and pushing, elevation of the body, forced inspiration and expiration, and even weight-bearing as in crutch-walking or hand stands. The extensive mobility is provided by the six moving areas:

1. Bony articulations
   a. Sternoclavicular
   b. Acromioclavicular
   c. Glenohumeral
2. Functional joints
   a. Scapulothoracic
   b. Suprahumeral (or subacromial)
   c. Bicipital groove

Mobility, however, is at the expense of structural stability. The only attachment of the upper extremity to the trunk is at the sternoclavicular joint, and the head of the humerus hangs loosely on the inclined plane of the glenoid fossa. Thus, support and stabilization of the shoulder primarily depend on muscles and ligaments.

219

BONES

The osseous parts participating in movements of the upper extremity in relation to the trunk are:

Sternum (breast bone)   (Gr. *sternon*, chest)
Costae (ribs)   (L. *costa*, rib)
Clavicle (collar bone)   (L. *clavicula*, dimin. of *clavus*, key)
Scapula (shoulder blade)   (L. *scapula*, shoulder blade)
Humerus (bone of upper arm)   (L. *humerus*, shoulder)

PALPATION

STERNUM. The sternum may be palpated anteriorly on the thorax from the *xiphoid process* at its lower end to the *manubrium sterni* at its upper end (Gr. *xiphos*, sword, and *eidos*, appearance; L. *manubrium*, handle).

CLAVICLE. The sternal portion of the clavicle is prominent where it articulates with the manubrium sterni (sternoclavicular joint). From this point, the clavicle may be followed laterally to its acromial end. The curved shape of this bone should be noted—it is convex forward medially and concave forward laterally. The acromial end, like the sternal end, is enlarged and may be palpated as a protuberance.

SCAPULA. At the tip of the shoulder, the broad *acromion process*, which extends like a shelf over the shoulder joint, is palpated (Gr. *acron*, tip, and *omos*, shoulder). Anteriorly, its free edge may be felt. Its junction with the clavicle (acromioclavicular joint) lies somewhat protected, being covered by the acromioclavicular ligament; hence, it is difficult to palpate with accuracy. In most individuals, two bony enlargements may be felt in this region, one on the acromion, the other on the clavicle; in the area between these two prominences is the joint.

By following the acromion process posteriorly, the *spine of the scapula* is palpated; it is continuous with the acromion process. The spine of the scapula may be followed transversely across the scapula to the medial (vertebral) border of the scapula where it flattens out to form a smooth triangular-shaped area. The *supraspinous fossa* of the scapula, above the spine, and *infraspinous fossa*, below the spine, should be identified; but since both are filled with muscles, their depths cannot be appreciated. This applies particularly to the supraspinous fossa, which is not accessible to palpation in its deeper parts. The *medial* (vertebral) *border* of the scapula and its *lateral* (axillary) *border* are easily palpable if the scapular muscles are relaxed. The *inferior angle* of the scapula is the lowest part of the scapula where the medial and lateral borders join. The *superior angle* of the scapula is well covered by muscles and therefore more difficult to palpate. Anteriorly, below the clavicle, where the roundness of the shoulder begins, the *coracoid process* is palpated (Gr. *korax*, raven, curved door handle, and *eidos*, appearance).

The *glenoid cavity* of the scapula (Gr. *glene,* a socket), which receives the head of the humerus, cannot be palpated. This also applies to the *supraglenoid tubercle,* which serves as origin for the long head of the biceps, and to the *infraglenoid tubercle,* where the long head of the triceps originates.

HUMERUS. The name *anatomic neck* is applied to a narrow area distal to the articular surface of the humeral head. Fractures in this region tend to occur at the *surgical neck,* below the tubercles. If the humerus is internally rotated while the arm is at the side of the body, the *greater tubercle* of the humerus may be palpated just distal to the acromion process. Once this tubercle has been identified, the palpating fingers may follow its changing position as the shoulder is rotated externally. In full external rotation, this tubercle is no longer palpable because it disappears under the heavy portion of the deltoid muscle. The greater tubercle has three facets, serving as points of attachment for muscles, but these facets cannot be distinguished by palpation. The *lesser tubercle* is best felt when the shoulder is externally rotated and may be followed during internal rotation. The proximal portion of the humerus may also be approached from the axilla, but palpation must be done gently because of the many nerves and vessels in this area.

On the proximal portion of the shaft of the humerus, the *crest of the greater tubercle* and the *crest of the lesser tubercle* should be noted. Between the two crests is the *intertubercular (bicipital) groove.* These structures should be studied on the skeleton, as they are difficult to palpate through the muscles. Note the changing position of the intertubercular groove during humeral rotation; in complete external rotation, the groove is in line with the acromion process.

JOINTS

The bones of the shoulder region are joined together at three articulations: the clavicle articulates with the manubrium sterni at the *sternoclavicular joint;* the clavicle and the scapula join at the *acromioclavicular joint;* and the humerus articulates with the scapula at the *glenohumeral joint.* During movements of the upper extremity, the scapula also slides freely on the thorax (scapulothoracic "joint"). In motions of flexion and abduction, the head of the humerus slides beneath the acromion (suprahumeral "joint"), and the tendon of the long head of the biceps brachii slides in the bicipital groove. Pain or limitation of motion in *any* of these true or functional joints will lead to shoulder dysfunction.

DEFINITION OF SHOULDER GIRDLE MOVEMENTS

Special terminology is used to describe the motions of the scapula (scapulothoracic joint) and the clavicle (sternoclavicular joint):

Elevation—The distal end of the clavicle and the acrominion process of the scapula (acromioclavicular joint) move superiorly (toward the ear) approximately 60 degrees (Kapandji, 1970a).

Depression—Motion of the acromioclavicular area distally. From a sitting resting position, only 5 to 10 degrees of depression can be achieved. The importance of the movement, however, is in stabilization of the scapula and elevation of the body as in crutch-walking or wheelchair transfers for paraplegic patients. From a position of maximum elevation, the movement of shoulder depression can elevate the trunk 4 to 6 inches (10 to 15 cm).

Protraction—The clavicle and scapula move anteriorly, and the medial borders of the scapula move away from the midline 5 to 6 inches (13 to 15 cm). This motion is also referred to as *abduction* of the scapula.

Retraction—The clavicle and scapula move posteriorly, and the medial borders of the scapula approach the midline. This motion is also called *adduction* of the scapula. At the sternoclavicular joint, the total range for protraction and retraction is approximately 25 degrees (Kapandji, 1970a).

A circling movement may be performed by moving the shoulder girdle upward-forward-downward-backward (involving a combination of elevation, protraction, depression, and retraction) or in the opposite direction. During these movements, the sternoclavicular joint is the pivot point, and the tip of the shoulder moves in a circular path. The scapula, because it articulates with the clavicle at the acromioclavicular joints, adjusts its position and stays close to the thorax.

Scapular motions are further described by the rotations that occur at the acromioclavicular joint:

Upward rotation is a movement of the scapula in which the glenoid fossa faces superiorly and the inferior angle of the scapula slides laterally and anteriorly on the thorax. Maximum range of upward rotation is seen with full shoulder flexion.

Downward rotation of the scapula is a movement of the glenoid fossa to face inferiorly. Complete range of downward rotation occurs when the hand is placed in the small of the back. The total range of upward and downward rotation is approximately 60 degrees.

STERNOCLAVICULAR JOINT

The sternoclavicular joint is the only joint that connects the upper extremity directly with the thorax. The shoulder girdle, together with the entire upper extremity, is suspended from the skull and the cervical spine by muscles, ligaments, and fascia. The position of this hanging structure is determined partly by the action of gravity and partly by the clavicle, which restricts shoulder girdle movements in all directions, particularly in a forward direction. Cases of absence of the clavicle have been reported in medical literature—these individuals were able to move their shoulders so far forward that the tips of the shoulders almost met in front of the body. If fractures of the clavicle heal with overriding fragments, the posture of the shoulder is permanently altered.

TYPE OF JOINT. The sternoclavicular joint is a sellar joint with three degrees of freedom. The enlarged sternal end of the clavicle and the articular notch of the sternum are separated by an articular disk. Motions thus take place both between the clavicle and the disk and between the disk and the sternum. Although the bony articulations appear slight, the ligamentous attachments are strong, and the clavicle will usually fracture before the joint dislocates. A major part of the motions of shoulder flexion and abduction occurs at the sternoclavicular joint (60 degrees).

AXES OF MOTION AND MOVEMENTS. The axis for *elevation and depression* of the shoulder girdle is an oblique one that pierces the sternal end of the clavicle and takes a backward-downward course. Movement about this axis takes place between the sternal end of the clavicle and the articular disk. Owing to the obliquity of this axis, shoulder girdle elevation occurs in an upward-backward, and depression in a forward-downward, direction.

The joint between the articular cartilage and the sternum is involved mainly in *retraction-protraction* of the shoulder girdle. These motions take place about a nearly vertical axis, which pierces the manubrium sterni close to the joint. Scapular excursion accompanies retraction and protraction, and the movement descriptions may refer to that excursion. *Scapular adduction* or scapular movement toward the spinal column occurs with retraction. *Scapular abduction* away from the spine accompanies protraction.

TRANSVERSE ROTATION OF THE CLAVICLE. In addition to elevation-depression and protraction-retraction, the clavicle also rotates at the sternoclavicular joint approximately 40 degrees around its long axis (Inman et al, 1944). This transverse rotation occurs after the shoulder has been abducted or flexed to 90 degrees, and is essential for complete upward rotation of the scapula and shoulder flexion or abduction.

ACROMIOCLAVICULAR JOINT

TYPE OF JOINT. The acromioclavicular joint is a single arthrodial joint involving the medial margin of the acromion and the acromial end of the clavicle that binds the scapula and the clavicle in similar motions and at the same time accommodates individual motions of the bones. These functions are provided by two strong ligamentous structures: the anterior and posterior ligaments of the joint and the more proximately located coracoclavicular ligaments (conoid and trapezoid) that limit separation of the clavicle and scapula.

MOVEMENTS PERMITTED. The joint effect of acromioclavicular and sternoclavicular motions is to permit scapular rotation so that the glenoid cavity may face forward and upward, or downward, as the need may be, while its costal surface remains close to the thorax. Motions of the acromioclavicular joint are small and not measurable by goniometry. These few degrees of motion are nonetheless essential for normal shoulder motion and function.

GLENOHUMERAL JOINT

TYPE OF JOINT. The glenohumeral joint is a ball-and-socket joint (also called spheroid or universal joint) possessing three degrees of freedom of motion (see Fig.

1-5, A). The hemispheric-shaped head of the humerus articulates with the shallow inclined plane of the glenoid cavity, which faces somewhat upward as well as forward and laterally. A rim of cartilage, labrum (lip), surrounds the periphery of the glenoid and serves to deepen the cavity. The joint capsule is loose to permit a wide range of motion. The loose capsule and shallow glenoid cavity permit relatively large accessory motions. For example, the head of the humerus can be passively distracted 1 to 2 cm on the glenoid fossa. Such movement capability is essential for normal range of shoulder flexion. Congruency of the joint surfaces (closed packed position) occurs at the end of the ranges of abduction and external rotation. This position of joint stability would occur when supporting an object overhead or in hand stands.

AXES OF MOTION AND MOVEMENTS PERMITTED. Conventionally, the movements of the glenohumeral joint are described as occurring about three axes perpendicular to each other, all of which pass through the center of the head of the humerus. Flexion takes place in the sagittal plane about a transverse axis through the head of the humerus. Approximately 90 degrees of motion is permitted (Kapandji, 1970a). At this point the coracohumeral ligaments become taut and limit further motion.

Extension is the reverse of flexion. When the arm passes behind the body, the movement is called *hyperextension*. The range of motion is 40 to 60 degrees and is limited again by the coracohumeral ligaments.

Abduction occurs in the frontal plane about a horizontal axis directed dorsoventrally. The amount of abduction permitted depends on rotation at the glenohumeral joint. When the joint is in full internal rotation, active abduction is limited to approximately 60 degrees, because the greater tubercle strikes the acromion process and the coracoacromial ligament (Cailliet, 1966). With external rotation, active abduction increases to 90 degrees as the greater tubercle goes behind and under the acromion. Here the limiting structures are the glenohumeral ligaments.

Adduction is the reverse of abduction. When performed strictly in the frontal plane and the arm is lowered to the side, adduction is arrested by contact with the body. With the arm slightly in front or in back of the body, the movement range increases and is functionally important, but is not classified as pure adduction.

The term *horizontal abduction* is often used to indicate a movement in the horizontal plane, starting with 90 degrees flexion and moving laterally to 90 degrees abduction. *Horizontal adduction* is the reverse movement.

External (lateral) rotation takes place about an axis longitudinally through the head and the shaft of the humerus in the horizontal plane. If the arm is hanging at the side of the body, external rotation causes the medial epicondyle of the humerus to move anteriorly. When the glenohumeral joint is placed in the standard goniometric position of 90 degrees of shoulder abduction and 90 degrees of elbow flexion (American Academy of Orthopedic Surgeons, 1965), the normal range of external rotation is approximately 90 degrees. Functionally, full range of external rotation is needed to place the hand behind the neck.

Internal (medial) rotation occurs in the same plane as external rotation. When the arm is at the side of the body, the medial epicondyle of the humerus moves posteriorly. Conventionally, internal rotation is considered to be 90 degrees. When, however, shoulder girdle movements are prevented, internal rotation is usually found to be approximately 70 to 80 degrees. A functional check for maximum range of internal rotation is the ability to place the hand behind the back and touch the opposite scapula.

DIFFERENTIATION OF GLENOHUMERAL AND RADIOULNAR ROTATIONS. Together the shoulder and elbow provide a full circle of motion for hand placement: glenohumeral rotation of approximately 180 degrees plus radioulnar supination and pronation of approximately 180 degrees. Functionally, internal rotation and pronation occur together, and external rotation occurs with supination. When the elbow is extended, it is impossible to differentiate between glenohumeral and radioulnar rotations. Therefore, in order to evaluate the range of motion at either joint, the elbow must be flexed to 90 degrees.

SCAPULOHUMERAL RHYTHM IN SHOULDER FLEXION AND ABDUCTION

Clinically, the ability to elevate the arm overhead is called shoulder flexion (sagittal plane) or shoulder abduction (frontal plane). Normal range of motion for each movement is conventionally given as 180 degrees (see Appendix B). This is a measurement of the angle between the *arm and trunk* rather than between the humerus and scapula. Thus, the terms shoulder flexion and abduction refer to a combination of scapulothoracic, scapulohumeral, and trunk motions. Scapular movement occurs because of motions permitted at the sternoclavicular, acromioclavicular, and scapulothoracic joints and contributes approximately 60 degrees to shoulder flexion or abduction (Kapandji, 1970a). Ninety to 100 degrees of shoulder flexion (or abduction) occur at the glenohumeral joint. Attainment of this range of motion requires that the joint externally rotate *fully* during the movement (internal rotation at the glenohumeral joint decreases the range of flexion or abduction by approximately 40 degrees). The remaining 20 to 30 degrees of shoulder flexion or abduction are produced by motions of trunk extension or lateral flexion (Kapandji, 1970a).

Normally, shoulder flexion and abduction occur in a precisely coordinated series of synchronous motions described as *scapulohumeral rhythm*. These relationships were first recorded by Braune and Fisher (1887) using x-ray photographs to determine the relationships between scapular and glenohumeral motions during abduction (cited by von Lanz and Wachsmuth, 1935):

Arm-Trunk Angle (degrees)	Scapular Contribution (degrees)	Glenohumeral Contribution (degrees)
45	17	28
90	36	54
135	57	78
155	60	95

Inman and associates (1944) substantiated these findings that both scapular and humeral segments participate throughout the motion. The early phase of shoulder abduction was variable, but after 30 degrees of motion, a *two-to-one ratio* occurred: for every 15 degrees of motion between 30 and 170 degrees of abduction, 10 degrees occurred at the glenohumeral joint and 5 degrees occurred at the scapulothoracic joint. More recently, other investigators (Freedman and Munro, 1966; Doody et al, 1970) found only slight differences from the earlier studies on the synchrony of humeral and scapular motions. With resistance, Doody and associates (1970) found that the major contribution of scapular motion occurred in the earlier phase of abduction (60 to 90 degrees) and that total scapular rotation increased slightly.

Clinical treatment of shoulder problems, therefore, requires a careful assessment of all the motions permitted at each joint: scapulothoracic, sternoclavicular, acromioclavicular, and glenohumeral, as well as the moving surfaces of the suprahumeral and bicipital groove areas.

MUSCLES OF THE SHOULDER REGION

The muscles of the shoulder region give fixation to, and produce movements of, the shoulder girdle and control scapulohumeral relationships. All joints previously discussed, to a variable extent, participate in such movements. The resulting mobility of the shoulder is largely responsible for the ability of using the hand in all desired positions—in front of the body, overhead, behind the body, and so forth. The muscles of the shoulder girdle also participate significantly in skilled movements of the upper extremity, such as writing, and are essential in activities requiring pulling, pushing, and throwing, to mention only a few of the important activities of the upper extremity.

The shoulder region muscles are divided in three groups for study:

Group I.   Muscles connecting the shoulder girdle with the trunk, the neck, and the skull.

Group II.   Muscles connecting the scapula and the humerus.

Group III.   Muscles connecting the trunk and the humerus, having little or no attachment to the scapula.

Group I.   Muscles From Trunk to Shoulder Girdle

SERRATUS ANTERIOR

Serratus anterior (L. *serra*, saw) is one of the most important muscles of the shoulder girdle. Without it, the arm cannot be raised overhead. *Proximal attachment:* By nine muscular slips from the anterolateral aspect of the thorax, from the first to the ninth ribs—hence its name, the saw muscle. The lowest four or five slips interdigitate with the external oblique abdominal muscle. Lying close to the thorax, the muscle passes underneath the scapula with the *distal attachment* occurring along the medial border of the scapula. The lowest five digitations converge on the inferior angle of the scapula, attaching to its costal surface. This is the strongest portion of the muscle. *Innervation:* Long thoracic nerve.

Inspection and palpation: On well-developed individuals, the lower digitations may be seen and palpated near their *proximal* attachment on the ribs when the arm is overhead (Fig. 7-1). The middle and upper portions of the muscle are largely covered by the pectoral muscles but may be palpated in the axilla close to the ribs, posterior to the pectoralis major. For palpation of the muscle in the axilla, the subject first elevates the arm to a horizontal position halfway between flexion and abduction, then reaches forward so that the scapula slides forward on the thorax.

TRAPEZIUS

The trapezius is a superficial muscle of the neck and upper back and is accessible for observation and palpation in its entirety. Because of its shape, it has been called the "shawl" muscle. Early anatomists named it "musculus cucullaris" (shaped like a monk's hood). The name presently used refers to a geometrical figure. *Proximal attachment:* Occipital bone, ligamentum nuchae, and spinous processes from C7 to T12. From this widespread origin, the muscle fibers converge to their *distal attachments* on the acromial end of the clavicle, the acromion, and the spine of the scapula. The fibers of the upper portion course downward and laterally, those of the middle portion more horizontally, and those of the lower portion obliquely upward. *Innervation:* Spinal accessory nerve.

Inspection and palpation: For observation of the entire muscle in action bilaterally, the subject abducts the shoulders and retracts the shoulder girdles, as seen in Figure 7-2. This position requires the action of all parts of the trapezius: retraction of the shoulder girdle by the entire muscle, and upward rotation of the scapula by the upper and lower portions of the muscle. If the trunk simultaneously is inclined forward or the subject lies prone, the muscle has to act against the force of gravity to hold the

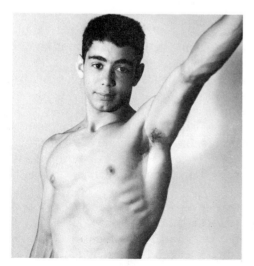

FIGURE 7-1. Lower digitations of serratus anterior near their origins on the ribs. The upper portion of the muscle is covered by the pectoralis major.

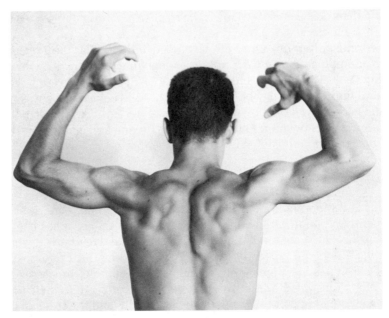

FIGURE 7-2. All portions of the trapezius in contraction. For strong action of this muscle, the subject inclines trunk forward. Note also the contraction of posterior deltoid, infraspinatus, and teres minor.

shoulders back, and the intensity of the contraction increases. The upper portion of the trapezius should also be observed and palpated as it performs its functions of shoulder elevation, and the lower portion, also, as it carries out its function of shoulder depression.

RHOMBOIDEUS MAJOR AND MINOR

The rhomboids (Gr. *rhombos*, a lozenge-shaped figure), which connect the scapula with the vertebral column, lie underneath the trapezius. The upper portion is known as the *rhomboideus minor*; the lower (larger) portion, as *rhomboideus major*. *Proximal attachment:* Ligamentum nuchae and the spinous processes of the lowest two cervical and the upper four thoracic vertebrae. *Distal attachment:* Medial border of scapula. The oblique direction of the muscles indicates that they serve to elevate as well as retract the scapula. The rhomboideus major also has the important function of downward rotation of the scapula since it attaches to the inferior angle of the scapula. The rhomboids are made up of parallel fibers, the direction of which is almost perpendicular to those of the lower trapezius. *Innervation:* Dorsal scapular nerve ("the nerve to the rhomboids").

Inspection and palpation: Since this muscle is covered by the trapezius, it is best palpated when the trapezius is relaxed. The subject's hand is placed in the small of the back. The investigator places the palpating fingers underneath the medial border of the scapula, which can be done without causing discomfort to the subject provided that the muscles in this region are relaxed (Fig. 7-3). If now the subject raises the hand just off the small of the back, the rhomboideus major contracts vigorously as a downward rotator of the scapula and pushes the palpating fingers out from underneath the medial border of the scapula (Fig. 7-4). If the lower trapezius is not too bulky, the direction of the contracting fibers of the rhomboids may be seen under the skin. In the case of trapezius paralysis, the course of the rhomboids is even better observable (Fig. 7-5).

PECTORALIS MINOR

The pectoralis minor (L. *pectus*, breast bone, chest) is located anteriorly on the upper chest, being entirely covered by the pectoralis major. *Proximal attachment:* By four

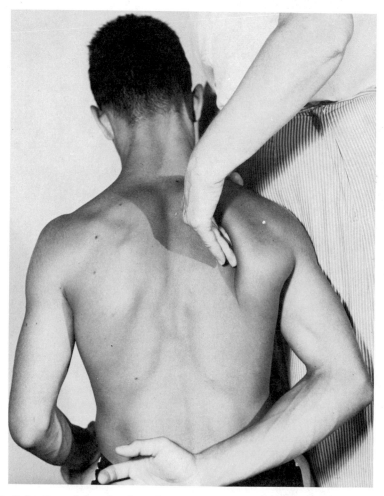

FIGURE 7-3. Palpation of rhomboids. When trapezius and rhomboids are relaxed, examiner's finger may be placed under medial border of scapula.

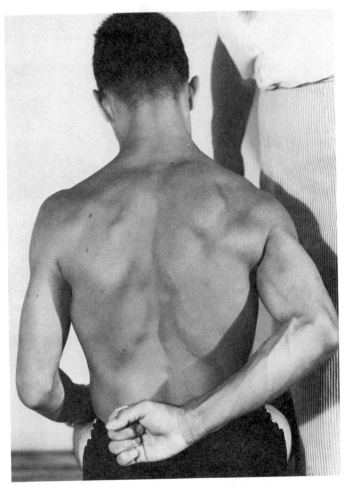

FIGURE 7-4. Palpation of rhomboids. As subject raises hand off the back, examiner's fingers are pushed out from underneath the scapula by the contraction of the rhomboideus major. Note also the contraction of teres major.

tendomuscular slips from the second to the fifth ribs. These muscular slips converge with their *distal attachment* into the coracoid process of the scapula. This gives the muscle a triangular shape. *Innervation:* Anterior thoracic nerve.

Inspection and palpation: The forearm is placed in the small of the back. In this position, the pectoralis major is relaxed, a prerequisite for palpation of the pectoralis minor. The examiner places one finger just below the coracoid process of the scapula, as seen in Figure 7-6, pressing down gently so as to let the finger sink in as far as possible.

In this position, the finger lies across the tendon of the pectoralis minor, which muscle is relaxed as long as the forearm rests in the small of the back. When the subject raises the forearm off the back, the pectoralis minor contracts, and its tendon

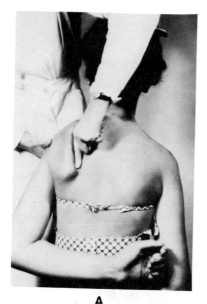 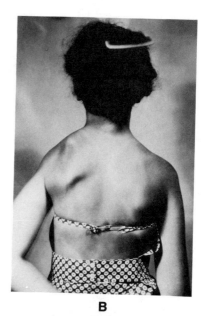

A   B

FIGURE 7-5. Testing the rhomboids in a subject with trapezius paralysis. *(A)* The examiner's finger lies along medial border of scapula. *(B)* When subject raises hand off back, the lower border of the rhomboideus major is well visible. (From Brunnstrom, S: *Muscle testing around the shoulder girdle.* J Bone Joint Surg [Am] 23:263, 1941, with permission.)

becomes tense under the palpating fingers. The muscle can also be palpated in its important function of shoulder depression (trunk elevation). The palpating fingers should be placed distal to the coracoid process, and the subject (sitting on a table) should be asked to push down on the table with the hands as if to elevate the body (actual trunk elevation or sitting pushup will cause other muscles to contract and obscure palpation of the muscle).

LEVATOR SCAPULAE

The levator scapulae, as its name indicates, is an elevator of the scapula, an action it shares with the upper portion of the trapezius and with the rhomboids. *Proximal attachment:* Transverse processes of the upper cervical vertebrae. *Distal attachment:* Medial border of the scapula, above the spine, near the superior angle. *Innervation:* Dorsal scapular nerve.

Inspection and palpation: The levator is covered by the upper trapezius and in its upper portion also by the sternocleidomastoid muscle. Posteriorly, its border extends to the rhomboideus minor and the splenius muscle of the neck. Ordinarily, in elevation of the shoulder girdle, the upper trapezius and the levator contract together. The levator is difficult to isolate and palpate. To bring out levator action with a minimum of trapezius participation, the subject places the forearm in the small of the back, then

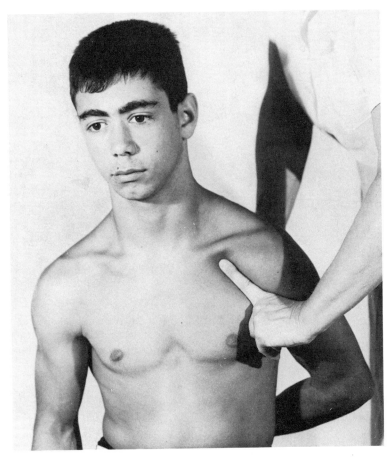

FIGURE 7-6. Palpation of pectoralis minor. With the subject's hand resting in the lumbar region of the back, both pectoralis major and pectoralis minor are relaxed. The tendon of pectoralis minor is palpated below the coracoid process when the subject raises the hand off the back.

shrugs the shoulder. The levator may then be palpated in the neck region, anterior to the trapezius but posterior to the sternocleidomastoid muscle.

Note that the line of action of the upper trapezius produces *elevation and upward rotation of the scapula;* whereas the levator, at least in a certain range, has a *downward-rotary* action on the scapula. Therefore, the levator muscle will more likely be used as an elevator when elevation is carried out with the scapula in a downward-rotated position, as in shrugging the shoulder when the hand is behind the body. A comparatively isolated action of the levator may be obtained if the shrug is made briefly and quickly and in short range. If much effort is exerted in raising the shoulder and if the elevated position is maintained, the trapezius will contract in spite of above precautions.

Inspection and palpation of the sternocleidomastoid muscle will be discussed in Chapter 11.

Group II.   Muscles From Shoulder Girdle to Humerus

DELTOID

The deltoid (Gr. *delta*, the letter Δ, and *eidos*, resemblance) is a superficial muscle of the shoulder consisting of three parts: *anterior, middle,* and *posterior.* The muscle fits over the glenohumeral joint like the upper portion of a sleeve, covering the joint on all sides except in the axillary region. *Proximal attachment:* The acromial end of the clavicle, the acromion process, and the spine of the scapula. From this widespread origin, the three portions of the muscle converge to have their *distal attachment* onto the deltoid tuberosity, a rather rough area about halfway down the shaft of the humerus. *Innervation:* Axillary nerve.

Inspection and palpation: The muscle is covered by skin only and may therefore be observed and palpated in its entirety. The characteristic roundness of the normal shoulder is due to the deltoid muscle. All parts of the deltoid are easily identified in Figures 5-9 and 5-10.

The *anterior deltoid* may be observed and palpated when the arm is held in a horizontal position (Fig. 7-7). Note that its inferior border lies close to the upper portion of the pectoralis major. The anterior deltoid contracts strongly when horizontal adduction is resisted.

The *middle deltoid* has the best anatomic position for abduction and is seen contracting whenever this movement is carried out or the abducted position is maintained.

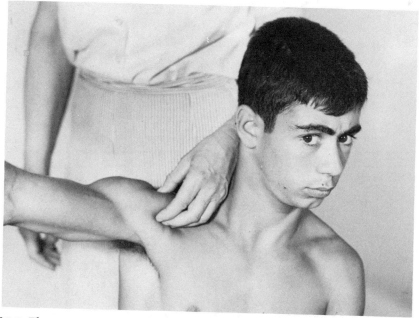

FIGURE 7-7. The examiner grasps around the anterior portion of the deltoid, separating it from the middle deltoid and from the pectoralis major.

The *posterior deltoid* contracts strongly when the shoulder is hyperextended against resistance, or resistance is given to *horizontal abduction*. The inferior border of the posterior portion of the deltoid has a close relation to the long head of the triceps and to the teres muscles (see Figs. 5-10, 7-12). Isolated action of the posterior deltoid may be seen in Figure 7-8. The patient (postpoliomyelitis) had extensive paralysis of the shoulder muscles, including the middle and anterior portions of the deltoid, while the posterior portion was more or less preserved.

The three portions of the deltoid should be observed in action while horizontal abduction and adduction are performed and in pulling and pushing activities. It will then be seen that the anterior and posterior portions often act antagonistically—the anterior portion exerting traction forward, the posterior portion backward—on the arm.

SUPRASPINATUS

As its name indicates, the supraspinatus muscle is located above the spine of the scapula. It is hidden by the trapezius and the deltoid, the trapezius covering its muscular portion, the deltoid its tendon. *Proximal attachment:* Supraspinous fossa of the scapula, which it completely fills. The muscle fibers converge toward the tip of the shoulder to form a short tendon which passes underneath the acromion and which adheres to the capsule of the shoulder joint. *Distal attachment:* The uppermost facet of the greater tubercle of the humerus. *Innervation:* Suprascapular nerve.

Palpation: The deepest portion of the supraspinatus lies too deep in the supraspinous fossa to be palpated, but its more superficial fibers may be felt through the trape-

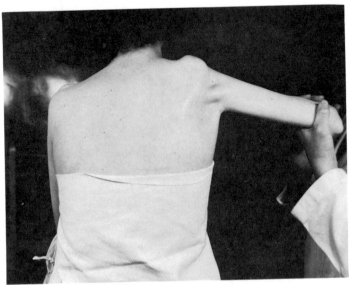

FIGURE 7-8. Isolated action of posterior deltoid in postpoliomyelitis patient. Examiner holds arm abducted while patient pushes back against resistance.

zius. The spine of the scapula is first identified, and the palpating fingers are placed above the spine (they should be moved to various positions so that the best spot for palpation is located). A quick abduction movement in short range is carried out and a momentary contraction of the muscle is felt. In wider range of abduction the supra-spinatus is more difficult to palpate because the trapezius becomes increasingly tense and it is then not easy to distinguish one muscle from the other.

Palpation of the supraspinatus may also be done with the subject prone and the arm hanging over the edge of the table. In this position, the scapula has moved forward on the rib cage by the weight of the arm and is already partially upwardly rotated. When abduction is carried out in this position, a contraction of the supraspinatus muscle may be felt with little or no interference by the trapezius. The supraspinatus may also be palpated when the subject lifts a heavy briefcase or the like, preferably with the trunk inclined forward. As the weight of the object exerts its downward traction, the supraspinatus becomes tense, apparently for the purpose of preventing excessive sep-aration of the glenohumeral joint.

INFRASPINATUS AND TERES MINOR

These two muscles, although supplied by two different nerves, are described together because they are closely related in location and action. *Proximal attachment:* Infraspi-nous fossa and lateral border of the scapula. The infraspinatus lies closest to the spine of the scapula and occupies most of the infraspinous fossa. The teres minor (L. *teretis,* round and long) is attached mainly to the lateral border of the scapula. *Distal attach-ment:* The greater tubercle of the humerus, the infraspinatus into its middle facet, the teres minor into its lower (posterior) facet. The tendons of both muscles are adherent to the capsule. *Innervation:* Infraspinatus by the suprascapular, teres minor by the axillary, nerve.

Inspection and palpation: The largest parts of the infraspinatus and the teres minor are superficial and may be palpated; some portions are covered by the trapezius and the posterior deltoid. In order to have as large parts of the muscles as possible avail-able for palpation, the arm must be away from the body and the posterior deltoid must be relaxed. This is accomplished if the subject lies prone or stands with the trunk inclined forward and if the arm hangs vertically (Fig. 7-9). The margin of the posterior deltoid is first identified. The palpating fingers are placed below the deltoid on the scapula, near its lateral margin. While the subject maintains the arm in a vertical position, the subject externally rotates the shoulder by turning the palm forward. The two muscles then rise under the palpating fingers, the teres minor being felt next to the infraspinatus, but further away from the spine of the scapula than the infraspina-tus. External rotation in this position requires only a mild contraction of these mus-cles, and consequently they do not show beneath the skin in the illustration. A more vigorous contraction is seen in Figure 7-2, where a large number of other muscles are also activated.

The distal attachments of these muscles (as well as the supraspinatus) as they blend into the joint capsule are a frequent site of injury and cause of shoulder pain. These

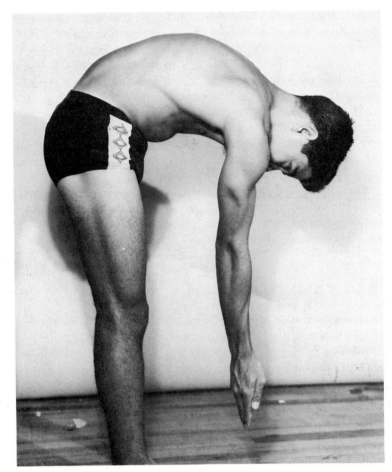

FIGURE 7-9. Infraspinatus and teres minor may be felt contracting near the lateral border of the scapula when the shoulder is externally rotated. Vertical position of arm allows activation of these two muscles in a rather isolated fashion.

attachments can be palpated on the head of the humerus if the glenohumeral joint is passively hyperextended.

SUBSCAPULARIS

The subscapularis is located underneath the scapula, close to the rib cage, but it is not attached to the rib cage. The smooth connective-tissue covering of the subscapularis provides a sliding surface for the scapula on the rib cage. *Proximal attachment:* Costal surface of scapula. Fiber bundles converge toward the axilla to form a broad tendon, which passes over the anterior aspect of the capsule of the glenohumeral joint. *Distal attachment:* The lesser tubercle of the humerus and the shaft below the tubercle. *Innervation:* Subscapular nerves.

Palpation: With the subject in the erect standing position, the muscle cannot very well be reached for palpation, but if the trunk is inclined forward so that the scapula slides forward on the rib cage by the weight of the hanging arm, a portion of this muscle may be palpated. The fingers are placed in the axilla anterior to the latissimus dorsi and, with gentle pressure, are moved in the direction of the costal surface of the scapula. With the arm hanging vertically, the subject internally rotates the shoulder by turning the palm backward and laterally (Fig. 7-10). The firm, round belly of the subscapularis can then be felt rising under the palpating fingers. If a person wishes to

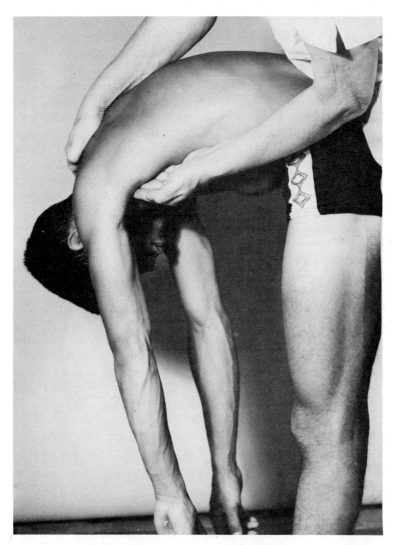

FIGURE 7-10. Subscapularis is palpated in internal rotation of the shoulder. The palpating fingers are placed in the axilla and are moved in direction toward the costal surface of the scapula.

feel the muscle on oneself, the thumb is used for palpation. As far as can be ascertained by palpation, the size of the muscle varies considerably from person to person. According to Fick (1911, p 82), the subscapularis has a cross section approximately equal to that of the middle deltoid, which indicates that it is a muscle of considerable size.

TERES MAJOR

The teres major is located at the axillary border of the scapula near the teres minor. It is round like the minor, but larger. *Proximal attachment:* Inferior angle of scapula. The muscle fibers course upward and laterally to have their *distal attachment* to the crest of the lesser tubercle of the humerus by means of a strong broad tendon. *Innervation:* Subscapular nerves.

Inspection and palpation: The muscular portion of the teres major is well accessible to palpation, but the tendon of its distal attachment is not. There are many ways of demonstrating and palpating the teres major. It acts in most pulling activities when the shoulder is extended or adducted against resistance. If the examiner gives manual resistance to adduction, as seen in Figure 5-10, the muscle may be palpated lateral to the inferior angle of the scapula. In this illustration, resistance is given simultaneously to extension of the elbow and adduction of the shoulder so that the triceps as well as the teres major contracts. (The teres major is also seen in Figure 7-12.) In most subjects, it is difficult to isolate the teres major from the adjacent teres minor and latissimus dorsi muscles.

CORACOBRACHIALIS

Proximal attachment: Coracoid process of scapula. *Distal attachment:* Medial surface of humerus, about halfway down the shaft of the humerus. *Innervation:* Musculocutaneous nerve.

Inspection and palpation: Part of this muscle is covered by the deltoid and the pectoralis major. The coracobrachialis may be palpated in the distal portion of the axillary region if the arm is elevated above the horizontal, as seen in Figure 7-11. It emerges from underneath the inferior border of the pectoralis major where it lies medial to, and parallel with, the tendon of the short head of the biceps. The biceps is first identified by supination of the forearm; the palpating fingers then follow the short head of the biceps proximally until the muscle tapers off, and this is the height best suited for palpation of the coracobrachialis. In the illustration, the subject is bringing the arm in a direction toward the head.

BICEPS AND TRICEPS

These two muscles do not belong to the scapulohumeral group, since they do not have their distal attachments on the humerus; however, the two heads of the biceps and the long head of the triceps cross the shoulder joint and therefore act on it. It should be recalled that the heads of the biceps originate from the supraglenoid tubercle and from

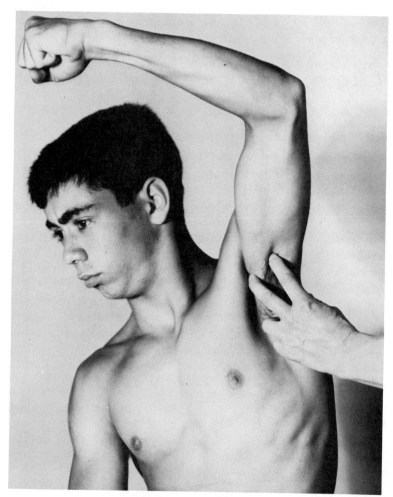

FIGURE 7-11. Identification of coracobrachialis. This muscle emerges from underneath the inferior border of the pectoralis major, where it lies close to the tendon of the short head of the biceps.

the coracoid process, respectively, and that the triceps originates from the infraglenoid tubercle.

Group III. Muscles From Trunk to Humerus

These muscles have their proximal attachments on the trunk and their distal attachments on the humerus, having little or no attachment to the scapula. They act primarily on the humerus, but also indirectly affect the position of the shoulder girdle. There are only two muscles in this group, the *latissimus dorsi* and the *pectoralis major*, which perform multiple actions at the shoulder including adduction, extension, internal rotation, and depression.

LATISSIMUS DORSI

The name is derived from the Latin *latus*, meaning broad, *latissimus* being the superlative of *latus*. This muscle is the broadest muscle of the back and the lateral thoracic region. It lies superficially, except a small part that is covered by the lower trapezius. *Proximal attachment:* Spinous processes of the thoracic vertebrae from T6 downward, dorsolumbar fascia, crest of ilium (posterior portion), and the lowest ribs, here interdigitating with the external oblique abdominal muscle. The fibers converge toward the axilla, some fibers passing over or near the inferior angle of the scapula, often adhering to it. The *distal attachment* is by a tendon that courses in the axilla and attaches to the crest of the lesser tubercle of the humerus, proximal to that of the teres major. *Innervation:* Thoracodorsal nerve.

Inspection and palpation: The largest part of this muscle is thin and sheetlike, which makes it difficult to distinguish from the fascia and from the deeper muscles of the back. Laterally, in the axillary line and where the fibers converge, the muscle has considerable bulk, and here it is easy to observe and palpate (Fig. 7-12). The latissimus and the teres major contract when adduction or extension of the shoulder is resisted as seen in the illustration, where the subject is pressing down on the examiner's shoulder. The latissimus forms the posterior fold of the axilla. Its relation to the teres major and the long head of the triceps in this region should be noted.

PECTORALIS MAJOR

Its name (L. *pectus*, breast bone, chest) indicates that the pectoralis major is a large muscle of the chest. It has an extensive origin but does not cover nearly as large an area as the latissimus dorsi. *Proximal attachment:* Clavicle (sternal half), sternum and costal cartilages of the second to seventh ribs, and the aponeurosis over the abdominal muscles. The muscle is usually described as consisting of three parts: the clavicular, sternocostal, and abdominal. From the standpoint of action, the muscle has an *upper portion* (clavicular) and a *lower portion* (sternocostal and abdominal). Because of its wide origin and the convergence of its fibers toward the axilla, the muscle takes the shape of a fan. *Distal attachment:* Crest of the greater tuberosity of the humerus, on an area several inches long. Before reaching its attachment, the tendon bridges the intertubercular (bicipital) groove. The manner in which the muscle fibers approach their distal attachment should be noted—the tendon appears to be twisted around itself, so that the uppermost fibers attach lowest on the crest and the lower fibers more proximally. *Innervation:* Medial and lateral anterior thoracic nerves.

Inspection and palpation: The muscle is easily observed and palpated since it is superficial and of considerable bulk. It is best palpated where the fibers converge toward the axilla. The entire muscle contracts when horizontal adduction is resisted, as in pressing the palms together in front of the body.

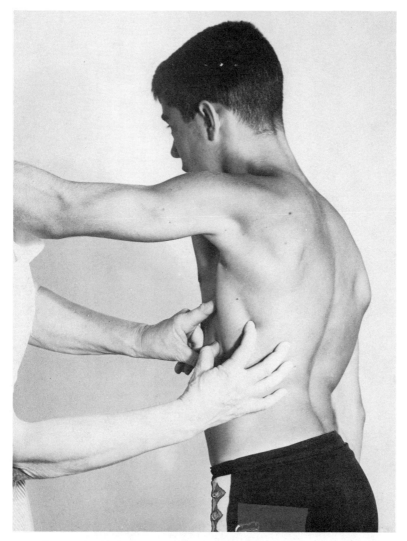

FIGURE 7-12. Palpation of the lower portion of the latissimus dorsi. The subject presses downward on the examiner's shoulder. The teres major may also be seen contracting strongly.

The *upper portion* acts separately if the arm is brought obliquely upward toward the head against resistance, as seen in Figure 7-13. A pencil has been placed across the lower portion of the muscle to show that it is not contracting. The *lower portion* contracts separately when the arm is adducted in a lower position (Fig. 7-14). The examiner's fingers are placed across the upper portion to show that it is relatively relaxed. The external oblique abdominal muscle is also seen contracting (note its interdigitations with the serratus anterior).

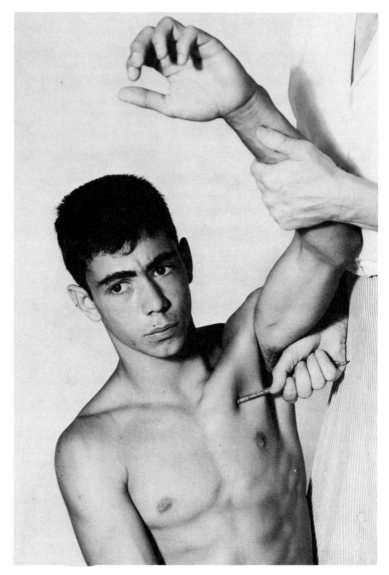

FIGURE 7-13. The upper portion of the pectoralis major is seen contracting as the subject is pulling the arm in direction toward the head against resistance. A pencil has been placed across the lower portion of pectoralis major to show that it is relaxed.

Function of Muscles of Group I

SUPPORT OF THE UPPER EXTREMITY

As previously described, the shoulder girdle is suspended from the skull and neck by means of muscles and fascia. The only joint connecting the upper extremity with the

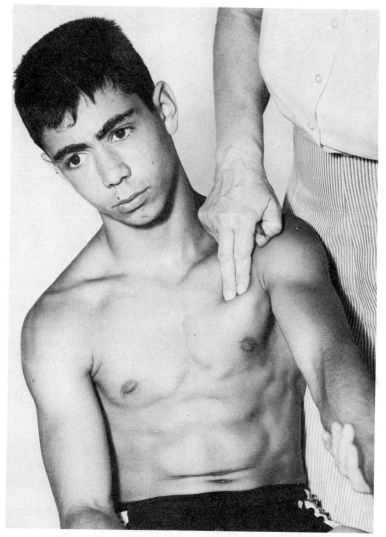

FIGURE 7-14. The lower portion of the pectoralis major contracts as the subject adducts the arm against resistance. The examiner's fingers are separating the lower portion from the upper.

trunk is the sternoclavicular joint. Several muscles are involved in this suspension, and the same muscles also act in elevation of the shoulder girdle.

TRAPEZIUS. Those portions of the trapezius that attach to the acromial end of the clavicle and to the acromion process normally support the shoulder girdle and prevent sagging of the shoulder. When the trapezius is paralyzed, this support is missing, and the shoulder slopes down more than it would normally (Brunnstrom, 1941). The weight of the arm tends to draw the tip of the shoulder down, causing the scapula to rotate downward beyond its normal hanging position (Fig. 7-15, A). The glenohu-

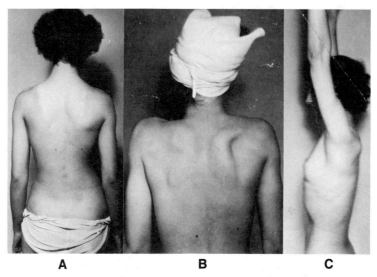

A   B   C

FIGURE 7-15. Left trapezius paralysis of long duration owing to injury to spinal accessory nerve. *(A)* In the relaxed standing position, the scapula has a downward-rotated position. The superior angle of the scapula is seen as a protuberance under the skin. The distal portion of the clavicle is visible. *(B)* In spite of the loss of the upper trapezius, the shoulder girdle can be elevated quite well (by the levator scapulae and the rhomboids). Note neck contour. *(C)* The serratus anterior without the aid of the trapezius is capable of rotating the scapula upward full range so that the arms may be elevated above the head. This patient experienced no difficulty in doing so.

meral joint is in slight abduction, and the glenoid fossa is perpendicular rather than inclined superiorly. In this position, the weight of the arm may lead to stretching of the capsular ligaments and subluxation at the glenohumeral joint. Subluxation is a common problem in patients with cerebrovascular accidents (hemiplegia) and is difficult to prevent. The leverage action of the weight of the arm on the clavicle also may cause a subluxation of the sternoclavicular joint (Fig. 7-16).

In spite of paralysis of the trapezius, the shoulder girdle can be elevated without difficulty (Fig. 7-15, B). The levator scapulae and the rhomboids are capable of doing so without the aid of the upper trapezius.

DEPRESSION OF THE SHOULDER GIRDLE

In the upright position, when the elevators of the shoulder girdle release their tension, the shoulder is lowered by the weight of the limb. Some additional lowering may be brought about by deliberately depressing the shoulder, and when this is done, a considerable tension is experienced in muscles of the trunk, both in front and in back. The *lower portion of the trapezius* then springs into action, and simultaneously the *pectoralis minor*, the *latissimus dorsi*, and the *lower portion of the pectoralis major* are felt contracting. These two latter muscles apply their action not to the scapula but to the humerus.

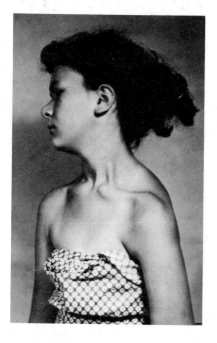

FIGURE 7-16. Paralysis of trapezius. Note subluxation of sternoclavicular joint and sharp outline of posterior border of clavicle; also note skin fold in anterior axillary region, characteristic of trapezius paralysis. (From Brunnstrom, S: *Muscle testing around the shoulder girdle.* J Bone Joint Surg [Am] 23:263, 1941, with permission.)

Such action of depression is used in pushups on parallel bars, in crutch-walking, and in getting up from the sitting position when the arms aid the motion by pushing down on the chair.

PROTRACTION OF THE SHOULDER GIRDLE

This movement is effected mainly by the *serratus anterior*, which pulls the scapula forward on the rib cage, and also by the *pectoralis major* exerting its pull on the humerus. In protraction of the shoulder girdle with the arms at the side of the body, the action of the two muscles can hardly be isolated. The two muscles also act simultaneously in reaching forward with the arm elevated to a horizontal position. If the reaching is done obliquely outward, however, the pectoralis ceases to contract, and the serratus assumes the responsibility alone. This isolated action of the serratus occurs at approximately 135 degrees of shoulder flexion and abduction. When the serratus is paralyzed and forward reaching is attempted (Fig. 7-17, A), a typical "winging" of the medial border of the scapula is seen, and the scapula fails to slide forward on the rib cage (Brunnstrom, 1941).

RETRACTION OF THE SHOULDER GIRDLE

Retraction of the shoulder girdle is carried out by the combined action of the *trapezius* and the *rhomboids*. The upward rotary action of the trapezius is counteracted by the downward rotary action of the rhomboids, and by the weight of the arm applied to the tip of the shoulder. The tendency of the upper trapezius and the rhomboids to elevate

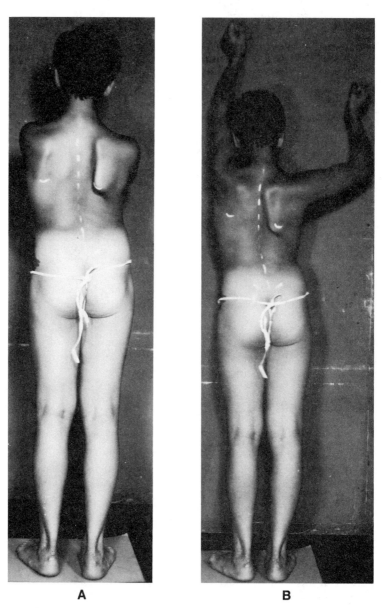

A   **B**

FIGURE 7-17. Isolated paralysis of serratus anterior. *(A)* Forward reach is poor. The scapula fails to slide forward on the rib cage, and there is a typical winging of its medial border. *(B)* In retraction of the shoulder girdle, the medial border of the scapula does not stay close to the rib cage. The right arm cannot be raised overhead since the trapezius does not provide sufficient upward rotation of the scapula. (From Brunnstrom, S: *Muscle testing around the shoulder girdle.* J Bone Joint Surg [Am] 23:263, 1941, with permission.)

the shoulder girdle is checked by the depressor action of the lower trapezius and by the weight of the arm. The result is that the scapula moves backward on the rib cage, with the medial border remaining approximately parallel to the vertebral column. Normally, the serratus anterior also plays a part in this motion by keeping the medial border of the scapula close to the rib cage. That this is so may be deduced from observing the effect of serratus paralysis on retraction of the shoulder girdle (Fig. 7-17, B).

When the arms are elevated to a horizontal position (i.e., the scapula is rotated partially upward) and the trunk is inclined forward, retraction of the shoulder girdle requires strong action by the trapezius (see Fig. 7-2). A subject with trapezius paralysis is unable in this position to hold the scapula back (Fig. 7-18).

The effect of loss of the trapezius as a retractor of the shoulder girdle is also seen in erect standing with the arms hanging at the sides. The shoulder girdle then tends to slide somewhat forward, causing a fold in the skin near the axilla (Fig. 7-19). Such a fold is particularly noticeable on obese individuals.

UPWARD ROTATION OF THE SCAPULA

In the erect position with the arms at the sides, the medial border of the scapula is more or less parallel to the vertebral column. When the arm is raised overhead, the scapula rotates upward while simultaneously sliding forward on the rib cage, so that its medial border assumes an oblique position and its inferior angle comes to lie approximately in the axillary line. The serratus anterior and the trapezius work together to bring about this movement. These muscles also act together to give fixation to the scapula in any partially upward rotated position that the occasion may demand.

The serratus and trapezius both have definite functions to fulfill but, as far as upward rotation of the scapula is concerned, the serratus appears to be the more important of the two. When the serratus is paralyzed, the subject is unable to raise the arm overhead, as the trapezius cannot bring about enough upward rotation for complete abduction (see Fig. 7-17, B). On the other hand, when the trapezius is paralyzed and

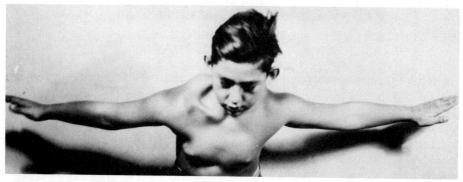

FIGURE 7-18. Paralysis of the right trapezius. Subject is unable to retract the shoulder girdle when the trunk is inclined forward. (From Brunnstrom, S: *Muscle testing around the shoulder girdle.* J Bone Joint Surg [Am] 23:263, 1941, with permission.)

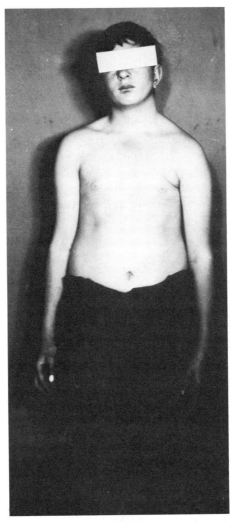

FIGURE 7-19. Partial paralysis of left trapezius. Note fold in skin anterior to axilla.

the serratus intact, the arms can be raised overhead without difficulty (see Fig. 7-15, C).

If both trapezius and serratus are paralyzed, the scapula has lost its most important stabilizing muscles, and its position will be determined mainly by the weight of the arm acting at the tip of the shoulder. When such a subject stands with the arms relaxed at the sides, the scapula assumes a downward-rotated position and also tips forward so that its inferior angle protrudes backward (Fig. 7-20). The effect of bilateral paralysis of the trapezius and the serratus on abduction of the shoulders is seen in Figure 7-21. When flexion or abduction of the shoulders is attempted, satisfactory *glenohumeral* motion takes place, but the scapula rotates *downward* instead of upward. The

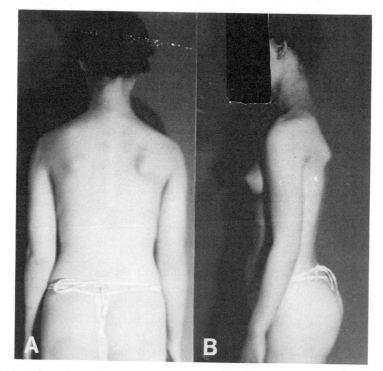

FIGURE 7-20. Bilateral paralysis of trapezius and serratus anterior. The scapulae assume downward-rotated positions *(A)* and also tip forward so that the inferior angles protrude backward *(B)*.

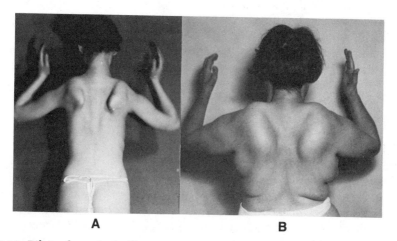

A   B

FIGURE 7-21. Bilateral paralysis of trapezius and serratus. Maximum elevation of the arms of which these subjects are capable is demonstrated. Note downward-rotated position of scapulae. (*A* from Brunnstrom, S: *Muscle testing around the shoulder girdle.* J Bone Joint Surg [Am] 23:263, 1941, with permission.)

result, in terms of arm elevation, is extremely poor. The deltoid in this instance becomes a downward rotator of the scapula as it exerts traction on the acromial process in a distal direction. Such action of the deltoid, of course, never occurs under normal conditions owing to synergic action of the upward rotators of the scapula.

DOWNWARD ROTATION OF THE SCAPULA

When resistance to the downward movement of the arm is encountered (as in swimming the crawl, pulling down a window, using an overhead pulley to lift a weight, or chinning oneself), the downward rotators of the scapula (together with the shoulder adductors and extensors) come into action. Manual resistance may also be applied to bring out action of the downward rotators. Ideally, such resistance should be applied to the scapula, but if this proves difficult, shoulder adduction may be resisted.

The most important muscle for downward rotation of the scapula is the *rhomboideus major*. This muscle, because of its attachment to the lower portion of the medial margin of the scapula, maintains a downward rotary action throughout the range of motion. When the scapula is already upwardly rotated (as in reaching overhead) the rhomboideus minor is a strong downward rotator of the scapula. The rotary effect decreases as the movement progresses: when the medial border of the scapula is vertical, the rotary effect becomes *nil*; beyond this point, the rhomboideus minor retracts and elevates the scapula without rotation. The *levator scapulae*, like the minor rhomboid, has a downward rotary action in the early range, then loses it to become an elevator of the scapula exclusively.

In the last portion of the range of motion, downward rotation proceeds beyond the vertical position of the medial border of the scapula. In this range, the scapula also tips forward by the combined actions of the rhomboideus major in back and the *pectoralis minor* in front, the latter exerting downward traction on the coracoid process.

The *latissimus dorsi*, to a greater or lesser extent, attaches to the inferior angle of the scapula; sometimes this angle is held in place by a pocket formed by the fascia around the latissimus. Thus, the latissimus may act on the scapula in the sense of downward rotation as it contracts in adduction and extension of the shoulder.

Function of Muscles of Groups II and III

Muscles of group II (connecting the scapula and humerus) are concerned with movements of the glenohumeral joint and may be thought of as primarily moving the humerus in relation to the scapula, although the reverse may also take place (see Fig. 7-20). In moving the humerus, the muscles of group II work *synergically* with muscles of group I that stabilize or move the scapula in relation to the thorax. Observation of the relative length of lever arms of scapular and humeral muscles shows those of the deltoid and supraspinatus to be small, while those of the caudal portion of the serratus anterior and the cranial part of the trapezius are considerably longer. This suggests scapular muscles are organized for force and that the deltoid and supraspinatus are organized for movement of greater range (Doody, Freedman, and Waterland, 1970).

The effect of length-tension relationships of these muscles is apparent also. The gleno-humeral joint can only flex or abduct 90 degrees, and at this point the muscles are in their shortest and therefore weakest position on their length-tension curve. Simultaneous movement of the scapula by the scapulothoracic muscles (scapulohumeral rhythm) extends effective length-tension relationships for the scapulohumeral muscles (group II) throughout full shoulder flexion or abduction (approximately 160 to 180 degrees).

Muscles of group III (the pectoralis major and latissimus dorsi) act mainly on the humerus, having a firm fixation on the trunk. They are particularly important in resisted adduction and extension of the shoulder, as in the crawl stroke in swimming or pulling down a window. When the hand and thus the humerus are fixed, these muscles move the trunk toward the humerus, as in a pullup or climbing a rope. In addition, the latissimus is active in forced expiration and coughing when the humerus is stabilized.

GLENOHUMERAL ABDUCTION

The *deltoid* and the *supraspinatus* are the most important muscles acting in abduction of the glenohumeral joint. *Both muscles* are active throughout the motion of abduction and their electromyographic activity increases progressively to become maximal between 90 and 180 degrees of shoulder flexion (Basmajian, 1978). When the shoulder is fully externally rotated, the *long head of the biceps* may also aid in abduction.

The effectiveness of the deltoid and the supraspinatus in abduction and flexion of the shoulder depends largely upon synergic action of the serratus anterior and the trapezius. Without the action of at least one of the latter muscles, a contraction of the deltoid and supraspinatus would cause the scapula to rotate downward, and these muscles would become so shortened that their ability to produce tension would diminish markedly, or even become exhausted. Fortunately, under normal conditions, this does not occur because of the strong linkage with their scapulothoracic synergists. The devastating effect of paralysis of the shoulder blade fixators is illustrated in Figure 7-21.

DELTOID PARALYSIS. Most patients with paralysis or marked weakness (paresis) of the deltoid cannot perform glenohumeral abduction. Instead, the arm is raised slightly by upward rotation of the scapula and lateral flexion of the trunk. Patients with isolated deltoid paralysis can frequently appear to perform the motion of abduction by externally rotating the glenohumeral joint (to use the biceps) and by a slight motion toward flexion at around 90 degrees of abduction. These "trick" motions are effective in getting the hand overhead, but they cannot be performed with resistance or at all points in shoulder abduction. Unless therapists are carefully observant, they may miss paralysis or paresis of the deltoid in their evaluation. During World War II, Brunnstrom (1941) observed three patients with gunshot injuries to the axillary nerve, with resulting paralysis of the deltoid and teres minor. All three men were capable of abducting the shoulder full range. One of these cases is illustrated in Figure 7-22. Note the normal contour on the right side and the flaccidity of the deltoid on the left side.

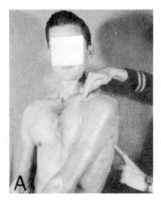 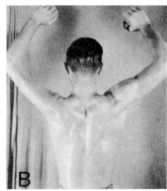

FIGURE 7-22. Deltoid and teres minor paralysis caused by gunshot injury to axillary nerve. *(A)* Examiner is indicating points of entry and exit of projectile. Note flaccidity of left deltoid. *(B)* Subject was able to abduct arm full range. (From Brunnstrom, S: *Muscle testing around the shoulder girdle.* J Bone Joint Surg [Am] 23:263, 1941, with permission.)

SUPRASPINATUS PARALYSIS (DELTOID INTACT). When the supraspinatus is paralyzed and atrophied, the region above the spine of the scapula becomes flat or even hollow (Fig. 7-23). In the case illustrated (postpoliomyelitis), the trapezius was also partially affected, which accounts for the marked emptiness in the supraspinous region. The serratus functioned satisfactorily and the subject experienced no difficulty in raising the arm overhead.

Van Linge and Mulder (1963) observed the effect of a temporary and complete paralysis of the supraspinatus following suprascapular nerve block by local anesthesia. All subjects (10 healthy males) experienced no difficulty in raising the arm overhead, but a decrease in strength and endurance resulted. The authors conclude that loss of abduction as seen in patients with rupture of the supraspinatus tendon is due to pain, possibly impingement of the tendon between the humeral head and the acromion, not primarily to absence of supraspinatus function.

The cases discussed in the previous paragraphs demonstrate that either of the two abductors can perform an unresisted motion of glenohumeral abduction with the other, although the strength and functional use in abduction is reduced; but if both deltoid and supraspinatus are not functioning, shoulder abduction is seriously affected. No true abduction is then possible unless the shoulder is fully externally rotated. In the externally rotated position, the long head of the biceps, coursing in the intertubercular groove, has a good line of action (but poor leverage) for abduction. That this muscle is capable of abduction was demonstrated by a patient whose deltoid and supraspinatus were paralyzed (Brunnstrom, 1946). Abduction was performed in external rotation but was lost in the internally rotated position.

FLEXION OF THE SHOULDER

When the shoulder is flexed (that is, the arm is raised forward in the sagittal plane), the *anterior deltoid,* the *clavicular portion of the pectoralis major,* the *coracobrachi-*

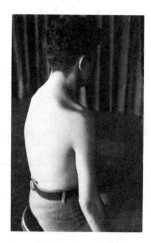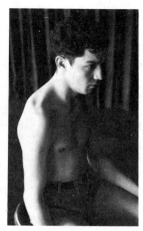

FIGURE 7-23. The emptiness in the supraspinous region is well observable in this boy who had involvement of the trapezius and the supraspinatus following an attack of poliomyelitis. The subject experienced no difficulty in raising arm over head.

alis, and the *biceps brachii* (both heads) have a favorable line of action. The first two muscles are the most important flexors, capable of carrying out a full range of flexion. The other muscles act mainly in the first 90 degrees of flexion, and their actions decline or cease altogether in flexion beyond 90 degrees. Terminal range of shoulder flexion is the same as terminal abduction, and both motions normally depend on the scapular-thoracic motions of abduction and upward rotation as well as external rotation at the glenohumeral joint. Arthrokinematically, the head of the humerus must be able to move distally so that these motions can occur.

THE ROLE OF THE INFRASPINATUS, TERES MINOR, AND SUBSCAPULARIS IN FLEXION AND ABDUCTION OF THE SHOULDER

So far, those muscles that are primarily responsible for abduction and flexion of the shoulder have been discussed. Electromyograms of the shoulder muscles in these two movements reveal that the infraspinatus, teres minor, and subscapularis act continuously during flexion and abduction (Inman and associates, 1944). Their function as a group is to *depress the humerus* to prevent the compression or stabilizing component of the deltoid muscle force from causing the head of the humerus to jam against the acromion process. This rotator muscle action accompanying shoulder abduction and flexion has been likened to a mechanical force couple (Inman and associates, 1944). Vertical upward pull of deltoid fibers is opposed by the downward pull of the rotator muscles. The humeral head presses against the glenoid, and resultant forces cause rotation about the joint center, and shoulder flexion or abduction occurs. The infraspinatus and teres minor also produce the necessary *external rotation* for complete elevation of the arm.

ADDUCTION AND EXTENSION OF THE SHOULDER

The main muscles involved in these movements are the *latissimus dorsi, teres major,* lower portion of the *pectoralis major,* the *posterior deltoid,* and the *long head of the triceps.*

When the arm is brought down to the side of the body from the overhead position *against a resistance,* it may be lowered laterally (adducted) or forward (extended), and these movements require essentially the same muscles, although in variable proportions.

The latissimus and pectoralis major have firm attachments to the trunk, whereas the teres major requires simultaneous action of the scapula-fixators, mainly the rhomboideus major. The rhomboids and the teres major in their synergic actions are comparable to the combination of the serratus anterior and the deltoid. In each case, relative elongation of the scapulohumeral muscles, with maintenance of their strength, is achieved. Without the rhomboids, the teres major would rotate the scapula upward and lose its effectiveness on the humerus, which is indeed the case when the rhomboids are paralyzed. In such a case, resistance to adduction of the shoulder causes the inferior angle of the scapula to slide forward owing to the action of the teres major. A similar position of the scapula is seen in a normal individual in Figure 7-24. Breaking up the strong linkage between the rhomboids and the teres major requires a coordination of which few individuals are capable.

The latissimus and the teres major adduct and extend the shoulder, drawing the arm backward; the pectoralis major, mainly its lower portion, draws the arm forward as it adducts. The coracobrachialis appears to be active during the first half of the movement of extension—from overhead position to the horizontal position of the arm—but its activity is difficult to assess by palpation.

When the movement of extension continues into *hyperextension,* the activity of the pectoralis declines, and the *posterior deltoid* springs into action. If the posterior deltoid is paralyzed, hyperextension is of very limited range (Brunnstrom, 1946).

EXTERNAL ROTATION OF THE SHOULDER

The *infraspinatus, teres minor,* and *posterior deltoid* are responsible for external rotation. The first two muscles contract in a fairly isolated fashion when the arm hangs vertically, and external rotation is performed without much effort (see Fig. 7-9). The posterior deltoid, if acting alone in external rotation, would simultaneously hyperextend the shoulder. In resisted external rotation, all three muscles act in variable proportions, depending upon the position of the joint.

FUNCTIONAL ASSOCIATION: EXTERNAL ROTATION AND SUPINATION. The external rotators of the shoulder and the supinators of the forearm are strongly linked. When the elbow is extended, these two muscle groups serve the same purpose, namely, to cause the palm to face upward, or forward, and they tend to be innervated together. This is well demonstrated if the forearm is supinated while the arm is hanging at the side of the body, in which case external rotation of the shoulder occurs

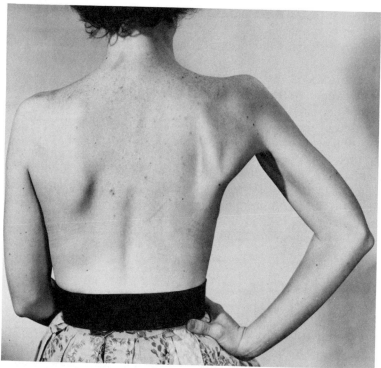

FIGURE 7-24. Contraction of the teres major without synergic action of the rhomboids results in upward rotation and forward sliding of the scapula on the rib cage. Movement performed by a normal individual capable of breaking up the strong linkage between the teres major and rhomboids.

invariably with supination. Good concentration is required to perform an isolated supination of the forearm whenever the elbow is extended.

INTERNAL ROTATION OF THE SHOULDER

There are five muscles for internal rotation: the *subscapularis, teres major, latissimus dorsi, pectoralis major,* and *anterior deltoid.* Of these, the subscapularis is the only one that comes close to being a pure internal rotator.

With the trunk and hip flexed to a right angle and the arm hanging relaxed (see Fig. 7-10), the subscapularis can usually perform internal rotation of the shoulder with little or no assistance from the other four muscles. This can be ascertained by palpation. Note that comparatively little effort should be used if the subscapularis is to act alone.

The pectoralis major combines internal rotation with adduction of the shoulder so that its action carries the arm in front of the body; the anterior deltoid flexes the shoulder as it internally rotates; the latissimus and teres major combine internal rotation with adduction and extension.

FUNCTIONAL ASSOCIATION: INTERNAL ROTATION AND PRONATION. Internal rotation and pronation are closely linked and tend to occur simultaneously for the purpose of turning the palm downward or backward. Isolated pronation seldom takes place.

Internal rotators and pronators often combine with other muscle groups in typical fashions. For example, in throwing a ball or in serving a ball in tennis, protraction of the shoulder girdle, internal rotation and adduction of the shoulder, extension of the elbow, pronation of the forearm, and trunk rotation combine. In preparing for the throw, exactly the reverse movement combination is used as that needed for the throw itself. Thus, preceding the throw are retraction of the shoulder girdle, external rotation and abduction of the shoulder, flexion of the elbow, supination of the forearm, and trunk rotation to the side of the raised arm. The muscles responsible for the throw are first elongated, which contributes materially to the effectiveness of the throw. If the movement analysis is carried to the hips and the lower extremities, it will be seen that the entire body contributes to an effective throw and that all muscles needed for the throw are first elongated.

ROTATOR CUFF

The distal attachments of the *supraspinatus, infraspinatus,* and *teres minor* muscles (SIT muscles) are blended with and reinforce the glenohumeral joint capsule. The tendon of the *subscapularis,* although separated from the capsule, protects the joint anteriorly. These four muscles, which attach close to the joint into the greater and lesser tubercles of the humerus, are called the *rotator cuff* muscles. The rotator cuff muscles play an intricate part in shoulder motions. The supraspinatus is essential for normal shoulder abduction; the teres minor, infraspinatus, and subscapularis depress the head of the humerus in the glenoid; and the teres minor and infraspinatus externally rotate the glenohumeral joint during shoulder flexion and abduction. When these muscles cannot perform their precise functions owing to fatigue or weakness, repetitive impingement of suprahumeral joint tissues occurs as the head of the humerus strikes the acromion process and the coracoacromial ligament. This acute injury, which is usually labeled as "bursitis," is common in the weekend painter who is tired but just wants to finish out the last bit of paint or to the end of the room.

An equally important function of the rotator cuff muscles is the prevention of glenohumeral joint subluxation in the erect position or when carrying a load in the hand (Basmajian, 1978). It was once thought that the vertical lines of pull of the deltoid, triceps, and biceps brachii stabilized the humerus to the scapula. These muscles, however, have been found to be electromyographically silent even with heavy pulls and loads of 25 lb (11 kg) in the hand (Basmajian, 1978; Bearn, 1961). Instead, electromyographic activity is found in the more horizontally directed muscles such as the supraspinatus and infraspinatus; with the absence of a load in the hand, there may not be any electromyographic activity of the muscles crossing the glenohumeral joint.

The theory for this remarkable mechanism is based on the principle of the force needed to keep a ball (head of the humerus) on an inclined plane (glenoid fossa). In the schematic illustration (Fig. 7-25, A), the weight of the ball (W) can be maintained in equilibrium by an equal and opposite vertical force Q. If, however, the force Q is directed more horizontally (Fig. 7-25, B, C), the ball is compressed against the plane by the resultant of the two forces (composition of forces). Since electromyographic activity is absent in vertically directed muscles and present in horizontally directed muscles, it appears that the body maintains coaptation (L. co-, together, plus *apere*, to bind or join) of the glenohumeral joint by horizontal forces. In the erect position without a load in the hand, the horizontal forces of the capsule and coracohumeral ligaments prevent descent of the head of the humerus (Basmajian, 1978). When a load is held in the hand, the horizontally directed muscles (rotator cuff) contract to stabilize the humeral head against the glenoid. With weakness or paralysis of the upper trapezieus, the scapula assumes a downwardly rotated posture and the glenoid fossa becomes vertical (Fig. 7-25, D). The angle between W and Q becomes larger (relative abduction), and compared with Figure 7-25, C, the resultant force becomes less. This force may not be sufficient to maintain coaptation of the joint, and in time subluxation of the glenohumeral joint may occur.

LATISSIMUS DORSI AS AN ELEVATOR OF THE PELVIS

The latissimus dorsi is attached, in part, to the crest of the ilium. When the arms are stabilized as in pushing down on crutch handles, this muscle aids in lifting the pelvis so that the foot clears the ground in walking. This function is of particular importance to the paraplegic patient, whose lower extremity muscles, including the hip-hikers, are paralyzed owing to an injury of the spinal cord. It should be recalled that the latissimus dorsi is innervated by the thoracodorsal nerve, derived from C6, C7, and C8, and therefore is not involved in injuries to the spinal cord below C8.

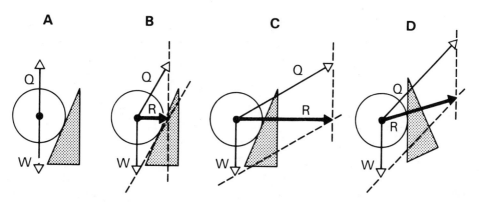

FIGURE 7-25. Schematic diagram to illustrate the mechanism thought to hold the head of the humerus (ball) on the glenoid fossa (inclined plane) at the shoulder. W = weight of the arm; Q = force required to counteract the weight of the arm; R = resultant of Q and W (composition of forces). See text for explanation.

SYNERGISM AND ANTAGONISM OF SHOULDER MUSCLES

Previous discussions in this section indicate that muscles and muscle groups of the shoulder region (as elsewhere) can combine their actions in many different ways. In other words, two muscles acting on the scapula (or the shoulder joint) in opposite directions are antagonistic for a particular movement only—they may act as synergists in other combinations. For example:

The *trapezius and serratus anterior* act as synergists in upward rotation of the scapula, but as antagonists in retraction and protraction of the shoulder girdle.

The *trapezius and rhomboids* act as synergists in retraction of the shoulder girdle, but as antagonists in upward and downward rotation of the shoulder blade.

The *upper and lower portions of the trapezius* act synergically in upward rotation of the scapula, but antagonistically in elevation and depression of the shoulder girdle.

The *anterior and posterior portions of the deltoid* act synergically in abduction of the arm in the frontal plane, the flexor component of the anterior deltoid being balanced by the extensor component of the posterior deltoid. The two portions of the muscle act antagonistically in flexion and extension, as in swinging the arm forward and backward in the sagittal plane.

The *subscapularis and the infraspinatus* act together to depress the head of the humerus in shoulder abduction, but they are antagonistic as far as internal and external rotation of the shoulder is concerned.

CHAPTER 8

HIP AND
PELVIC REGION

The pelvis (L., a basin) consists of the *sacrum, coccyx*, and the two *innominate bones,* which are formed by a fusion of the ilium, ischium, and pubis. The pelvic basin, or pelvic girdle, provides support and protection to the abdominal organs and transmits forces from the head, arms, and trunk to the lower extremities. Seven joints are formed by the pelvic bones: *lumbo-sacral, sacro-iliac* (two), *sacro-coccygeal, symphysis pubis,* and the *hip* (two). While motions at the sacro-iliac, symphysis pubis, and sacro-coccygeal joints are small, the ability to have movement at these joints is very important. These joints are subject to injury, and they may become hypomobile or hypermobile with resulting pain and dysfunction. These joints also play an important role in permitting childbirth.

The hip joint (acetabulo-femoral) is the most structurally stable, yet mobile, single joint in the body. In addition to transmitting large forces between the trunk and the ground, the hip region is a major component of the locomotor system; it participates in elevating and lowering the body, as in climbing or rising from a chair; and it is important in bringing the foot toward the body or hands, as in putting on a shoe. With every step, the hip abductor muscles (on the stance leg) must create a force to balance about 85 percent of the body weight (head, arms, trunk, and opposite leg). The hip joint serves as the fulcrum in this system and therefore sustains more than twice the body weight with each step.

Palpable Structures

Palpation may conveniently begin by placing the thumbs laterally on the *crests of the ilia,* one on the right and one on the left side. Under normal conditions, these two points are level in the standing position. Clinically, a lateral tilt of the pelvis is discovered by checking the height of the crests of the ilia. The symmetry of the pelvis may also be checked from the front by placing the thumbs on the *anterior superior spines of the ilia* which, in most individuals, are easily located, often being visible under the skin. In obese individuals, it may be best to start palpation on the crests of the ilia laterally, and to follow the downward curve of the crests anteriorly until the anterior superior spines are located.

If the crests are followed in a posterior direction, the *posterior superior spines of the ilia* are located. The subject in Figure 8-1 is palpating them with the thumbs. These prominences are broader and sturdier than the anterior spines and feel rough under the palpating fingers. Below each posterior spine is a depression, which is the posterior landmark for the *sacro-iliac joint.*

To locate the *greater trochanter of the femur,* the subject places the thumb on the crest of the ilium laterally and reaches down on the thigh as far as possible with the middle finger. The greater trochanter is a large bony prominence, over which the fingers may slide from side to side and upward and downward. If the subject stands on the opposite leg and the examiner passively rotates the femur, the greater trochanter can be palpated with more certainty. In the standing position, the height of the greater trochanter should be the same for both legs.

Other points on the pelvis, such as the pubic symphysis, the rami of the pubic bones, and the rami of the ischia, may also be palpated, at least in part. The *tuberosities of the ischia* (the "sit bones") are easy to locate when the subject is sitting on a hard chair or when the subject is lying on the side with hips and knees flexed. Once located in these positions, the tuberosities should also be palpated in the standing position. They are then approached below the gluteal fold and are best palpated when the gluteus maximus and the hamstrings are relaxed. Such relaxation is achieved by having the subject standing in front of a table or in parallel bars. The subject bends forward at the waist and flexes the hips while supporting the weight of the trunk on the hands. The ischial tuberosities can be palpated when the hips are flexed and then followed as the subject returns to the erect posture by pushing the trunk up with the arms. This technique of palpation is used clinically to determine the relationship of the ischial tuberosities to the posterior brim of a prosthesis or the thigh cuff of an orthosis.

Nonpalpable Structures

A disarticulated set of bones and anatomic atlases should be used to identify the articulating surfaces of the *sacro-iliac joint;* the *acetabulum* (L. a shallow vinegar vessel or cup), the socket of the hip joint, into which the head of the femur fits; the *posterior, anterior, and inferior gluteal lines* on the outer surface of the ilium, which separate the areas of attachment of the three gluteal muscles; the *anterior inferior iliac spine,* located below the superior spine and separated from it by a notch; the *posterior inferior iliac spine;* the *greater sciatic notch;* the *spine of the ischium;* the *head and neck of the femur;* and the *lesser trochanter of the femur.*

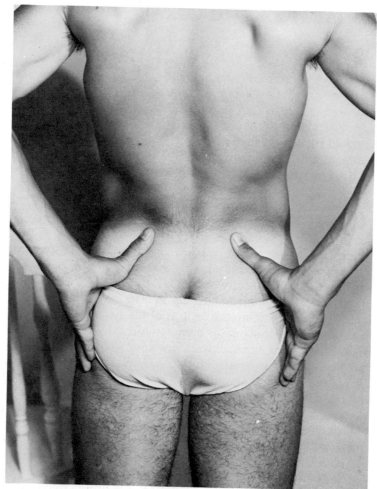

FIGURE 8-1. The subject's thumbs are palpating the posterior superior spines of the ilia. The spines are best located by following the crests of the ilia in a posterior direction.

The sacrum and the innominate bone have extensive and strong ligamentous connections including the *anterior and posterior sacro-iliac, sacro-spinous (ischium), and sacro-tuberous (ischium) ligaments*. The acetabulum is deepened by the fibrocartilaginous labrum, which further surrounds the head of the femur and assists in holding it in the acetabulum. The strong ilio-femoral ligament lies on the anterior side of the hip joint. This ligament is frequently called the *Y ligament* because it resembles an inverted Y as it courses from the lower aspect of the anterior inferior iliac spine and spreads to attach along the intertrochanteric line of the femur. The Y ligament severely limits hyperextension of the hip joint (0 to 10 degrees). Medially, the joint is covered by the *pubo-femoral ligament* and posteriorly by the *ischio-femoral ligament*. The ischio-femoral ligament strongly reinforces the joint capsule and the fibers are twisted so that hip flexion is free but medial rotation is limited (Kapandji, 1970b).

HIP JOINT (ARTICULATIO COXAE)

Type of Joint

The hip joint is the best example of a ball-and-socket joint in the human body. The joint surfaces of the head of the femur and the acetabulum correspond better to each other and have firmer connections than the joint surfaces of the glenohumeral joint. This promotes stability but limits range of motion. The hip joint has three degrees of freedom of motion: *flexion-extension*, *abduction-adduction*, and *internal-external rotation*. In most activities, combinations of these three types of movements occur, and hip motions are accompanied by movements of the lumbar spine for total mobility.

Axes of Motion

At the hip joint, movement may take place about any number of axes, all passing through the center of the femoral head; but for descriptive purposes, three axes perpendicular to each other are usually chosen.

In standing, the *axis for flexion and extension is transverse* (horizontal, in a side-to-side direction). A line connecting the centers of the two femoral heads is called the *common hip axis*. Movement about the common hip axis takes place when, for example, the pelvis rocks forward and backward in standing or when, in a back-lying position, both knees are pulled up toward the chest. Unilateral hip flexion with the knee flexed can be carried out until the thigh contacts the anterior surface of the trunk. When the knee is extended, hamstrings muscle length limits hip flexion to 70 to 90 degrees. Hyperextension of the hip is limited to 0 to 10 degrees by the ilio-femoral ligament. As further motion is attempted, the lumbar vertebrae extend (lordosis) and may give a misleading impression of the amount of true hip extension present.

The axis for *abduction and adduction* (in standing) is *horizontal*, in a front-to-back direction. The limb may move in relation to the pelvis, as in lifting the limb laterally, or the pelvis may move in relation to the limb, as in inclining the trunk to the side of the stance leg (see Fig. 1-3). In each instance, whether the limb or the pelvis moves, the correct term to use is abduction or adduction of the hip. Hip abduction is approximately 45 degrees (see Appendix B) and is usually accompanied by elevation of the pelvis (hip hiking). Hip adduction is frequently given as contact of the two legs or 0 degrees. The legs may be crossed, however, to adducted positions of 30 to 40 degrees. While this is not pure planar motion (since one hip must be in flexion and the other in extension), it is an important motion in running and turning and crossing the thighs.

The *axis for internal and external rotation* (in standing) is *vertical* and this axis is identical with the mechanical axis of the femur (Fig. 8-2). In internal rotation, the greater trochanter moves forward in relation to the front part of the pelvis or, conversely, the front part of the pelvis moves toward the greater trochanter. External rotation is a movement in the opposite direction. When the knee is flexed to 90 degrees, hip rotation can be observed by the motion of the tibia from the neutral position.

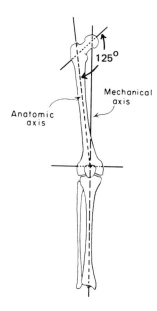

FIGURE 8-2. The anatomic and the mechanical axes of the femur.

External rotation in the adult is approximately 40 to 45 degrees, and internal rotation is usually less (30 to 35 degrees).

ANATOMIC AND MECHANICAL AXES OF FEMUR

The *anatomic axis* of the femur is represented by a line through the femoral shaft (see Fig. 8-2). However, the *mechanical axis* is represented by a line connecting the centers of the hip and knee joints. In the erect position, the mechanical axis is usually vertical. The neck of the femur forms an angle of approximately 125 degrees with the anatomic axis of the femur.

Deformities of Femur at the Hip

Coxa vara is a pathologic condition characterized by a decrease in the neck-shaft angle of the femur (see Fig. 8-2) so that this angle becomes smaller than 125 degrees, that is, approaches 90 degrees. As a result, there is an overall shortening of the limb.

Coxa valga presents the opposite changes, that is, an increase in the size of the neck-shaft angle which becomes larger than 125 degrees, resulting in a lengthening of the limb.

Coxa plana is caused by a pathologic condition (osteochondritis) resulting in a flattening of the spheric surface of the femoral head, a deformity that occurs mainly in children.

MUSCLES

Posterior Muscles

The posterior muscles are the gluteus maximus; the biceps femoris, the semitendinosus, and the semimembranosus (collectively called the hamstrings); and the posterior portion of the adductor magnus. In addition, there is a deeply located group consisting of six small muscles, all external rotators of the hip.

Gluteus Maximus

The *gluteus maximus* (Gr. *gloutos*, buttock) is the large, superficial muscle that is responsible for the roundness of the buttock region. *Proximal attachment:* Posterior portion of the crest of the ilium, lumbo-dorsal fascia, parts of the sacrum and coccyx, and sacro-tuberous ligament. The fibers take a downward and lateral course and have their *distal attachments* (1) into the iliotibial tract and (2) into the gluteal tuberosity of the shaft of the femur, on the posterior aspect of the femur. *Innervation:* Inferior gluteal nerve.

INSPECTION AND PALPATION. The gluteus maximus may be observed when the subject is prone or standing erect. Like the quadriceps, it can be tightened by simply "setting" it without any joint motion being carried out. For stronger activation of the muscle, the hip is extended and externally rotated (Fig. 8-3), in which case the muscle acts in its two functions simultaneously. If palpated when the limb is in this potition, the muscle feels very firm. Strong contraction of the gluteus maximus may also be observed in climbing stairs and in running and jumping.

Hamstrings

The *hamstrings* have their proximal attachments on the ischial tuberosity and their distal attachments on the proximal shaft of the tibia (see Chapter 9 for more details). They should now be observed and palpated in their function as hip extensors.

PALPATION IN PRONE POSITION. If the hip is extended and simultaneously internally rotated (Fig. 8-4), the hamstrings and part of the adductor magnus, all with attachments on the tuberosity of the ischium, may be felt contracting while the gluteus maximus, at least in part, ceases contracting. Note that this inner extensor group of muscles cannot raise the limb as high as when the gluteus maximus participates in the movement. The shift from one muscle group to the other should be observed by maintaining the hip extended while alternating internal rotation with external rotation.

PALPATION IN STANDING ERECT. In standing, the hamstrings may be palpated close to their proximal attachments on the ischial tuberosity. First, the subject inclines the trunk somewhat backward so that the center-of-gravity line of the upper part of the

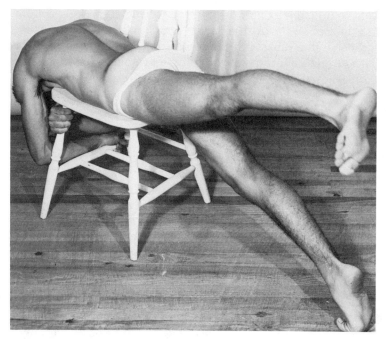

FIGURE 8-3. The gluteus maximus is strongly activated when the hip is extended and externally rotated.

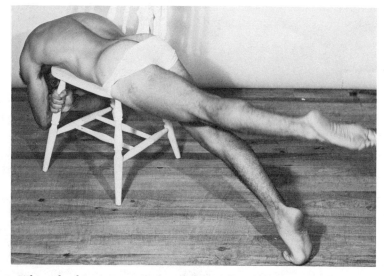

FIGURE 8-4. When the hip is extended and internally rotated, the inner extensor group of muscles contracts while the gluteus maximus markedly decreases its contraction.

body falls well behind the axis of the hip joint. This secures relaxation of the hip extensors, and the ischial tuberosities may then be palpated more easily. The finger tips are placed below the tuberosities, but close to them, and as deeply as the tissue will allow. The subject now reverses the trunk movement, that is, inclines the trunk slightly forward. The instant the center-of-gravity line passes anterior to the common hip axis, a contraction of the hamstrings, acting as hip extensors, is felt. By swaying the trunk slightly forward and backward, alternating contraction and relaxation of these muscles are brought about.

When the same trunk movements are repeated while the buttocks are being palpated, very little, if any, contraction of the gluteus maximus can be detected. The hamstrings, rather than the gluteus maximus, appear to be used in small-range antero-posterior balance of the pelvis. On the other hand, if a large range of hip flexion is performed by inclining the trunk forward and then quickly returning the trunk to the erect position, a strong contraction of the gluteus maximus may be felt. These clinical observations have been substantiated by electromyography (Joseph, 1960).

The *six external rotators* are small muscles, located in the posterior gluteal region and covered by the gluteus maximus. They have *proximal attachments* both inside and outside the pelvis, have a more or less horizontal direction, and have *distal attachments* in the region of the greater trochanter in such a fashion that they have an external rotary action at the hip.

The uppermost of the six external rotators is the *piriformis*; the lowermost is the *quadratus femoris*; these two can be palpated with fair accuracy. Palpation of the piriformis will be described with that of the lateral group with which this muscle is closely associated. The quadratus femoris is palpated in the area between the tuberosity of the ischium and the greater trochanter, and it may be felt contracting when the hip is externally rotated. The other four, the *gemellus superior*, the *gemellus inferior*, the *obturator internus*, and *obturator externus* are located between the piriformis and the quadratus femoris. They can be palpated as a group but not very well individually.

Anterior Muscles

This group of muscles includes the *rectus femoris*, the *sartorius*, the *tensor fasciae latae*, the *iliopsoas*, and the *pectineus*. The tensor has an antero-lateral location, and the pectineus has an antero-medial location.

Rectus Femoris and Sartorius

The proximal attachment of the *rectus femoris* on the anterior inferior spine of the ilium of the acetabulum and its distal attachment on the patella will be described in Chapter 9. *Palpation of its proximal attachment as the muscle acts in flexion of the hip will be described under the tensor fasciae latae.*

The *sartorius* (L. *sartor*, a tailor) is a superficial, band-like muscle extending obliquely down the thigh from the anterior to the medial side of the thigh. *Proximal attachment:* Anterior superior spine of the ilium. *Distal attachment:* Medial surface of the tibia close to the crest of the tibia (anterior to the distal attachments of the gracilis and semitendinosus tendons). *Innervation:* Femoral nerve.

INSPECTION AND PALPATION. When the hip is flexed and externally rotated, the sartorius may be observed and palpated from its proximal attachment down almost to its distal attachment (Fig. 8-5). In many subjects, the lower portion of the muscle cannot be well observed but may be followed by palpation if the subject alternately contracts and relaxes the muscle. This is best accomplished if the examiner carries the weight of the limb with the hip flexed and externally rotated and the knee flexed (muscle relaxed), then asks the subject to hold the limb in position actively (muscle contracts).

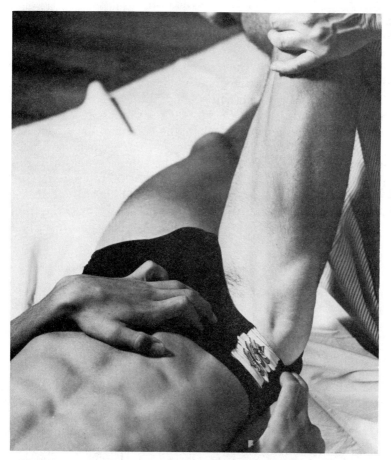

FIGURE 8-5. Near the hip (flexed and externally rotated), the sartorius and the tensor form a V, the sartorius taking a medial direction, the tensor a lateral direction. The tendon of the rectus femoris may be palpated in the V between the other two muscles. The muscular portion of the rectus is seen further down the thigh.

The perpendicular distance from the axis for flexion and extension of the hip to the line of action of the sartorius is considerable. Therefore, even though the muscle's cross section is relatively small, it can exert a comparatively large torque. Note that, as the muscle contracts, it rises from the underlying structures, and this mechanically enhances its action. Because of its great length, the sartorius muscle can shorten a long distance.

The sartorius is a two-joint muscle, passing on the flexor side of the knee where it is in close relation to the tendons of the gracilis and the semitendinosus muscles.

Tensor Fasciae Latae

The *tensor fasciae latae,* like the sartorius, has effects both on the hip and the knee. *Proximal attachment:* Crest of the ilium and adjacent structures, laterally to the *proximal attachment* of the sartorius. *Distal attachment:* Ilio-tibial tract, about one third of the way down the thigh. *Innervation:* Branch of the superior gluteal nerve.

INSPECTION AND PALPATION. The tensor fasciae latae is palpated near the hip, but more laterally than the upper portion of the sartorius. A strong contraction is brought out by resisting flexion of the internally rotated hip (Fig. 8-6). The relation of the tensor to the sartorius and the rectus femoris is seen in Figure 8-5. The tensor forms the lateral border of the V-shaped area where the tendon of the rectus femoris is palpated. The relation of the tensor to the anterior portion of the gluteus medius should be noted—the two muscles lie side by side in the antero-lateral hip region.

The *ilio-tibial tract* extends on the lateral side of the thigh, from the ilium above to the tibia below. The gluteus maximus and the tensor both have their distal attachment to this tract, the gluteus maximus from behind, the tensor from the front. The ilio-tibial tract is seen in Figure 9-6 as it approaches its distal attachment on the tibia.

Iliopsoas

The *iliopsoas* consists of two parts, the *iliacus* and the *psoas major,* which have separate *proximal attachments* but a common *distal attachment.* That portion of the iliopsoas which lies below the hip joint is located medial to, and is partially covered by, the upper portion of the sartorius.

The *iliacus* has *proximal attachments* on the iliac fossa and the inner sides of the anterior spines of the ilium. The muscle covers the anterior side of the hip joint and the femoral neck. It winds around the neck in a medial and posterior direction and has its *distal attachment* on the lesser trochanter of the femur. *Innervation:* Branches of the femoral nerve.

The *psoas major* (Gr. *psoa,* the loins) is located in the posterior wall of the abdominal cavity, close to the lumbar vertebrae and the ilium. *Proximal attachment:* Vertebral bodies, intervertebral disks, and transverse processes of T12 to L5. The muscle fibers form a round, rather long belly that lies medial to the iliacus. *Distal attachment:* Lesser trochanter of the femur. *Innervation:* By branches directly from the lumbar plexus.

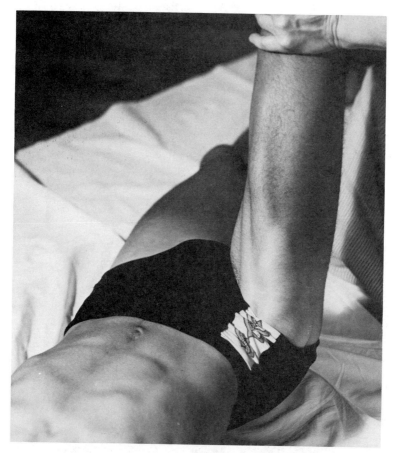

FIGURE 8-6. The tensor fasciae latae is seen contracting as resistance is given to flexion of the internally rotated hip. The rectus femoris and the sartorius are also seen.

PALPATION OF THE ILIACUS AND PSOAS MAJOR. The *iliacus* is difficult to palpate since it lies behind the abdominal viscera and is rather flat. It follows, and partly fills out, the iliac fossa.

The *psoas major*, in spite of its deep location, may be palpated as follows: In the sitting position, the subject inclines the trunk slightly forward to secure relaxation of the abdominal muscles. The palpating fingers are placed at the waist, between the lower ribs and the crest of the ilium, and with gentle pressure are made to sink in as deeply as possible toward the posterior wall of the abdominal cavity, near the vertebral column. In some subjects, this meets with no difficulty. The subject now flexes the hip, raising the foot just off the floor (Fig. 8-7), and the round firm belly of the psoas major may be felt as the muscle contracts.

It is suggested that the student first palpate the psoas major on oneself before attempting to do so on another person. Palpation is best done if the bowels are fairly empty and should not be attempted if it causes discomfort.

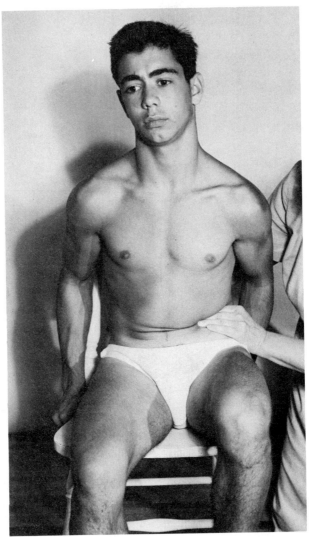

FIGURE 8-7. Palpation of psoas major. If the subject's abdominal muscles are relaxed, the examiner may place the palpating fingers deep enough to feel the contraction of the psoas major when the subject lifts the foot off the floor, flexing the hip beyond 90 degrees.

Pectineus

The *pectineus* is a rather flat muscle bordering laterally to the iliopsoas and medially to the adductor longus. *Proximal attachment:* Superior ramus of the pubic bone and neighboring structures. *Distal attachment:* Along a line (pectineal line) on the upper postero-medial aspect of the femur, below the lesser trochanter. The area of the distal attachment of this muscle is approximately as wide as its proximal attachment, giving the muscle a quadrangular shape. *Innervation:* Femoral nerve.

The pectineus belongs essentially to the adductor group of muscles, its fibers running approximately parallel to those of the adductor longus. *Palpation* of the pectineus as a separate muscle is difficult, but it may be felt contracting together with other muscles. It is suggested that the student palpate this muscle on oneself, as follows: In the sitting position, the palpating fingers are placed in the crotch where some of the adductor tendons can be grasped from front to back. The hip is now flexed further with adduction and external rotation, and the motion is continued until the legs are crossed. The tendon of the adductor longus is prominent and easily recognized; the pectineus lies just lateral to the adductor longus.

Lateral Muscles

The muscles of this group—the *gluteus medius*, the *gluteus minimus*, the *tensor fasciae latae*, and the *piriformis*—are located laterally, on the abductor side of the hip. The tensor, described with the flexors, lies antero-laterally and the piriformis postero-laterally.

Gluteus Medius

The *gluteus medius* is the largest of the lateral hip muscles. It is covered, in part, by the gluteus maximus and by the tensor, but its upper middle portion is superficial, covered only by thick fascia. *Proximal attachment:* In a fan-shaped fashion from the crest of the ilium and from a large area on the outer surface of the ilium, as far down as the anterior gluteal line, a line which separates its origin from that of the gluteus minimus. From this wide proximal attachment, the fibers converge to have their *distal attachment* on the greater trochanter, near its tip. This muscle, like the deltoid in the upper limb, has anterior, middle, and posterior portions, but these portions are not clearly separated from each other. The posterior portion is comparatively small and supplemented by the piriformis muscle. *Innervation:* Superior gluteal nerve.

INSPECTION AND PALPATION. The *middle portion* of the gluteus medius is palpated laterally below the crest of the ilium when the hip is abducted, either in the side-lying position (subject lying on the side opposite to the muscle palpated), or in the standing position (Fig. 8-8). In the illustration, the subject is standing on the left foot while abducting the right hip by raising the limb laterally.

The *anterior portion* is palpated when the hip is internally rotated either in the supine position or in standing. This portion lies close to the tensor fasciae latae and acts together with the tensor in internal rotation. If the posterior margin of the tensor is first identified by the tests previously described, the gluteus medius may be palpated posterior to the tensor. The two muscles may also be identified by making them alternately contract and relax and by following the palpated muscle distally. If the muscle takes a direction toward the greater trochanter, it is the anterior portion of the gluteus medius; if the muscle takes a more anterior course, it is the tensor fasciae latae.

In palpating the anterior portion of the gluteus medius, it should be remembered that the gluteus minimus, which is covered by the medius, also participates in inter-

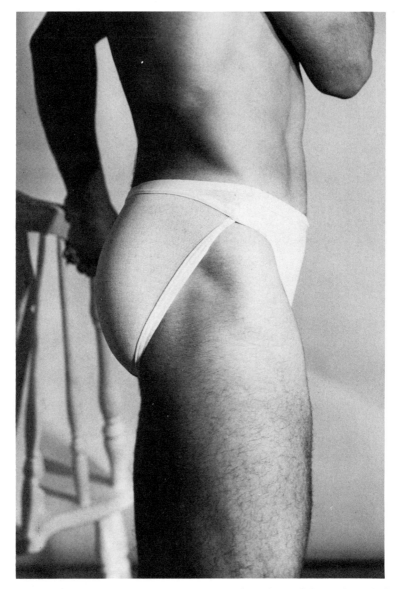

FIGURE 8-8. The gluteus medius is seen contracting as the subject abducts the right hip, raising the right foot off the floor.

nal rotation and that the muscle tissue palpated represents the combined contraction of the two muscles.

The *posterior portion* of the gluteus medius is palpated in back of the middle portion when the hip is abducted. A part of the posterior portion is seen in Figure 8-8. This portion contracts strongly if the hip is abducted and externally rotated at the same time. However, with external rotation, other muscles in this region become active, so that the gluteus medius cannot be palpated in an isolated fashion.

The entire gluteus medius may also be felt as it contracts in supporting body weight on one leg, palpation being carried out on the side of the stance leg. In this case, the gluteus medius furnishes lateral stabilization of the pelvis to *prevent dropping of the pelvis on the opposite side.* This is the *most important function of the gluteus medius.*

Piriformis

The *piriformis*, the pear-shaped muscle (L. *pirum*, pear), belongs to the second layer of muscles in this region, as does the gluteus medius, both of which are covered here by the gluteus maximus. *Proximal attachment:* Ventral surface of the sacrum, sciatic notch, and sacro-tuberous ligament. The fibers take a downward-lateral course, following the posterior border of the gluteus medius to have their *distal attachment* on the inner portion of the greater trochanter. *Innervation:* A branch derived directly from the first and second sacral nerves.

PALPATION. The muscle is palpated in external rotation, especially if the gluteus maximus is relaxed as when the limb is raised slightly forward. The palpating fingers are placed posterior to the greater trochanter and moved about somewhat until the best spot for palpation is located.

In palpating the piriformis, its close association with the posterior portion of the gluteus medius, in regard to location and action, should be kept in mind. The two muscles are likely to be felt contracting simultaneously.

Gluteus Minimus

The *gluteus minimus* belongs to the third and deepest layer of the muscles in the gluteal region. It lies close to the capsule of the hip joint and is covered by the gluteus medius. *Proximal attachment:* Fan-shaped, from the outer surface of the ilium, between the anterior and inferior gluteal lines, and from the septum between it and the medius. *Distal attachment:* Anterior border of the greater trochanter of the femur. *Innervation:* Superior gluteal nerve.

PALPATION. The gluteus minimus muscle cannot be very well differentiated from the medius since both muscles contract simultaneously in abduction and internal rotation. The anterior portion of the muscle is the thickest part and is felt, together with the medius, when the hip is internally rotated.

Medial Muscles (Adductor Group)

The adductor group is identified as the large muscular mass of the medial thigh, bordering anteriorly to the vastus medialis and the sartorius (see Fig. 8-5), posteriorly to the hamstrings. This group comprises the following muscles: *adductor magnus, adductor longus, adductor gracilis, adductor brevis,* and *pectineus.* The obturator externus, the quadratus femoris, and the lower portion of the gluteus maximus also are capable of adducting the hip but do not belong to the adductor group proper.

From the functional standpoint, it is not necessary to study the exact location of attachments of individual muscles of the adductor group. In general, these muscles have proximal attachments on the rami of the pubes and the rami of the ischia and distal attachments posteriorly on the linea aspera of the femoral shaft. The line of action of these muscles in relation to the axis changes when the hip flexes, so that the action of each muscle can be determined only for a specific position of the joint.

The *nerve supply* to the adductor group is mainly from the obturator nerve. The adductor magnus, however, is innervated by a branch from the sciatic nerve as well as by a branch from the obturator nerve, and the pectineus is supplied by the femoral nerve.

FUNCTION OF MUSCLES ACTING AT THE HIP

Weight-Bearing and Non-Weight-Bearing Functions of Hip Muscles

In the lower extremities, muscles must be studied in both non-weight-bearing and weight-bearing situations. Non-weight-bearing, or open chain, actions are important in the understanding of movements that can be produced by the muscles in the free extremity, limitations of motion produced by tightness or passive insufficiency of muscles, and positions used to elicit isolated contractions of muscles. Perhaps more important are the weight-bearing, or closed kinematic chain, functions such as standing on one leg, climbing, rising up from a chair, or performing a sit-up. In these activities, the muscles of the lower extremity are required to perform forceful contractions upon the fixed distal extremity (sometimes called reversed actions). Slight to moderate weakness of the muscles will be reflected by a decreased ability to perform closed chain functions, while unresisted open chain motions may still appear unimpaired.

PORTIONS OF A MUSCLE MAY HAVE DIFFERENT ACTIONS

Muscles such as the gluteus maximus and the gluteus medius cover large areas so that one portion of the muscle may be capable of an action different from another portion. Each of these muscles, however, has a main action that is shared by all portions of the muscle. The action of the gluteus maximus is extension, and that of the gluteus medius is abduction. The upper portion of the maximus is located so that it acts in abduction; the location of the lower portion permits action as an adductor. The anterior portion of the medius is located well for internal rotation, while its posterior portion acts in external rotation.

CHANGE OF ACTION DUE TO JOINT ANGLE

The leverage of the muscles of the hip about the three axes changes with the joint angle so that the effectiveness (torque) of a muscle, for a certain motion, may increase or decrease. These leverage changes are commonly found in the hip because of the large range of motion and the relative long distances of the muscle force arms (perpendicular distance from the line of pull of the muscle to the axis of joint motion). The gluteus medius and the tensor fasciae latae are considered internal rotators of the extended hip, but their leverage for internal rotation increases when the hip is flexed to 90 degrees. In some positions of the hip, the line of pull of a muscle may change so markedly (i.e., from a position anterior to the axis of motion to one in which it is posterior to the axis) that the muscle can perform antagonistic muscle actions (Steindler, 1955). The piriformis is an external rotator when the hip is extended, but the same muscle becomes an internal rotator when the hip is flexed (Steindler, 1955; Kapandji, 1970b). The best example of inversion of action occurs in the hip adductors. The line of pull of the muscles is anterior to the hip joint axis when the hip is in extension and posterior to the joint axis when the hip is in flexion. When the hip is in a position of flexion, as in climbing, the hip adductors are forceful hip extensors; and when the hip is extended, the adductors are flexors. The change from flexor to extensor action varies with the individual muscles between 50 and 70 degrees of hip flexion (Steindler, 1955).

Two-Joint Muscles Acting at the Hip

The hip muscles are either one-joint muscles acting at the hip only, or they pass two or more joints and have actions, or potential actions, over all these joints.

LENGTH-TENSION RELATIONS

The efficiency of a two-joint muscle is substantially influenced by the positions of the two joints, in accordance with the laws governing length-tension relations of muscle (see Chapter 4). Therefore, the *rectus femoris* is more effective as a hip flexor if the knee flexes simultaneously with the hip, because this permits the muscle to contract within a favorable range. For the same reason, the rectus is more efficient as a knee extensor if the hip extends simultaneously with the knee. The *hamstrings* are more efficient as hip extensors when the knee extends simultaneously with the hip; the hamstrings are more efficient as knee flexors when the hip flexes simultaneously with the knee.

Muscles Acting in Flexion of the Hip

HIP FLEXION IN ERECT STANDING. When a subject is standing with one hip flexed, that is, the knee pulled up toward the chest, it may be ascertained by palpation that the iliopsoas, the rectus femoris, the sartorius, and the tensor spring into action. The internal rotary action of the tensor appears to be compensated by the external rotary action of the sartorius, and the knee extensor action of the rectus appears to be checked by gravity and perhaps also by the action of some of the knee flexors. Both internal and external rotary actions have been ascribed to the iliopsoas, but for all practical purposes, this muscle should be considered as a pure flexor. The combined action of the iliopsoas, rectus femoris, sartorius, and tensor muscles (in proper proportion) results in pure flexion. The adductor muscles also act in hip flexion in the early part of the motion, and particularly when resistance is applied. Maximum isometric torque of the hip flexors is greatest when the muscles are stretched (hip is extended) and decreases with hip flexion (see Fig. 4-10).

HIP FLEXION IN SITTING POSITION. Since, in the sitting position, the hip is already flexed to about 90 degrees, additional flexion necessitates actions by the hip flexors in the shortened range of their excursion. When flexion to an acute hip angle is carried out, the sartorius and the tensor can be felt contracting strongly, but in this range these muscles have lost much of their ability to develop tension and are incapable of carrying out the motion without the aid of the iliopsoas. In fact, as may be concluded from observation of patients with isolated paralysis of the iliopsoas, this is the only hip flexor that can produce enough tension to flex the hip beyond 90 degrees in the sitting position. These patients can flex the hip sufficiently to walk, but when sitting, they must use their hands to lift and move the leg.

In the sitting position, the hip flexors—in particular, the iliopsoas—control the vertebrae and pelvis on the femur as the person leans back and returns to the upright position. If the iliopsoas muscles are paralyzed bilaterally, the subject will fall backward as soon as the center-of-gravity line of the head, arms, and trunk (HAT) falls behind the hip joint axis. Thus, paraplegic patients must use hand support to prevent falling over backward when sitting without a back rest.

A general principle, which may be confirmed by observing the postural adjustments made by patients with paralysis of muscles ordinarily engaged in balancing the body or body segments, is that in the erect position—sitting or standing—*the trunk tends to incline toward the weak or paralyzed muscles.*

A study of the actions of the hip flexors must also include an analysis of muscle action in sit-ups, and in raising one or both legs in the supine position. In these activities, the abdominal muscles act synergically with the hip flexors to furnish the necessary fixation to the pelvis and vertebrae. In the sit-up, the neck flexors and abdominal muscles perform concentric contractions until the trunk is flexed (scapula clears the surface), and then they maintain isometric contractions while the *iliopsoas* becomes the prime mover to raise the trunk and pelvis on the fixed femur. The torque produced by the head, arms, and trunk (HAT) is great and, in turn, requires that the iliopsoas muscles produce large forces. If the abdominal muscles are not strong enough to maintain lumbar flexion, the great force of the psoas major pulls the lumbar spine into hyperextension (lordosis). Repetitive performance can lead to microtrauma and back problems. Patients with back injuries should neither perform sit-ups as an exercise nor use the maneuver to rise from the supine position (Kendall et al, 1952). Rather, they should be taught to turn on the side and push up using the arms.

Straight leg raising, and in particular bilateral straight leg raising, creates similar forces on the lumbar vertebrae. In Figure 2-24, the torque to initiate unilateral straight leg raising is 360 inch-lb (30 ft-lb). Since the force arm distance for the iliopsoas is less than 1 inch, it can be appreciated that the muscle force will be great. Leg raising, therefore, should not be performed unless the subject's abdominal muscles are of sufficient strength to maintain the lumbar area in contact with the supporting surface (back flat).

Muscles Acting in Extension of the Hip

Five important muscles pass behind the axis for flexion and extension of the hip and serve as extensors in all positions of the joint, namely the *gluteus maximus*, the *biceps femoris* (long head), the *semimembranosus*, the *semitendinosus*, and the *adductors* (when the hip is in flexion). When the hip is flexed, as when the trunk is inclined forward in standing, the ischial tuberosities are carried backward in relation to the hip axis, and this improves the leverage of those extensor muscles that are attached to the tuberosities.

The hip extensors should be observed and palpated both when the lower extremities move in relation to the trunk and when the trunk moves in relation to the lower extremities. In many activities, both segments move simultaneously.

PRONE-LYING UNILATERAL HIP EXTENSION WITH KNEE EXTENDED. Palpation of the gluteus maximus and the inner extensor group in the prone position has already been described. To obtain a larger range of motion than seen in Figures 8-3 and 8-4, the subject should be prone on a table with the hips flexed over the edge of the table. A range of about 90 degrees in hip extension may then be observed. The changing muscular requirements when external or internal rotation is carried out simultaneously should again be observed: increased activity of the gluteus maximus in external rotation, decreased activity of the gluteus maximus in internal rotation, and increased activity of the inner extensor group in internal rotation.

PRONE-LYING UNILATERAL HIP EXTENSION WITH KNEE FLEXED. When the hamstrings are palpated in hip extension while the knee is flexed, they can be felt "bunching up," that is, they become short and thick. In this movement combination, length-tension relations are most unfavorable, and the muscles may come close to, or arrive at, the point of active insufficiency. Subjectively, an uncomfortable cramplike feeling is experienced in the posterior thigh region when full-range hip extension is attempted while the knee is maintained flexed to an acute angle. Children and young adults may not complain about discomfort, but in older subjects this movement may be extremely uncomfortable and may produce a cramp, and therefore should be used with caution or avoided.

Since very little tension can be produced by the hamstrings when they contract in their shortened range, hip extension with the knee flexed requires strong action of the gluteus maximus. This movement combination has been advocated as an isolated test for the gluteus maximus. While it is true that, in hip extension with the knee flexed, the gluteus maximus must be credited with doing most of the work, the hamstrings still contract to the best of their ability, so that an isolated action of the gluteus maximus is by no means achieved.

PRONE-LYING BILATERAL HIP EXTENSION, KNEES EXTENDED. In unilateral hip extension in the prone position, the pelvis remains comparatively stable; only mild synergic contraction of the extensors of the vertebral column is required and may be observed and palpated. But when both limbs are raised simultaneously, the leverage action on the pelvis (due to the contracting hip extensors and to the weight of the limbs) becomes marked. Therefore, the demand on the extensors of the vertebral column, and in particular on the lumbar extensors, is much increased. The strong tension in these muscles should be observed and palpated.

HIP EXTENSORS IN THE SITTING POSITION. Forward inclination of the trunk and pelvis in the sitting or standing position is controlled at the hip joint by the hip extensors. An eccentric contraction permits forward movement to retrieve an object on the floor, and a concentric contraction of the hip extensors produces return to the erect position. Patients with paralysis of the hip extensors will fall forward unless the upper extremities are used to control the pelvis on the fixed femur (see Fig. 2-26, B, C). Such hip extensor muscle activity can be seen in a more subtle form in ascending and descending stairs, in rising from a sitting position, and in walking. These activities are associated with simultaneous contraction of the quadriceps (acting as knee extensors) and the hamstrings (acting as hip extensors).

In these functional motions of leaning forward in the sitting position, bending over to touch the toes in the standing position, climbing the stairs, or rising from a chair, the hamstrings are primarily activated as hip extensors. When such motions are rapid or are accompanied by moderate or maximum resistance, the gluteus maximus is also activated (Basmajian, 1978).

Muscles Acting in Abduction of the Hip

SUPINE, UNILATERAL ABDUCTION. If in the back-lying position the hip is abducted by moving the limb sideward, the abductors on that side, mainly the gluteus medius and gluteus minimus, are activated. Synergic action of the hip-hikers (quadratus lumborum and lateral abdominals) on the same side occurs automatically, so that the crest of the ilium moves upward in a direction toward the rib cage. If these muscles were idle, contraction of the abductors would approximate the crest of the ilium and the greater trochanter by moving regions of proximal and distal attachments toward each other simultaneously. Thus, hip abduction, as far as side motion of the limb were concerned, would become rather ineffective. Owing to the action of the hip-hikers, the abductors are kept at a favorable length to produce abduction.

SUPINE, BILATERAL ABDUCTION. In bilateral abduction, the traction exerted on the ilium by the abductors on one side is counterbalanced by an equal traction on the opposite side; hence, the pelvis remains level and stable.

SUPINE, HIP-HIKING. If the hip-hikers are used first on one side and then on the other, without simultaneous contraction of the abductors, a lateral tilt of the pelvis to alternate sides takes place. The muscles of the extremities remain inactive, but the entire limb follows the motion of the pelvis, and the result is a shortening of the limb on alternate sides. When the hip-hikers on the right side contract, they cause *adduction* of the right hip and *abduction* of the left hip as the pelvis moves in relation to the limbs.

Electromyographic studies by Close (1964) have revealed that electric activity is present in the iliopsoas muscle when approaching the outer limit of hip abduction. As pointed out by the above investigator, in the neutral position of the hip, the distal portion of the iliopsoas muscle courses anteriorly and directly over the femoral head; but as abduction proceeds, the muscle slides over to the lateral side of the center of rotation of the hip joint and thus becomes mechanically capable of abduction. When the tendon of the iliopsoas muscle is surgically transferred to the greater trochanter (Mustard, 1952; Close, 1964), the muscle comes to lie lateral to the center of rotation of the hip joint in all positions of the joint. The transfer of this tendon has been found useful in assisting or replacing weak action of the gluteal muscles not only in voluntary abduction of the thigh with respect to the pelvis, but also in lateral stabilization of the pelvis in automatic activities such as walking.

Unilateral Stance

The *major function of the hip abductors* (gluteus medius, gluteus minimus, and tensor fasciae latae) is to *maintain a level pelvis during unilateral stance* (Fig. 8-9, B). In standing on one foot, which occurs with every step, 85 percent of the weight of the body (HAT and contralateral limb) must be balanced by the hip abductors around the femoral head (fulcrum), forming a first-class lever system (Figs. 8-10, 2-7). Since the lever arm (d) of the weight in Figure 8-10 is longer than the lever arm (l) of the muscles, the hip abductors are at a mechanical disadvantage and must produce a force greater than 85 percent of body weight to maintain equilibrium. The two downward forces (W and M) produce a high compression force (J) between the head of the femur and the acetabulum. The joint compression force in unilateral stance has been calculated to be approximately 2.5 times body weight (Inman, 1947; Le Veau, 1977; Frankel and Nordin, 1980).

The magnitude of joint reaction forces can be decreased by shifting HAT *over the supporting leg (Fig. 8-9, C), thus decreasing the force required of the abductor muscles to match the torque acting at the hip axis and thereby decreasing the joint com-

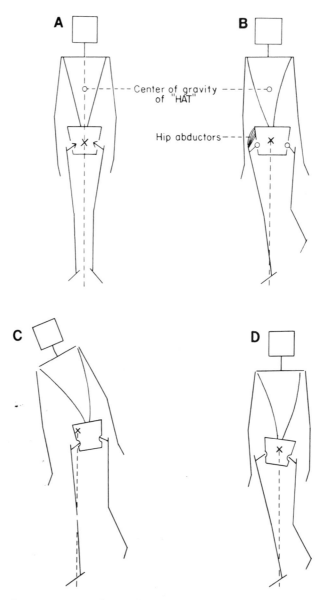

FIGURE 8-9. Body alignment in standing on both feet and in standing on one foot. *(A)* Standing on both feet. Pelvis is supported from both sides. Center-of-gravity line of head, arms, and trunk (HAT) and of the body as a whole (X) falls in the center of the base of support. *(B)* Standing on one foot. Body weight shifts over stance limb. Hip abductors on stance side become activated to balance the pelvis. *(C)* One-legged balance in the presence of hip joint pain or when abductors of hip are paralyzed. Upper part of body inclines toward side of paralysis. Weight of HAT counterbalances weight of raised leg, and the abductors at the stance hip are substantially relieved of their balancing function. *(D)* Trendelenburg sign in paralysis or weakness of hip abductors. Stance hip is adducted. Ligamentous tension is relied upon for hip balance.

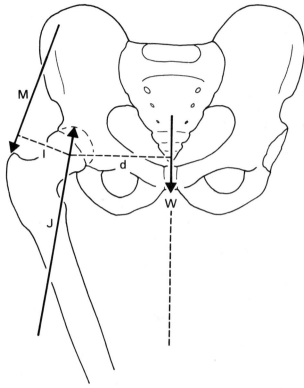

FIGURE 8-10. Forces on the pelvis when standing on one leg. W = weight of head, arms, and trunk, and opposite leg; M = force of the hip abductors to maintain a level pelvis; J = joint reaction force between the acetabulum and the head of the femur; d = lever arm distance for the weight; l = lever arm for the muscle force.

pression force. The maximum isometric torque curves (see Fig. 4-14) demonstrate that the hip abductors produce the greatest torque at 15 degrees of hip *adduction* where length-tension relationships are most favorable. This point coincides with the functional demands placed on the muscle in unilateral stance. As the center of gravity of the body is shifted laterally over the supporting foot, the hip assumes an adducted position, and the opposite foot can be raised from the floor.

HIP ABDUCTOR PARALYSIS

When the hip abductors are paralyzed, one-legged standing with the pelvis level, as in Figure 8-9, B, becomes impossible. However, the individual may still manage to balance on one foot, at least momentarily, and to do so well enough to permit walking. There are three common methods of compensating for the loss of the abductor muscles in one-legged standing and walking:

1. By skillful use of the weight of the upper part of the body; this means inclining the trunk laterally toward the stance side until the combined center of gravity of

HAT and the suspended limb comes to lie vertically over, or slightly lateral to, the hip joint. In the latter case, the adductors of the stance limb may aid in maintaining equilibrium. The arms, if free to move, may also assist in balancing. In order that the center of gravity of the entire body be maintained vertically over the base of support, the stance limb loses its slant (Fig. 8-9, C). It should be noted that lateral trunk inclination in abductor paralysis can be modified, even eliminated, if a weight of proper size is carried in the hand on the affected side. Such a weight helps to counterbalance the weight of HAT and the unsupported limb.

2. By allowing the pelvis to sag laterally toward the unsupported side until the hip on the stance side has been maximally adducted, at which point tension in capsule, ligaments, and ilio-tibial tract prevents further motion (Fig. 8-9, D). This hip posture is known as the *Trendelenburg sign*, a term originally employed to describe the asymmetric position of the pelvis in congenital dislocation of the hip, which renders the hip abductors ineffective. When the Trendelenburg sign is present, owing to the obliquity of the pelvis, the summit of the head comes to lie lower when the affected limb supports the body weight than when the weight is on the unaffected limb.

3. By placing a cane in the *opposite* hand to provide an upward force at a long distance from the joint axis, thereby counterbalancing the torque of HAT.

Muscles Acting in Adduction of the Hip

When adduction of the hip is carried out against resistance and with the thigh in a neutral position with respect to flexion, extension, and rotation, the five main adductors previously enumerated contract as a group. Their individual functional characteristics in various degrees of hip flexion have been described. Since some of these muscles, or parts of the same muscle, have opposite secondary actions, these actions counterbalance each other when pure adduction is carried out.

The total cross section of the adductors far surpasses that of the abductors. At first glance, it might appear illogical that this is the case, since in the erect position the hip abductors have to work against gravity, whereas gravity does the work for the adductors. Activities such as squeezing an object between the knees and climbing a rope, which require force in adduction, are relatively rare and hardly warrant such a large cross section. The explanation for the adductors' large bulk is found in their functions as flexors, extensors, and rotators and, in general, in their stabilizing action as co-contractors with the abductors. The electric activities of these muscles in walking are illustrated in Chapter 12.

Muscles Acting in Rotation of the Hip

From previous discussions, it is obvious that most of the muscles about the hip joint have rotary actions. Which of these muscles are used for rotation depend on the position of the joint with respect to flexion, extension, abduction, and adduction. For example, the gluteus maximus, when *extending the hip* fully, also *externally rotates* the hip; but when the hip is *flexed*, the upper fibers have a line of pull for *internal rotation* (Steindler, 1955). The six small external rotators (piriformis, gemellus superior, gemellus inferior, obturator internus, obturator externus, and quadratus femoris) have a good angle of pull for external rotation, but the external rotary components of these muscles decrease in flexion of the hip, and at 90 degrees of hip flexion they possess a considerable abductor component. The piriformis changes from an external rotator in hip extension to an internal rotator in hip flexion. (Kapandji, 1970b; Steindler, 1955). The anterior portions of the gluteus medius and minimus and the tensor fasciae latae increase their leverage for internal rotation when the hip is flexed.

ROTARY ACTION OF THE ADDUCTORS

In years past, the adductors were thought to be external rotators of the hip. Electromyographic studies, however, have shown them to act as internal rotators (Williams and Wesley, 1951; Basmajian, 1978). This action also can be identified by palpation with the subject in the sitting or standing position (careful attention should be paid to avoidance of active hip flexion). Even though the adductors attach on the posterior aspect of the femur (linea aspera), the axis of rotation does not go through the anatomic axis of the bone, but rather through the mechanical axis from the head of the femur to the medial femoral condyle (see Fig. 8-2). When the femur is rotated medially, the linea aspera approaches the pubis. With lateral rotation, the distance between these attachments becomes longer.

The maximum isometric torque for both the internal and external rotators occurs at their lengthened positions and decreases as the muscles contract in their shortened positions (May, 1966). Their forces were found to be equal when the leg was near the vertical (neutral) position. An interesting change in maximum torque of the internal rotators occurs when the hip is in flexion and extension. When the hip is flexed, the internal rotators can produce almost three times the torque that they can produce when the hip is extended (Jarvis, 1952; Woodruff, 1976). The external rotators show little difference with hip position. This large difference in the torque of the internal rotators is theorized to be the result of inversion of muscle actions, such as the increased internal rotation leverage of the gluteus medius, gluteus minimus, and piriformis when the hip is flexed. The conventional *sitting position* for testing the strength of the rotators of the hip may provide misleading information as to the functional strength of this group when the subject is actually using the internal rotators in the *erect position* for walking or pivoting on one foot. A person with weak internal rotators may appear to have good strength in the sitting position but inadequate strength for the functions to be performed in the standing position.

Pelvic Balance

The rigid sacral portion of the vertebral column, firmly connected with the ilia, is part of the pelvis. The pelvis, interposed between the lower extremities and the flexible portions of the vertebral column, possesses movements of its own. Owing to the firmness of the sacro-iliac and lumbosacral junctions, however, every pelvic movement is accompanied by a realignment of the spine, most marked in the lumbar region.

PELVIC INCLINATION

In erect standing, when the hip is flexed by a pelvic movement while the upper part of the body remains erect, the *inclination* of the pelvis is said to be *increased*—a *forward tilt* of the pelvis has occurred. When this movement takes place, the anterior superior spines of the ilia come to lie anterior to the foremost part of the pubic symphysis while these spines are normally in vertical alignment with, or lie slightly posterior to, the symphysis (Fig. 8-11, A). The opposite movement of the pelvis (in direction of extension) is referred to as a *backward tilt of the pelvis,* and the resulting position as a *decreased pelvic inclination.*

A determination of the pelvic inclination in degrees can be made by laying an oblique plane through the posterior superior spines of the ilia and the foremost portion of the pubic symphysis. The angle of this plane with the horizontal is said to be the *angle of pelvic inclination* (Fig. 8-11, A). This method of measuring the pelvic inclination was advocated by Fick (1911), who considered an angle of 50 to 60 degrees to be normal for adult men and a somewhat larger angle to be normal for women.

Fick's method of measuring the angle of pelvic inclination has been used by many investigators, but has not been adopted universally. Sometimes, the "plane of the inlet" (inlet to the lesser pelvis) is used as a reference plane. This plane, indicated by the line a–b in the illustration, passes through the lumbo-sacral junction and through the foremost portion of the pubic symphysis. If this plane is used, the angle of pelvic inclination will be greater than when determined by Fick's method.

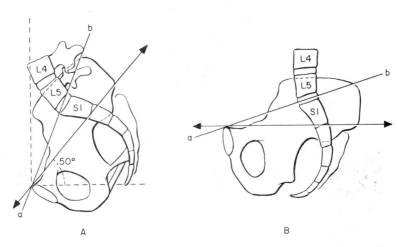

FIGURE 8-11. Pelvic inclination in standing *(A)* and in sitting *(B)*. Arrow shows plane of plevic inclination. Line a–b represents "plane of the inlet." (Redrawn from Fick, 1911, pp 438 and 439.)

The range of backward tilt of the pelvis in the erect standing position is determined by the tension of the capsule of the hip joints and the reinforcing ligaments, noticeably, the ilio-femoral or Y ligament. If further backward tilt is attempted, this can be accomplished only by flexing the knees simultaneously with the pelvic movement, which also causes hip flexion and slackening of the ligaments.

In the sitting position, these ligaments no longer restrict the pelvic movement, and the pelvis tilts backward so that the plane through the posterior superior spine of the ilia and the pubic symphysis becomes horizontal (Fig. 8-11, B). A backward tilt of the pelvis is accompanied by a decrease in, or obliteration of, the physiologic lumbar curve. Such flattening of the lumbar spine is particularly marked in sitting. A forward inclination of the pelvis is accompanied by an increase in the physiologic lumbar curve.

CLINICAL EVALUATION OF PELVIC INCLINATION

It is difficult to measure the angle of pelvic inclination in the living subject. Clinically, therefore, a more practical method to determine normal or abnormal inclination of the pelvis is needed. Because the anterior superior spines of the ilia and the front part of the pubic symphysis are superficial and easily located, the alignment of these points may be observed. When the subject is viewed from the side, the pelvic inclination may be considered normal if these two points are approximately in vertical alignment, as seen in Figure 8-11, A.

CHAPTER 9
KNEE REGION

The knee is a complex joint (Figs. 9-1, 9-2) with three bones (*femur, tibia,* and *patella*), *two degrees of freedom of motion,* and *three articulating surfaces:* the *medial tibio-femoral, lateral tibio-femoral,* and *patello-femoral articulations,* which are enclosed by a common *joint capsule.* Functionally, the knee can support the body weight in the erect position without muscle contraction; it participates in lowering and elevating body weight (up to 0.5 m) in sitting, squatting, or climbing; and it permits rotation of the body when turning on the planted foot as a football player does when avoiding a pursuing tackler. In walking, the normal knee reduces energy expenditure by decreasing the vertical and lateral oscillations of the center of gravity of the body (Inman, Ralston, and Todd, 1981) while sustaining vertical forces equal to two to four times body weight (Morrison, 1970). The multiple functions of the normal knee—to withstand large forces, to provide great stability, and to afford large ranges of motion—are achieved in a unique way. *Mobility* is primarily provided by bony structure, and *stability* is primarily provided by the soft tissues: ligaments, muscles, and cartilage. Athletic and industrial injuries to these stabilizing structures are common, and are frequently caused by the large torques developed by forces acting on the long lever arms of the femur and tibia.

Palpable Joint Structures

The superficial structures of the knee can be palpated best with the subject sitting on a table and with the knee relaxed in 90 degrees of flexion. The distal enlargements of the femur, the condyles (Gr. *kondylos,* knuckle; a rounded projection on a bone), can be felt anteriorly on both sides of the patella and followed proximally to the epicon-

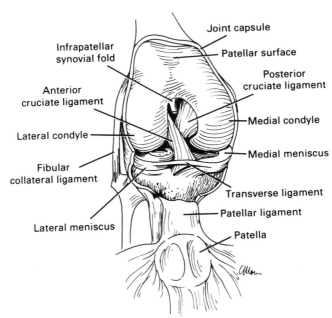

FIGURE 9-1. The right knee of a young adult flexed to about 90 degrees and viewed from the front. The anterior part of the capsule has been removed and the patella turned down. (Redrawn from *Acta Clinica: Osteoarthritis of the Knee*, Vol 1. Geigy Pharmaceuticals, Ardsley, NY, 1963.)

dyles (Gr. *epi*, upon). When the palpating fingers then move inferiorly from the femoral condyles, the depression for the *tibio-femoral joint line* is encountered. This line can be confirmed by *passively* rotating or extending the knee while feeling the motion of the tibial condyles on the femur. Anteriorly on the tibia, and below the tibial condyles, is a large roughened area, the *tuberosity of the tibia*, which is the distal attachment of the patellar tendon of the quadriceps femoris muscle. The sharp *crest of the tibia* may be followed distally to the ankle.

The *medial* (tibial) *collateral ligament* spans the tibio-femoral joint on the medial side and may be felt by palpating along the joint line. This broad fibrous band obliterates the joint line as the ligament courses from the medial epicondyle of the femur to the medial condyle and shaft of the tibia. If the palpating finger is placed on the joint line at the anterior margin of the medial collateral ligament, the edge of the *medial meniscus* may be palpated. The medial edge of the meniscus can be made more prominent by passively internally rotating the tibia. With passive external rotation, the meniscus will retract.

If the index finger is placed on the lateral epicondyle of the femur and the middle finger on the head of the fibula, the attachments of the *lateral* (fibular) *collateral ligament* can be identified. This smaller ligament is difficult to palpate as it crosses the joint line. It becomes readily palpable, however, if the foot is placed on the opposite knee and the hip is permitted to fall into external rotation. The lateral meniscus cannot be palpated.

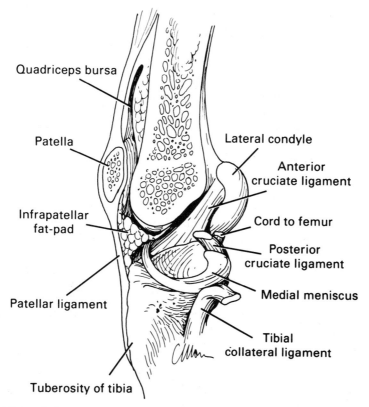

Quadriceps bursa

Patella

Infrapatellar
fat-pad

Patellar ligament

Tuberosity of tibia

Lateral condyle

Anterior
cruciate ligament

Cord to femur

Posterior
cruciate ligament

Medial meniscus

Tibial
collateral ligament

FIGURE 9-2. The right knee seen from the medial side. Femur and patella have been split in half sagittally. (Redrawn from *Acta Clinica: Osteoarthritis of the Knee,* Vol 1. Geigy Pharmaceuticals, Ardsley, NY, 1963.)

The patella is best palpated when the subject is supine with the knee extended and relaxed. The thick patellar ligament may be felt from the tuberosity of the tibia to the apex of the triangular patella. Normally, the patella can be easily mobilized laterally and distally and can be compressed on the femur without discomfort.

Nonpalpable Structures

Note the following nonpalpable structures on the skeleton, models, and in Figures 9-1 and 9-2: *articular surfaces and patellar surfaces of the condyles of the femur; intercondyloid fossa; lateral and medial supracondylar lines,* extending proximally from the condyles and enclosing an area which forms the floor of the popliteal fossa (L. *poples,* back of knee); *articular surfaces of the condyles of the tibia* ("tibial plateau"), separated by the *intercondylar eminence; lateral meniscus,* nearly circular in form (Gr. *meniskos,* crescent); *medial meniscus; anterior and posterior cruciate ligaments;* and *transverse ligament,* connecting the menisci anteriorly.

KNEE JOINT

Motions of the Knee

The knee joint (*Articulatio Genu*, L. *genua*, knee or any structure bent like the knee) possesses two degrees of freedom: flexion-extension and axial rotation. In the sagittal plane, *flexion* occurs from 0 to about 120 degrees (see Appendix B), depending on the size of the muscle mass of the calf in contact with the posterior thigh. When the hip is extended, knee flexion range decreases, owing to limitation by the rectus femoris muscle. Hyperextension is minimal and does not normally exceed 15 degrees.

AXES FOR FLEXION AND EXTENSION

The axis of motion is located a few centimeters above the joint surfaces, passing transversely through the femoral condyles. The curve of the condyles presents a changing radius that is smallest when the knee is flexed and increases with extension (Fig. 9-3). We owe much of our present knowledge of the mechanics of the knee to investigations by Fischer (quoted by Fick, 1911, pp 533, 534). He marked successive points of contact between the joint surfaces on a series of radiographs showing the profile of the femoral condyles at various knee angles, and for each point, he determined the center for the curve of the condyle. By connecting these centers, a curved line (the evolute) was obtained, representing the path of the moving axis (see Fig. 9-3). Smidt (1973) measured the axis as moving through a pathway of 3.2 cm from 0 to 90 degrees of knee

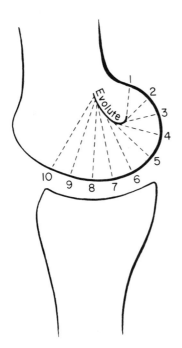

FIGURE 9-3. Changing radius of curves of femoral condyles. Axis of motion for flexion and extension moves along evolute. Number 1 represents the radius of curvature in flexion and number 10 the radius in extension. (Redrawn from Fick, 1911, p 538.)

flexion. The author used the method of Frankel, Burstein, and Brooks (1971) that produces an evolute which opens anteriorly as opposed to the posterior-opening evolute of Fick.

Because of the shifting axis of motion of the human knee, problems occur when devices with mechanical hinge joints such as a goniometer, isokinetic dynamometer, a knee-ankle-foot (long leg) orthosis, or a below-knee prothesis are applied to the knee. When the knee joint is moved from extension to flexion the anatomic axis of the knee moves about 2 cm, while the mechanical axis of the attached device remains fixed. Thus the arms of the mechanical device cannot remain parallel to the thigh and leg, and motions or pressures between the mechanical and anatomic parts will occur. Compromise and careful alignment are required to prevent discomfort and abrasions. Misalignment of an orthotic knee joint can cause pressure of cuffs on the extremity during knee flexion and gapping during knee extension (or vice versa).

Axial Rotation

Axial rotation occurs in the transverse plane when the knee is flexed. When the knee is fully extended, the medial and lateral collateral ligaments are relatively tense, which contributes materially to the stability of the joint. These ligaments slacken when the joint flexes, and this is one of the reasons a considerable amount of transverse rotation may take place in the flexed position. In Figure 9-4, the position of the medial epicondyle when the knee is extended (Me) is compared with its position when the knee is flexed (Mf). Note that the distance from the medial epicondyle to point A (representing the attachment of the medial collateral ligament) is less in flexion than in extension. During knee flexion, more slack is produced in the lateral than in the medial collateral ligament; hence, the movement between the femoral and tibial

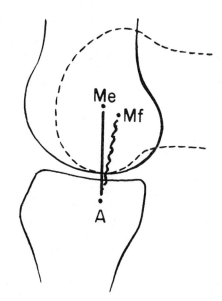

FIGURE 9-4. Slackening of medial collateral ligament in flexion of knee. Me = medial epicondyle in extension; Mf = medial epicondyle in flexion; A = point of attachment of medial collateral ligament. (Redrawn from Fick, 1911, p 542.)

condyles is more extensive laterally than medially. Transverse rotation takes place about a longitudinal axis located medial to the intercondylar ridge of the tibia so that, roughly, it may be stated that the lateral condyle rotates around the medial one.

Although many conflicting values are reported for this motion, the results of published studies indicate the average total rotation to be approximately 40 degrees (Ross, 1932; Ouellet et al, 1969). At 90 degrees of knee flexion, Mossberg and Smith (1982) found a mean total rotation of 40 degrees (standard deviation = ±8 degrees). External rotation was approximately twice as large as internal rotation. Axial rotation decreases with the angle of knee flexion and cannot be performed as the knee approaches extension. Rotation of the tibia on the femur can be performed voluntarily in the sitting position and can be useful in placing and positioning the foot. The major functional importance of the motion, however, is in closed chain motion where the femur rotates on the fixed tibia, as in turning from kneeling, sitting, or squatting positions and in sudden changes in direction while running.

TERMINAL ROTATION OF THE KNEE

Normally when the knee moves into extension, the tibia externally rotates about 20 degrees on the fixed femur. This motion can be observed in the last 20 degrees of knee extension and is called *terminal rotation of the knee* or the "screw home mechanism." It is purely a mechanical event that occurs with both passive and active knee extension and one that cannot be produced (or prevented) voluntarily. In closed chain motion such as rising from a chair, terminal rotation is seen as *internal rotation of the femur* on the fixed tibia. Although many species such as chimpanzees, orangutans, and birds walk on flexed knees, terminal rotation provides humans with an exquisite and energy-efficient mechanism for the extended knee. This screw mechanism provides a mechanical stability to withstand forces occurring in the sagittal plane. It permits humans to stand erect without quadriceps muscle contraction and to withstand anterior-posterior forces on the extended knee with reduced muscle force. Although the amount of terminal rotation of the knee is modest, it is, like axial rotation, a requisite for normal knee function. Both motions must be evaluated and regained for successful rehabilitation of the knee.

Anatomic Basis for Joint Motion

The tibio-femoral joints achieve their great stability and two degrees of freedom of motion in a remarkable way. The *medial and lateral femoral condyles* are convex both longitudinally and transversely. They are connected anteriorly by the patellar surface and separated distally and posteriorly by the intercondylar notch. These condyles articulate with the two smaller tibial condyles, which have only a slight concavity (the lateral tibial condyle is also convex anterior-posteriorly). The congruity of the articulations is increased slightly by the intercondylar eminence of the tibia and the wedge-shaped medial and lateral menisci (semilunar cartilages), which form an incomplete ring or crescent on each tibial condyle. Since the longitudinal articulating surface of the femoral condyles is approximately twice the length of the surface of the tibial condyles, it can be appreciated that the motions of flexion and extension could not be pure rolling or hinge motions (see Fig. 1-10). Instead, the condyles execute both rolling and sliding movements, with the ratio of each varying in the range of motion. Rolling is predominant at the initiation of flexion, and sliding occurs more at the end of flexion (Kapandji, 1970b). Since the length of the articular surface of the lateral femoral condyle is longer than that of the medial condyle, the movements of the two condylar surfaces will differ also.

The strong *medial and lateral collateral ligaments* prevent the knee from movement in the frontal plane. The attachments of the collateral ligaments on the femoral condyles are offset posteriorly and superiorly to the axis for flexion. This offsetting causes the ligaments to become taut when the knee moves into extension and to become slack as the knee flexes (see Fig. 9-4). The collateral ligaments thus provide stability to terminal rotation of the extended knee and yet permit axial rotation in the flexed knee. Axial rotation is also facilitated by a decrease in the congruency of the joint surfaces when the knee is flexed. The posterior aspects of the femoral condyles have a greater convexity and the intercondylar notch is wider at this point. Thus, when the knee is flexed, the mating surfaces with the tibial intercondylar tubercles and the menisci are reduced, and the condyles have more freedom to rotate.

The *anterior and posterior cruciate ligaments* (L. *crux*, cross) provide stability to the knee joint throughout its range of motion. These ligaments lie in the center of the joint within the femoral intercondylar fossa (see Figs. 9-1, 9-2). Although intimately related to the joint capsule, they are on the outside of the capsule and are considered extracapsular structures. The anterior cruciate ligament attaches to the anterior intercondylar fossa of the tibia. It courses laterally to attach on the *inside* of the lateral condyle of the femur. Severance of this ligament allows anterior dislocation of the tibia on the femur (anterior drawer sign; Hoppenfeld, 1976; McCluskey and Blackburn, 1980). The posterior cruciate attaches on the posterior intercondylar fossa of the tibia and runs medially to the inside of the medial femoral condyle. Severance of the posterior cruciate allows posterior dislocation of the tibia on the femur (posterior drawer sign).

The cruciate ligaments are strong and are attached so that they maintain a relatively constant length throughout flexion and extension. Thus, the cruciate ligaments *force* the sliding motions of the condylar surfaces to occur. In knee flexion, sliding is forced by the anterior cruciate; in knee extension, sliding is forced by the posterior cruciate. The cruciate ligaments also limit axial rotation and contribute to terminal rotation and stability of the extended knee.

The *medial and lateral menisci* are fibrocartilages that serve to increase the congruency of the tibio-femoral articulations and to distribute pressures (see Figs. 9-1, 9-2). The only bony attachments of the menisci to the tibia are through their horns at the anterior and posterior intercondylar fossae and through the coronary ligaments, which are part of the capsule and which attach the peripheral edges of the menisci to the margin of the tibia. These cartilages are not attached to the articulating surfaces of the tibia and are therefore movable. They do have numerous other attachments:

1. The transverse ligament connects the anterior horns of the two menisci.
2. Fibrous bands connect the anterior horns of both menisci to the retinaculum of the patellar tendon (menisco-patellar fibers).
3. The medial collateral ligament is attached to the medial meniscus.
4. The tendon of the semimembranosus muscle sends fibers to the posterior edge of the medial meniscus.
5. The popliteus muscle sends fibers to the posterior edge of the lateral meniscus.
6. The menisco-femoral ligament extends from the lateral meniscus (posteriorly) to the inside of the medial condyle near the posterior cruciate ligament.

The menisci are moved and controlled on the tibia by both passive and active forces. Passively, they are pushed anteriorly by the femur as the knee extends and the contact of the femoral condyles is more anterior on the tibial condyles. Conversely, the menisci move posteriorly with knee flexion. According to Kapandji (1970b), a total movement of 6 mm occurs in the medial meniscus and 12 mm in the lateral meniscus. In addition, the menisci move or deform according to the direction of movement of the femoral condyles during axial rotation. Edges of the menisci are moved by their ligamentous and muscular attachments. For example, anterior movement is caused by the menisco-patellar fibers of the extensor mechanism, and posterior movement is caused by their attachments to the knee flexors (the semimembranosus and the popliteus muscles). If a meniscus fails to move with the femoral condyles, as may occur with sudden twisting or forceful movement, the meniscus may be crushed or torn by the condyles.

The ligaments and the menisci of the knee perform complex, multiple, and overlapping functions to provide joint stability. For example, the medial collateral ligament is primarily responsible for limitation of lateral motion of the tibia on the femur. Equally important are the secondary functions in controlling terminal rotation, axial rotation, and hyperextension.

With compressive loading of the tibio-femoral joints, Hsieh and Walker (1976) found that joint laxity (L. *laxare*, to unloose or relax) decreased markedly, and that dislocation due to rotary forces did not occur even with removal of all ligaments and menisci. The authors present the theory that in weight-bearing the femoral condyles are forced to move "uphill" on the planted tibia. This structural restraint contributes to knee stability during weight-bearing activities. McLeod and Hunter (1980) add support to this theory from their findings that the tibial surface where most of the condylar contact occurs slopes posteriorly about 9 degrees.

Patello-Femoral Joint

The patello-femoral joint is a part of the *extensor or quadriceps mechanism*. The patella, a large sesamoid bone, is anchored distally to the tuberosity of the tibia by the patellar tendon, superiorly to the tendon of the quadriceps femoris muscle, and by the medial and lateral retinacula to the joint capsule. These structures form a strong fibrous and bony cap for the anterior compartment of the knee. The articular surface of the patella has a prominent vertical ridge dividing the medial and lateral articular surfaces, which articulate with the femoral condyles on the saddle-shaped patellar surface and the intercondylar groove.* The patella is anchored on all sides and is maintained at a constant distance from the tibial tuberosity during motion. If the tibia moves on the femur, the patella slides on the femoral condyles. When the femur moves on the fixed tibia, the femoral condyles slide on the patella.

The function of the patella is to increase the leverage of the quadriceps muscle and, as a part of the extensor mechanism, to restrain and distribute the forces on the femur. The leverage advantage provided by the patella changes within the range of motion of knee extension. When the knee is fully flexed, the patella lies in the intercondylar groove and thus is near to the axis of motion. (The quadriceps muscle is at this point stretched and has an advantageous length-tension position.) As the knee is extended, the patella moves out of the groove to reach a maximum lever arm distance at about 45 degrees of flexion. Thereafter, the lever arm distance decreases (Smidt, 1973). With patellectomy (removal of the patella), the quadriceps muscle force must be increased 30 percent to perform knee extension (Kaufer, 1971).

Knee Alignment and Deformities

An anterior view of the extended knee reveals an angle, open laterally, between the shafts of the femur and the tibia. The size of the angle is variable; about 170 degrees (as measured from the longitudinal axis of each bone) is regarded as average (Fig. 9-5). This angle is due to the adducted position of the shaft of the femur and the compensatory direction of the tibia to transmit weight perpendicularly to the foot and ground. Thus, during weight-bearing on one leg, forces are directed toward the medial side of the knee. If the angle becomes smaller than 170 degrees, the condition is referred to as *genu valgum*, or knock knee. Conversely, if the angle approaches 180 degrees or opens medially, the deformity is referred to as *genu varum*, or bowleg.

The tendons of the quadriceps femoris and the ligamentum patella also form an angle with the center of the patella. This is called the "Q angle" (Ficat and Hungerford, 1977; see Fig. 9-5). As this angle becomes greater than 15 degrees, the tendency for the contracting quadriceps muscle to exert lateral forces on the patella increases. Subluxation of the patella as it tracks on the femoral condyles is normally prevented by the congruence of the joint surfaces and by the more elevated lateral trochlear facet and the medial soft tissue stabilizers.

Normally, a person may stand with the knees extended, slightly flexed, or in slight hyperextension. The amount of hyperextension depends on the looseness of the capsule and ligaments that limit the motion. *Genu recurvatum* is an excessive hyperextension that develops from weight-bearing on an unstable knee. The deformity may be a result of ligamentous injury (e.g., anterior cruciate), muscle paralysis (e.g., quadriceps femoris), or limitation of motion at the ankle (e.g., spasticity of the plantar flexors).

---

*The patella actually possesses five surfaces that articulate with the femoral condyles at different points in the range of motion.

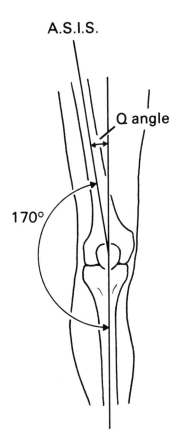

FIGURE 9-5. Alignment of the shaft of the femur with the tibia. The angle (on the lateral side) between the longitudinal axis of the femur and that of the tibia is usually about 170 degrees. The Q angle is formed by drawing a line from the tibial tuberosity through the center of the patella and drawing another line from the center of the patella to the anterior superior iliac spine (ASIS).

MUSCLES

Knee Extensors

The quadriceps femoris muscle group extends the knee and consists of four muscles: *rectus femoris, vastus lateralis, vastus medialis,* and *vastus intermedius.* These four muscles form a single strong distal attachment to the patella, capsule of the knee, and the anterior proximal surface of the tibia. In well-developed subjects where little adipose tissue is present, the rectus femoris, the vastus medialis, and the vastus lateralis may be observed as separate units (Figs. 9-6, 9-7), while in other subjects, the boundaries of these muscles are less distinct. The vastus intermedius is deeply located and cannot be observed from the surface.

Rectus Femoris

The *rectus femoris* occupies the middle of the thigh, is superficial, and takes a straight course down the thigh. *Distal attachment:* By two tendons: (1) the anterior or

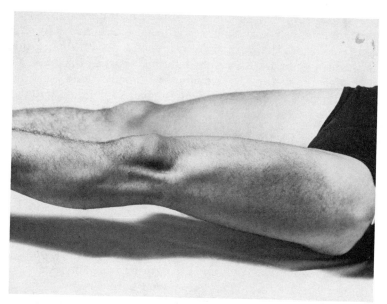

FIGURE 9-6. Vastus lateralis in contraction. Subject maintains knee extended while lifting heel off the floor. The iliotibial tract is seen as it approaches its attachment on the tibia.

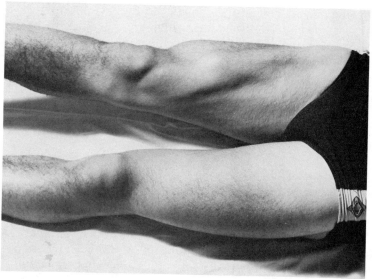

FIGURE 9-7. Vastus medialis in contraction. Subject's right knee is held extended while the heel is raised off the floor. Note the bulk of this muscle near the knee.

"straight" tendon, from the anterior inferior spine of the ilium; and (2) the posterior or "reflected" tendon from just above the brim of the acetabulum; as this tendon swings forward, it courses close to the hip joint and is blended with the capsule. The two tendons unite, covering part of the capsule anteriorly. *Distal attachment:* The muscle fibers attach to a deep aponeurosis narrowing to a broad tendon that attaches to the superior border of the patella and by means of the patellar tendon, into the tuberosity of the tibia. *Innervation:* Two branches of the femoral nerve. *Inspection and palpation:* When the hip is flexed, the tendon of origin may be observed and palpated in the V-shaped area between the sartorius and the tensor fasciae latae as seen in Figure 8-5. The muscular portion is superficial and may be followed down the thigh to its attachment on the patella (see Figs. 9-6, 9-7).

Vastus Lateralis

The *vastus lateralis* is the largest of the four muscles and is located on the lateral side of the rectus femoris. *Proximal attachment:* By a broad aponeurosis on the lateral and posterior aspects of the femur, as high up as the greater trochanter and as far posterior as the linea aspera. *Distal attachment:* The lateral border of the patella, the lateral patellar retinaculum, and by means of the patellar tendon, the tuberosity of the tibia. The fibers converge toward the patella at a 12- to 15-degree angle, which is even greater in distal portions (Lieb and Perry, 1968). *Innervation:* Branches of the femoral nerve. *Inspection and palpation:* The muscle may be seen and palpated from just below the greater trochanter down to the patella (see Fig. 9-6).

Vastus Medialis

The *vastus medialis* lies in a position medial to the rectus. *Proximal attachment:* Medial and posterior aspects of the femur, as high up as the intertrochanteric line and as far posterior as the linea aspera. *Distal attachment:* Medial portion of superior border of patella, medial patellar retinaculum, and, by means of the patellar tendon, the tuberosity of the tibia. *Innervation:* Branches of the femoral nerve. *Inspection and palpation:* The distal portion of the muscle is quite bulky and is palpated in the lower third of the thigh medially (see Fig. 9-7).

Vastus Intermedius

Vastus intermedius, located underneath the rectus, is partially fused with the two other vasti muscles. *Proximal attachment:* The anterior and lateral surfaces of the femur, as high up as the lesser trochanter and as far posterior as the linea aspera. The muscle fibers are aligned parallel to the long axis of the femur. *Distal attachment:* Superior border of the patella, fused with the tendons of the two other vasti muscles, and directly into the capsule of the knee joint. *Innervation:* Branches of the femoral nerve. *Palpation:* If the rectus is grasped and lifted somewhat, the vastus intermedius may be palpated underneath the rectus if approached from the medial or lateral side of the rectus.

The patella lies within the *common tendon of the quadriceps*, which extends above and on the sides of the patella as well as being attached to it. From the apex of the patella, the patellar ligament, the continuation of the quadriceps tendon, extends to the tuberosity of the tibia. On the sides of the patella, tendinous fibers spread out to form the *medial and lateral retinacula*, which attach to the condyles of the tibia.

Articularis Genu

The *articularis genu* (subcrureus) is a small flat muscle whose attachments are on the anterior lower portion of the shaft of the femur and the capsule of the knee joint or on the superior edge of the patella. The muscle lies beneath the vastus intermedius and is sometimes blended with it. This muscle is *innervated* by a branch of the nerve to the vastus intermedius. Neither the attachments of this muscle nor its purpose has been clearly described. The predominant theory is that the function of the articularis genu is to pull the joint capsule (and synovial membrane) superiorly as the knee extends, thereby preventing an impingement or crushing of these structures in the patello-femoral articulation. Perhaps more important than a controversy about the role of this muscle is the fact that the anterior-superior capsule must move and pleat with knee extension. When it does not do so, injuries to the capsule and plica (seams in the synovial membrane) may occur.

Knee Flexors

A number of muscles pass posterior to the axis for flexion and extension of the knee, contributing to a variable extent to knee flexion. The muscles are the biceps femoris, the semitendinosus, and the semimembranosus (collectively called the hamstrings); the gastrocnemius; the plantaris; the popliteus; the adductor gracilis; and the sartorius.

Biceps Femoris

The *biceps femoris* is a muscle of the posterior thigh, also known as the "lateral hamstring." *Proximal attachment:* By two heads: (1) The long head to the tuberosity of the ischium, having a common tendon of attachment with the semitendinosus; (2) the short head, to the lower portion of the shaft of the femur and to the lateral intermuscular septum. *Distal attachment:* The two heads unite to be attached to the head of the fibula, to the lateral condyle of the tibia, and to the fascia of the leg. *Innervation:* Branches of the sciatic nerve.

INSPECTION AND PALPATION. When knee flexion is resisted (subject prone), the long head of the biceps femoris may be observed and palpated from its attachment on the head of the fibula to the ischial tuberosity. (Fig. 9-8). The short head is covered largely by the long head and is, therefore, difficult to identify. The common tendon of the two heads also is seen in Figure 10-4 as it approaches its attachment to the head of

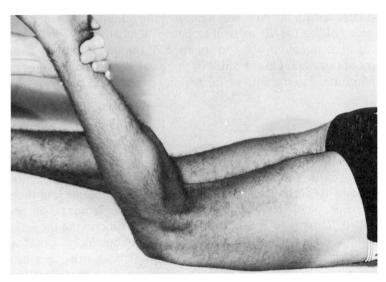

FIGURE 9-8. Tendon of biceps femoris is seen on lateral side of posterior knee region when knee flexion is resisted. Note also the two heads of the gastrocnemius.

the fibula. The biceps tendon is also easily palpated with the subject in the sitting position if the leg is externally rotated with respect to the femur.

Semitendinosus

The *semitendinosus* is one of the medial hamstrings, the muscular portion of which lies medial to that of the long head of the biceps in the posterior thigh. *Proximal attachment:* Tuberosity of the ischium, having a common tendon with the long head of the biceps. *Distal attachment:* The medial aspect of the tibia near the knee joint, distal to the attachment of the gracilis. *Innervation:* Branches of the sciatic nerve.

INSPECTION AND PALPATION. With the subject prone, the tendon may be observed and palpated posteriorly on the medial side of the knee when knee flexion is resisted (Fig. 9-9). Palpation of the tendon may also be done with the subject in the sitting position. The palpating fingers are placed in the "fold" of the knee, medially, where several relaxed tendons may be distinguished. If the muscles of this region are then tightened without joint movement, the tendon of the semitendinosus rises markedly from the underlying tissue, it being the most prominent tendon in the back of the knee. The tendon may be followed proximally toward the muscle belly as it proceeds obliquely toward the ischial tuberosity. Once the tendon of the semitendinosus has been identified, another small, firm, and round tendon may be palpated medial to the semitendinosus. This is the *tendon of the adductor gracilis*. The adductor gracilis may be distinguished from the semitendinosus by palpating the muscle belly toward its proximal attachment. The gracilis remains medial in its course toward the pubis. In

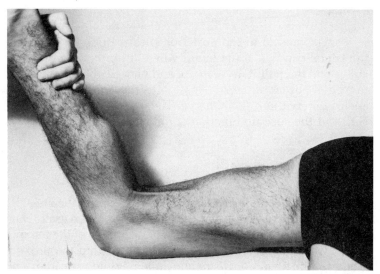

FIGURE 9-9. The prominent tendon of the semitendinosus is seen on the medial side of the posterior knee region when knee flexion is resisted.

the sitting position, internal rotation of the leg with respect to the thigh also brings out the tendons of both the semitendinosus and gracilis.

Semimembranosus

The *semimembranosus* has a *proximal attachment* on the tuberosity of the ischium and a *distal attachment* on the medial condyle of the tibia. *Innervation:* Branches of the sciatic nerve.

PALPATION. Although this muscle has the largest cross section of the hamstrings, it is not easily palpated as an individual muscle because it is to a large extent covered by the semitendinosus and, proximally, by the adductor magnus. Together with these muscles, the semimembranosus makes up the large muscular mass of the medial and posterior thigh. The muscular portion of the semimembranosus extends farther distally than that of the semitendinosus; therefore, its lower portion may be palpated on both sides of the semitendinosus tendon. As the semimembranosus approaches its distal attachment, its tendon lies deep and can be palpated only with difficulty.

Gastrocnemius

The two heads of the *gastrocnemius* (Gr. *gaster*, belly, and *kneme*, leg) have their proximal attachments above the femoral condyles and span the knee joint on the flexor side. The muscular portion of the gastrocnemius may be seen contracting in resisted flexion of the knee (see Figs. 9-8, 9-9). Since the gastrocnemius is more important as a plantar flexor of the ankle than as a knee flexor, it is discussed in more detail in Chapter 10.

Plantaris

The plantaris, a small muscle in the posterior knee region, has its proximal attachment above the lateral condyle of the femur where it lies between the lateral head of the gastrocnemius and the popliteus close to, and partially blended with, the capsule. Following the medial border of the soleus, it joins the Achilles' tendon and attaches into the calcaneus. *Innervation:* Tibial nerve. The muscle belly is at times large and at times atrophied, and the specific function is unknown.

Popliteus

The *popliteus* is the most deeply located muscle in the back of the knee. It lies close to the capsule, covered by the plantaris and the lateral head of the gastrocnemius. *Proximal attachment:* By a strong tendon from the lateral condyle of the femur. The muscle fibers take a downward-medial course and are attached into the proximal posterior portion of the body of the tibia. The *distal attachment* is widespread in a proximal-distal direction, giving the muscle a somewhat triangular shape. The location of the popliteus and the direction of its fibers are indicated in Figure 9-10. *Innervation:* Tibial nerve.

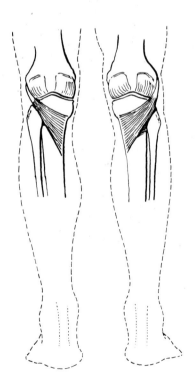

FIGURE 9-10. Location of the popliteus muscle.

Rotators

The muscles that act in *internal rotation* of the tibia with respect to the femur are the semitendinosus, semimembranosus, popliteus, gracilis, and sartorius.

External rotation of the tibia with respect to the femur is accomplished by the biceps femoris, possibly aided by the tensor fasciae latae. That the biceps femoris is a strong external rotator may be ascertained by applying resistance to the motion with the subject in the sitting position. Contraction of the biceps femoris may be isolated from the medial hamstrings by placing the subject prone with the knee flexed slightly beyond 90 degrees. The muscle will contract when performing external rotation of the knee.

The distal attachments of the tendons of the sartorius, gracilis, and semitendinosus are on the *anterior medial* surface of the tibia below the medial condyle, where they form the *pes anserinus* (L. *pes*, foot; *anserinus*, goose). Some of the fibers of these three tendons blend with each other and with the deep fascia of the legs. The three muscles are thought to be important for medial stabilization of the knee.

FUNCTIONS OF MUSCLES OF THE KNEE

Knee Extensors

The quadriceps femoris is a large and powerful muscle capable of generating in excess of 1000 lb (4450 N or 2200 kg) of internal force. Such great force is needed in closed chain motion to elevate and lower the body, as in rising from a chair, climbing, and jumping, and to prevent the knee from collapsing in walking, running, or landing from a jump. Here the quadriceps mechanism provides an active restraint to the femoral condyles on the tibial plateau to supplement passive restraints such as the posterior cruciate ligament and joint contours.

The rectus femoris crosses the hip and is a hip flexor as well as a knee extensor. As would be expected, the muscle becomes active as a knee extensor early in the range of motion when the hip is extended and the maximum torque output of the quadriceps is increased with hip extension. This effect can be observed when a seated subject is having difficulty extending the knee against resistance. If the subject leans back to place a stretch on the rectus femoris, increased torque will become available.

At one time it was thought that the vastus medialis was responsible for the last 20 to 30 degrees of knee extension. Electromygraphic studies have shown, however, that all four of the quadriceps muscles are active early and throughout the range of motion (Pocock, 1963; Lieb and Perry, 1971). Basmajian (1978) found that while the onset of electromyographic activity in the four muscles was variable when knee extension was performed against little or no resistance, working against resistance caused all four muscles to be activated by 80 degrees of knee flexion. Anatomically and functionally, Lieb and Perry (1968) further divide the vastus medialis into the vastus medialis longus (VML) and the vastus medialis oblique (VMO). The superior longitudinal fibers of the VML are directed 15 to 18 degrees medially from their attachment on the patella in the frontal plane. The prominent inferior fibers of the VMO are more obliquely directed to form an angle of 50 to 55 degrees. In a mechanical study on cadavers, the authors found that each of the quadriceps muscles *except the VMO* could extend the knee and that the vastus intermedius was the most efficient (required the least force). It was, however, impossible to extend the knee with the VMO regardless of the amount of force applied. The vastus medialis is believed to play an important role in keeping the patella on track in gliding on the femoral condyles (tracking mechanism). The medially directed forces of the VMO counteract the laterally directed forces on the vastus lateralis, thus preventing lateral displacement of the patella in the trochlear groove.

Knee Flexors

Open chain motions of knee flexion and rotation are important for placement and movement of the foot, but require little muscle force to execute (except deceleration of the leg in walking or running). Great forces are required of these muscles, however, as they act on other joints or in closed chain motion. The hamstrings muscles are primary hip extensors and contract strongly to stabilize the pelvis during trunk extension (prone), and to control the pelvis on the femur as the seated or standing subject leans forward to touch the feet and then returns to the upright position. The hamstrings, sartorius, and the gracilis muscles have rotatory actions at the hip and knee, and the popliteus is a rotator at the knee. After the foot is planted on the ground during the stance phase of walking, the knee and hip must rotate for forward motion of the body to occur over the supporting foot. The rotation is initiated and controlled by the rotator muscles. In activities such as running, turning, cutting, or maintaining balance on an unstable base of support (such as uneven ground or a rocking boat), the force required of the rotator muscles increases markedly. Activities carried out in the kneeling or squatting position (such as gardening, welding, mining, or playing football) require strong forces from the rotator muscles to initiate and control hip and knee motions on the fixed tibia in response to necessary twists of the trunk and upper extremities. Thus, injuries to the knee flexors (i.e., hamstring "muscle pull") are more commonly due to their actions as rotators or as decelerators of limb motion than as flexors of the knee.

FUNCTION OF THE POPLITEUS

The popliteus muscle is deep-set in the calf and difficult to palpate or study. Although considered a small muscle, it has a cross-sectional area larger than those of the gracilis or the sartorius muscles and an area approximately 70 percent as large as that of the semitendinosus (see Appendix A). Although the popliteus is classified as a knee flexor, its leverage is poor for this motion. Basmajian (1978) reported finding only 10 to 15 percent of maximum electromyographic activity of the popliteus associated with performance of knee flexion (prone) or knee extension (sitting). On the other hand, when these motions were performed with voluntary medial rotation of the knee, the activity of the popliteus increased to 40 to 70 percent of maximum activity. A greater amount of activity occurred during knee extension than during knee flexion!

One of the most important functions of the popliteus is considered to be its rotary action for unlocking the extended knee. Since terminal knee extension requires lateral rotation of the tibia on the femur, initiation of knee flexion requires the reverse action of medial rotation of the tibia on the femur. This action is thought to be performed by the popliteus muscle. An additional function of the muscle has been investigated electromyographically by Barnett and Richardson (1953). These investigators recorded large amounts of electromyographic activity from the popliteus when "knee bends" were performed from the standing position. When the knee approached a right angle, action potentials appeared in the popliteus, and the activity persisted as long as a crouching posture was maintained. The investigators point out that when the knee is bent, the weight of the body from above tends to cause the femoral condyle to slide forward on the tibial plateau, and "although the posterior cruciate ligament is generally credited with resisting this subluxation, it appears, in fact, that it has active support of the popliteus to stabilize the knee in this position."

The posterior cruciate ligament attaches to the medial condyle of the femur, while the popliteus—by means of its strong tendon—attaches to the lateral condyle. The action of the popliteus, therefore, is an important complement to that of the posterior cruciate ligament in preventing a forward sliding of the condyles in weight-bearing on flexed knees.

ONE-JOINT AND TWO-JOINT MUSCLES ACTING AT THE KNEE

Only five of the muscles that act on the knee are one-joint muscles: the three vasti, the popliteus, and the short head of the biceps femoris. The remaining muscles cross both the hip and knee (rectus femoris, sartorius, gracilis, semitendinosus, semimembranosus, long head of the biceps femoris, and the ilio-tibial tract of the tensor fasciae latae), or the knee and ankle (gastrocnemius). Thus, motions or positions of the hip and ankle influence the range of motion that can occur at the knee as well as the forces that the muscles can generate (passive and active insufficiency).

Under ordinary conditions of use, two-joint muscles are seldom used to move both joints simultaneously. More often, the action of two-joint muscles is prevented at one joint by resistance from gravity or the contraction of other muscles. If the muscles were to shorten over both joints simultaneously and to complete the range at both joints, they would have to shorten a long distance and would rapidly lose tension as the shortening progressed. In natural motions, however, the muscles are seldom, if ever, required to go through such extreme excursion. The two joints usually move in such directions that the muscle is gradually elongated over one joint while producing movement at the other joint. The result is that favorable length-tension relations are maintained.

TWO-JOINT MUSCLES OF THE KNEE

The action of the two-joint muscles will be considered in the following movement combinations:

KNEE FLEXION COMBINED WITH HIP EXTENSION. If the subject is lying prone or standing erect and flexes the knee while extending the hip, the hamstring muscles must shorten over both joints simultaneously, and difficulty is experienced in completing knee flexion. Some subjects complain of a cramp in the muscles of the posterior thigh when performing this motion. All subjects lose strength rapidly as knee flexion proceeds while the hip is extended (see Fig. 4-8). The range of useful excursion becomes almost exhausted. Another factor that often limits full excursion of the hamstrings is the inability of the rectus femoris, which is being stretched over the hip and knee simultaneously, to elongate sufficiently. When spasticity of the rectus femoris is present, the interference of this muscle becomes marked, resulting in a forward tilting of the pelvis; in the prone position the buttocks then become elevated in an awkward manner.

KNEE EXTENSION COMBINED WITH HIP FLEXION. In a supine or standing position, straight leg raising—consisting of hip flexion with the knee maintained extended—may be performed. The movement proceeds without strain throughout a certain range, then difficulty arises mainly from the inability of the hamstrings to elongate sufficiently and, to a lesser extent, from the decrease in strength of the rectus, which muscle has to shorten over the hip and knee simultaneously. By performing a passive movement of hip flexion, first with the knee extended and then with the knee flexed, the effect of hamstring interference in hip flexion becomes obvious. If straight leg raising is limited by contracture or spasticity (e.g., 30 degrees), normal step length will be diminished in walking. The knee may be extended fully on one side when the hip is extended, but the opposite leg will not be capable of reaching as far forward (hip flexion and knee extension) as usual. The subject will be limited to short steps and will usually walk with the knees flexed. By performing a passive movement of hip flexion, first with the knee extended and then with the knee flexed, the effect of hamstring interference in hip flexion becomes obvious.

KNEE FLEXION COMBINED WITH HIP FLEXION. This combination provides for elongation of the hamstrings over the hip while knee flexion is carried out, resulting in favorable length-tension relations. During hip-knee flexion, the hip flexors and the hamstrings act synergically to provide a functionally useful movement; whereas in other movement combinations, these two muscle groups may act as antagonists.

KNEE EXTENSION COMBINED WITH HIP EXTENSION. This is a most useful combination that occurs in activities such as rising from the sitting position, climbing stairs, running, and jumping. The hamstrings then act as hip extensors, while the quadriceps extends the knee and, by doing so, elongates the hamstrings over the knee. In this movement, as in the previous one, an effective portion of the length-tension curve is used.

KNEE FLEXION COMBINED WITH PLANTAR FLEXION OF THE ANKLE. The gastrocnemius is capable of performing these two motions simultaneously, but if full range at both joints is attempted, the muscle has to shorten a long distance and tension falls rapidly. It is not a very useful movement.

KNEE EXTENSION COMBINED WITH PLANTAR FLEXION OF THE ANKLE. The quadriceps extends the knee while the gastrocnemius (and soleus) plantar-flex the ankle. As the quadriceps extends the knee, the gastrocnemius becomes elongated over the knee, and optimal conditions for plantar flexion of the ankle result. This functional combination is commonly seen, as, for example, in rising on tiptoes, running, and jumping.

Torque of Muscles Acting at the Knee

Maximum isometric torque curves for the flexors and extensors of the knee (see Figs. 4-16 and 4-17) were investigated by Williams and Stutzman (1959). The torque exerted by the extensors was found to be much higher throughout the range than that of the flexors. In this investigation and subsequent studies (Mendler, 1963 and 1967; Haffajee et al, 1972; and Smidt, 1973), peak torque values for the extensors were found to occur at the 50- to 60-degree position of the knee (complete extension is at 0 degrees). The increase in torque output while the muscles are losing favorable length-tension relationships is due to the increase in patella lever arm distance. Radiographic measurements of the lever arm distance made by Smidt (1973) were greatest at the 30- to 60-degree position of the knee and decreased in distances above and below this position. In a cadaver study, however, Kaufer (1971) measured a consistent increase in patella force arm distance from knee flexion to extension. Functionally, the greater torque output at the 50- to 60-degree position is important in elevating the body, as in rising from a chair and climbing stairs. In these activities, a perpendicular line projected through the center of gravity of the body falls well posterior to the knee; therefore, the center of gravity exerts a large resistance torque that the quadriceps must match. Relatively little quadriceps torque is required in standing, since the center-of-gravity projection passes very close to the knee joint axis and the knees may be stabilized by the terminal rotation mechanism.

The shape of the maximum isometric knee flexor curve indicates that the length-tension factor predominates over the leverage factor. The highest torque values occur at the initiation of knee flexion where the muscles are elongated. The effect of the position of the hip to further lengthen the knee flexors is demonstrated by the markedly higher values when the hip is in a flexed position (see Fig. 4-17).

An example of maximum isokinetic torque for the quadriceps and hamstring muscles is shown in Figure 4-20. At slow speeds of motion (below about 30 degrees per sec), the maximum values at selected points in the range are similar to those obtained under isometric conditions. As the speed increases, the torque output decreases, and the peak torque occurs later in the range of motion. Analysis and comparison of the results of different testing conditions require careful measurement of joint positions as well as speed of motion. For the reader who is interested in more specific information on this topic, normative values for the isokinetic torque developed by the quadriceps

and hamstrings muscle groups of young adult subjects (nonathletes) have been reported recently by Wyatt and Edwards (1981).

JOINT FORCES

Even in normal activity, the articulating surfaces of the knee sustain forces that far
exceed body weight and are thus subject to microtrauma and its subsequent degenera-
tive results (Davies, Wallace, and Malone, 1980). While walking on level surfaces, the
femoro-tibial joint forces momentarily reach three times body weight (Morrison,
1970). Maximum isometric knee extension was calculated by Smidt (1973) to produce
a femoro-tibial compression force of 1.6 times the body weight when the knee was
extended and three times the body weight when the knee was in a position of 60
degrees. In Figure 2-19, the joint force was calculated as 350 lb when holding a 30-lb
weight on the foot. Symptomatic inflamatory responses may occur when these forces
are accompanied with sudden overuse of the knee (e.g., gardening, jogging, or roof-
ing) and with hypermobility or hypomobility of joint structures from the foot to the
spine, which call for compensatory motion or stabilization at the knee during weight-
bearing activities (Davies et al, 1980). For example, excessive pronation at the ankle

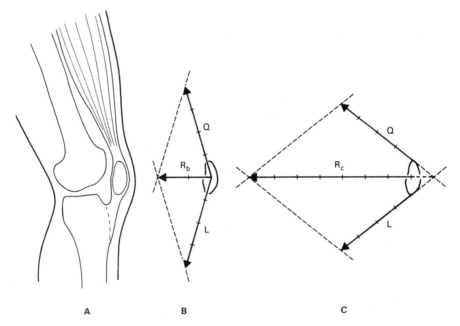

FIGURE 9-11. Patello-femoral joint compression forces. Lateral view of the patello-femoral articulation (A). Graphic composition of the forces on the patella during *active contraction of the
quadriceps muscle group* when the knee is in slight flexion (B) and when in marked flexion (C).
Q = quadriceps muscle force; L = force of the patellar ligament; R = resultant of Q and L, or the
patello-femoral compression force. Even with a similar force in Q, R is seen to increase with the
joint angle ($R_c > R_b$).

produces increased medial rotation of the tibia and repetitive abnormal stresses on knee joint structures.

The *patello-femoral* joint surfaces are a common source of knee pain and dysfunction. Biomechanically, the patella can be considered to act like a pulley as it receives forces from the quadriceps tendon and the patellar tendon (Fig. 9-11). The resultant of these two forces is the patello-femoral joint reaction force. The large forces that can be created by the quadriceps muscle (e.g., 380 lb with a 30-lb boot in Fig. 2-19) also produce *large compression forces between the patella and the femur.* When the knee is in *extension,* the resultant force is *small* since the forces of the tendon and the ligament are almost on a straight line. When the knee is *flexed,* the resultant force becomes *large* and can easily *exceed the force of the muscle.* Smidt (1973) calculated patello-femoral joint reaction force in maximum isometric quadriceps contractions as 0.8 times body weight when the knee was in the 15-degree position. The force increased to 2.6 times body weight when the knee was at a 90-degree angle. During level walking, the joint reaction forces were calculated by Reilly and Martens (1972) to be one half or less of body weight. Patients with patello-femoral dysfunction find that pain is increased in ascending or descending stairs and in activities requiring kneeling and squatting. Quadriceps resistive exercises through a full arc of knee extension may be impossible to complete because of pain. When pain is present, quadriceps muscles may be strengthened by applying resistance with the knee in an extended position, or through a short arc of terminal extension (e.g., 20 degrees).

CHAPTER **10**
ANKLE AND FOOT

The ankle, foot, and toes consist of a complex of 34 joints that, by bony structure, ligamentous attachments, and muscle contraction, can change in a single step from a flexible structure conforming to the irregularities of the ground to a rigid weight-bearing structure. The flexible/rigid characteristics of the ankle/foot complex provide multiple functions, including:

1. Support of superincumbent weight.
2. Control and stabilization of the leg on the planted foot.
3. Elevation of the body, as in standing on the toes, climbing, or jumping.
4. Shock absorption in walking, running, or landing from a jump.
5. Operation of machine tools.
6. Substitution for hand function in persons with upper extremity amputations or muscle paralysis.

Ankle injuries and foot pain and dysfunction are common and stem from the large forces that occur in the foot and ankle even in standing (see Fig. 2-13). Ankle joint forces up to 4.5 times body weight were calculated by Stauffer and associates (1977) to occur while walking on a level surface. As the foot sustains these large forces, it is also making the final adjustment to the ground and must compensate for motions or deviations at the knee or hip to keep the center of gravity within the small base of support. When the foot is not protected by a shoe, the structures are subjected to trauma and temperature extremes. If the foot is enclosed in a shoe, the structures may be subjected to abnormal pressures and friction, as well as a warm, humid environment conducive to bacterial and fungal growth and infection.

311

Palpable Structures

The malleoli of the ankle, like the epicondyles of the knee, serve as landmarks for their respective regions. The *medial malleolus* (L. diminutive of *malleus*, hammer) is a prominent process on the enlarged distal portion of the tibia on the inner side of the ankle. The *lateral malleolus* is found on the outer side of the ankle. It is the most distal portion of the fibula.

Palpation of the malleoli reveals that the lateral malleolus projects further distally than the medial one. Thus, lateral motion of the ankle is more limited than medial motion. If the subject stands with the knee cap pointing straight forward (knee axis in frontal plane), palpation also reveals that the lateral malleolus has a more posterior location than the medial one.

PALPATION ON THE MEDIAL SIDE OF THE FOOT

Just distal to the tip of the medial malleolus, the edge of the *sustentaculum tali* (L. *sustentaculum*, a support) may be felt as a slight protuberance (about the distance of a finger-width). The sustentaculum tali is like a shelf of the calcaneus, which supports the inferior medial aspect of the talus and where the two bones form one of their three articulations. If the finger is moved toward the toe, again about a finger-width, the more prominent *tuberosity of the navicular* (L. *navicula*, diminutive of *navis*, ship) can be felt. The strong calcaneo-navicular or *spring ligament* runs from the sustentaculum tali to the tuberosity of the navicular. This ligament supports the head of the talus and, when overstretched, permits the talus to move medially and plantarward, thus reducing the amount of longitudinal arch and producing a flat foot deformity. If the palpating finger is placed between the tuberosity of the navicular and the distal end of the medial malleolus, the talus can be felt. The bone becomes more prominent when the foot is passively everted and then disappears as the foot is inverted. Immediately posterior to the distal end of the medial malleolus, the small prominence of the *medial tubercule of the talus* can sometimes be palpated.

These four landmarks (the medial malleolus, the tuberosity of the navicular, the sustentaculum tali, and the medial tuberosity of the talus) are the attachments of the medial collateral or *deltoid ligament* of the ankle. Within this triangle, the deltoid ligaments may be palpated. Identification in the normal subject is difficult; pain or tenderness in this area may be indicative of ligamentous tear or strain (Hoppenfeld, 1976). The deltoid ligament is composed of both deep and superficial layers, and it prevents lateral motion of the ankle or talo-crural joint (talus-tibia-fibula). The deltoid ligaments are so strong that eversion sprains are unusual; with severe lateral motion, avulsion (L. *avulsio*, from *a-*, away, plus *vellere*, to pull) of the ligamentous attachments or fracture may occur before ligamentous tears.

As the palpating finger proceeds from the tuberosity of the navicular toward the toe on the medial side of the foot, the *first cuneiform* is palpated followed by a prominence of the *first tarso-metatarsal joint*, the concave shaft of the *first metatarsal*, and the prominence and joint line of the *first metatarso-phalangeal joint*.

PALPATION ON THE LATERAL SIDE OF THE FOOT

A large area of the lateral surface of the *calcaneus* may be palpated. The posterior portion feels relatively smooth, but below and slightly anterior to the tip of the lateral malleolus a small process may be felt. This process is an attachment for a lateral collateral ligament (calcaneo-fibular) and separates the tendons of the peroneus longus and brevis. More anteriorly, the *tuberosity at the base of the fifth metatarsal bone* may be felt as a large, easily identified prominence on the lateral side of the foot near the sole. The *cuboid bone* may be palpated between the calcaneus and the tuberosity of the fifth metatarsal bone and may be followed dorsally toward its articulations with the lateral cuneiform and with the navicular bones. The cuboid extends dorsally to about the middle of the foot, but this area is covered by ligaments and tendons, and the various bones are difficult to distinctly recognize.

The three *cuneiform bones* (L. *cuneus*, wedge), lying across the instep of the foot, form the arched part of the dorsum of the foot. The height of this arched portion varies considerably in different individuals. The *medial cuneiform bone* is identified by its medial position between the tuberosity of the navicular bone and the base of the first metatarsal bone. The *intermediate and lateral cuneiform bones* lie in line with the second and third metatarsal bones, respectively, articulating proximally with the navicular bone.

The *tarsal-metatarsal articulations* can be palpated on their dorsal surfaces if the metatarsal bones are passively moved up and down or rotated. The second tarso-metatarsal joint is strongly mortised into the recess formed by the three cuneiforms and the third metatarsal, and thus forms a very rigid part of the arch.

The *heads of the metatarsal bones* are felt both on the dorsal and the plantar sides of the foot. By manipulating the toes in flexion and extension, the heads of the metatarsal bones are particularly well palpated from the plantar side. Their plantar surfaces constitute the ball of the foot on which weight is carried when standing on tiptoes. In the region of the head of the first metatarsal bone, the sesamoid bones, which are imbedded in the tendon of the flexor hallucis brevis, can sometimes be palpated and moved slightly from side to side. The *shafts of the metatarsal bones* are best palpated on the dorsum of the foot. The phalanges of the toes are easily recognized. The *interphalangeal joints* should be palpated and manipulated.

The *talus* (astragalus)—articulating with the tibia and the fibula above, with the calcaneus below, and with the navicular bone in front—has only small palpable areas. If the finger is placed on the anterior side of the lateral malleolus, the *trochlea* (dome) of the talus becomes prominent with plantar flexion. Slightly distal to this point is a depression that lies over the *sinus tarsi*, which is a channel that runs between the articulations of the talus and the calcaneus. If the foot is inverted, the neck of the talus may become more prominent. Over the sinus tarsi lies the *anterior talo-fibular* ligament, one of the three lateral collateral ligaments of the ankle. The *calcaneo-fibular* ligament courses from the distal end of the lateral malleolus to the lateral aspect of the calcaneus, and the *posterior talo-fibular* ligament runs horizontally from the posterior portion of the lateral malleolus to the talus. The lateral collateral ligaments limit medial motion of the talus and calcaneus. The anterior talo-fibular ligament is commonly sprained in inversion injuries of the ankle.

Nonpalpable Structures

Because of the joint capsules and the many ligaments (short, long, transverse, longitudinal, and oblique) that cross the various joints of the foot, the shape of each individual bone cannot be palpated in detail. Shapes of the articulating surfaces should be studied on a disarticulated bone set. The attachments and course of the long plantar ligament should be noted from the plantar surface of the calcaneus (anterior to the tuberosity) to the bases of the third, fourth, and fifth metatarsals. The tarsal canal (between the talus and the calcaneus) should be explored and the strong interosseous (talo-calcaneal) ligament visualized. This ligament becomes a major limiting factor in the motion between the two bones.

It is of interest to note that several of the bones of the foot have grooves to accommodate tendons. A groove on the inferior surface of the cuboid bone contains the tendon of the peroneus longus; the tendon of the flexor hallucis longus is lodged in a groove on the talus, then courses below the sustentaculum tali of the calcaneus; the same tendon, nearing its distal attachment on the distal phalanx, passes through an osteofibrous groove on the plantar surface of the big toe.

JOINTS

Talo-crural Joint (Upper Ankle Joint)

TYPE OF JOINT

The talo-crural joint, between the talus and the crus (L. leg), is a hinge joint with one degree of freedom of motion. The talo-crural joint is usually referred to as the "ankle joint," although "upper ankle joint" is more specific. The trochlea of the talus possesses a superior weight-bearing surface that articulates with the distal end of the tibia, and medial and lateral surfaces that articulate with the medial malleolus of the tibia and the lateral malleolus of the fibula. The tibia and fibula are bound together by the anterior and inferior talo-fibular ligaments. Thus, the malleoli form a strong mortise for the trochlea of the wedge-shaped talus.

AXIS OF MOTION

A line connecting points just distal to the tips of the malleoli identifies the approximate direction of the upper ankle joint axis (Fig. 10-1). It is oblique to the long axis of the leg, and it is inclined, in the frontal plane, posteriorly and laterally (Inman, 1976). Inman states that the axis is obliquely oriented in the transverse plane also. He has demonstrated that the upper ankle axis is not horizontal, as frequently described, but

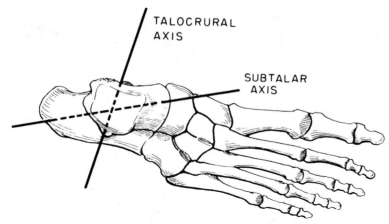

TALOCRURAL
AXIS

SUBTALAR
AXIS

FIGURE 10-1. Axes of upper ankle joint (talocrural) and lower ankle joint (subtalar). (Redrawn from Elftman, 1960.)

that it is inclined laterally and downward to a varying amount. His detailed investigations showed, too, that in 20 percent of the specimens studied, the ". . . axis may be a changing one . . .", but for all practical purposes it can be considered a single axis. Since the lateral malleolus extends further posteriorly than the medial one, the upper ankle axis is not parallel to the axis for flexion and extension of the knee. The amount of deviation of the ankle axis from the frontal plane may be measured (see Appendix C). Individual variations of this external rotation of the ankle axis with respect to the knee axis are considerable. Knee-ankle-foot orthoses in which the transverse mechanical axes of the knee and ankle are in the same plane cause deviation of the extremity within the orthosis and may lead to further deformity (Lusskin, 1966).

MOVEMENTS OF THE UPPER ANKLE JOINT

These movements are best described as dorsiflexion, toward the dorsal side of the foot, and plantar flexion, toward the plantar side of the foot. If the terms flexion and extension are used, misunderstandings may arise. Functionally, plantar flexion of the ankle may be called extension, since it is part of a general extension movement of hip, knee, and ankle. From the anatomic standpoint, dorsiflexion may be called extension, since the movement occurs toward the extensor side of the limb. To avoid this dilemma, it is customary to use the terms dorsiflexion and plantar flexion because these terms are descriptive and cannot be misunderstood.

Role of the Tibio-fibular Joints in Ankle Motion

The dome of the talus is wider anteriorly than posteriorly in most anatomic specimens; yet the malleoli maintain congruence with the talus throughout the range of plantar flexion and dorsiflexion (Inman, 1976). Such disparity requires motion to occur at the malleoli. The motion occurs either by rotation or by abduction of the fibula at the distal tibio-fibular syndesmosis (Gr. *syndesmos*, band or ligament), and is in turn reflected at the proximal tibio-fibular joint. In the normal subject, this motion can be detected by palpation of the head of the fibula as it is accompanied by a small proximal movement with dorsiflexion of the ankle. In addition, dorsiflexion can be limited by forceful compression of the malleoli. The importance of the tibio-fibular joints are described by Helfet (1974), and their clinical relevance in knee and ankle dysfunction is presented by Radakovich and Malone (1982) as the "forgotten joint."

Terminology for Denoting Motions at Joints of the Foot

Study of the motions of the joints of the foot is complicated by nomenclature designed to describe planar motion or gross motion of the structure as a whole—inversion-eversion, supination-pronation, abduction-adduction, and flexion-extension. In the foot, the axes of joint motions are not in perpendicular planes, and joint motions are interdependent, particularly with weight-bearing. Clinically, *inversion* is a rotation at the tarsal joints to turn the sole of the foot inward or to raise the medial border of the foot. *Eversion* is an elevation of the lateral border of the foot. *Pronation* is a depression of the medial longitudinal arch, and *supination* is an elevation of the arch. *Adduction* and *abduction* are medio-lateral motions. *Flexion* and *extension* are motions in a plantar or dorsal direction. Since these motions occur at several joints and may have common elements (e.g., inversion and supination), use of these terms to describe *individual joint motion* may vary with authors. Morton (1952) describes the motion at the subtalar joint as supination and pronation. Cailliet (1983) describes subtalar motion as inversion, adduction, and plantar flexion, which, if complete, produces supination. Inman (1976) rarely used this terminology to describe subtalar motion, but when he did, the words are used synonymously, that is, eversion (pronation). The reader is cautioned to be aware of these semantic problems and to seek out the definitions being used.

Subtalar Joint (Lower Ankle Joint)

The inferior surface of the talus presents three articular facets that rest on corresponding areas of the calcaneus to form the subtalar joint, or lower ankle joint. Anteriorly, the talus articulates with the navicular bone. This complex set of articulations allows movements about an oblique axis, allowing the foot to be turned in (*inversion*) and turned out (*eversion*).

AXIS OF MOTION

The axis of motion for inversion and eversion is represented by a line that begins on the lateral-posterior aspect of the heel and proceeds in a forward-upward-medial direction, as seen in Figure 10-1 (Manter, 1941; Hicks, 1953; Elftman, 1960; Inman, 1976).

Transverse Tarsal Joint

The transverse tarsal joint is also called the *midtarsal joint*. A disarticulation at the transverse tarsal joint is known as *Chopart's amputation* (after the French surgeon, François Chopart), and the joint itself is sometimes referred to as *Chopart's joint*. The bones which go into the formation of this joint are the *talus* and *calcaneus* proximally, and the *navicular* and *cuboid* distally. Functionally, with respect to this joint, the navicular and cuboid bones may be considered as one segment since very little movement is permitted between them.

At the *talo-navicular joint*, the convex head of the talus fits into the concave surface of the navicular bone. The *calcaneo-cuboid joint* is saddle-shaped. When the foot skeleton is viewed from above, the joint line of the transverse tarsal articulation has the shape of an S (see Fig. 10-1). The character of this rather complicated joint with its shifting axes of motion, its relation to the upper and the lower ankle joints, and its muscular control has been discussed by Elftman (1960).

MOVEMENTS OF THE TRANSVERSE TARSAL JOINT

This joint permits movement of the front part of the foot in relation to the back part, called pronation when the arch of the foot becomes lowered and supination when the arch is raised (Elftman, 1960). Motion at this joint occurs in combination with subtalar and tarso-metatarsal joint motions.

For a comprehensive and classic review of anatomy, biomechanics, and application to orthopedics, as well as a discussion of areas for further clinical research concerning the upper (talo-crural) and lower (subtalar) ankle joints, read Inman's *The Joints of the Ankle* (1976).

Tarso-metatarsal Joints

The cuboid and the three cuneiform bones articulate with the bases of the five metatarsals to form the *tarso-metatarsal joints* (see Fig. 10-1). The strong mortising of the second metatarsal by the cuneiforms and the adjacent metatarsals permits only slight motions of flexion and extension. The other metatarsal joints permit slight rotary motions and can be moved in arcs around the more rigid second segment.

Metatarso-phalangeal Joints

These joints correspond to the metacarpo-phalangeal joints of the hand, and like the latter, they permit a considerable range of motion. In the hand, metacarpo-phalangeal flexion is approximately 90 degrees while hyperextension is 0 to 30 degrees. At the metatarso-phalangeal joints of the foot, these relationships are reversed. Hyperextension is 90 degrees and flexion is only 30 to 45 degrees (see Appendix B). This fact is related to the weight-bearing function of the foot, as in rising on the toes and just before toe-off in walking. In these important motions, the metatarso-phalangeal joints are in hyperextension, while the flexor muscles of the toes are contracting strongly and press the toes against the ground.

TYPE OF JOINT AND AXES OF MOTION

The metatarso-phalangeal joints, like their counterparts in the upper extremity, possess two degrees of freedom of motion and permit flexion-extension and abduction-adduction movements, the latter being less important and less well under control than in the hand. The axes of motion for these movements pass through the center of the head of the metatarsal bone—that for flexion-extension in a transverse direction and the one for abduction-adduction in a dorsal-plantar direction. Orientation for abduction-adduction is a line through the second toe, while the corresponding line in the hand goes through the third finger.

Interphalangeal Joints

The interphalangeal joints of the toes are similar to those of the fingers, the great toe possessing one such joint, the four lesser toes having two such joints.

Deformities of the Foot

Foot deformities may develop from various causes, such as congenital malformations of bones, muscular paralysis or spasticity, stresses and strains in weight-bearing and poorly fitting shoes, or from a combination of several of these, as follows:

PES VALGUS. A more or less permanent pronation-eversion of the foot, the body weight acting to depress the arch. Several stages may be recognized, the last stage being known as *pes planus* or structural, rigid, flat foot.

PES VARUS (CLUB FOOT). A more or less permanent supination-inversion of the foot so that the weight is transferred to the outside of the foot and the medial border of the foot is off the ground.

PES CALCANEUS. Subject walks on heel. The front part of the foot does not touch the ground.

PES EQUINUS. In pes equinus (L. *equinus*, relating to a horse), subject walks on ball of foot with the heel off the ground.

PES CAVUS. Exaggerated high arch, or hollowness of the foot.
    Combination of two of the above deviations also occurs, such as *calcaneo-valgus*, *equino-varus*, and *equino-cavus*.

HALLUX VALGUS. A lateral deviation of the great toe at the metatarso-phalangeal joint. This condition is often accompanied by a *bunion*, or inflammation of the bursa on the medial side of the toe joint.

MUSCLES OF THE ANKLE AND FOOT

The muscles that pass over the ankle joints have proximal attachments on the tibia and the fibula, except the gastrocnemius and the plantaris, which are attached to the femur. Since no muscles attach to the talus, the muscles passing from leg to foot act simultaneously on both the upper and the lower ankle joints. The toes are activated both by *long muscles*, that is, those which originate above the ankle joints, and by *short muscles*, originating below these joints.

The muscles that act on the ankle, or on the ankle and the toes, and that have proximal attachments mainly on the shank may be divided into three groups: posterior, lateral, and anterior.

Posterior Group of Muscles

Gastrocnemius

The *gastrocnemius* (G. *gaster*, belly, and *kneme*, knee) makes up the major portion of the muscles of the calf. *Proximal attachment*: By two tendinous heads, the *medial* and the *lateral*, from above the condyles of the femur, these attachments being partly adherent to the capsule of the knee joint. The medial head is the largest of the two and its muscular portion descends further distally than that of the lateral head. (Fig. 10-2). The muscle fibers of the two heads converge to have *distal attachments* on a broad tendon-aponeurosis, which begins as a septum between the two heads and which fuses with the aponeurosis over the soleus muscle. Distally, this tendon-aponeurosis narrows to form the *tendo-calcaneus* (Achilles' tendon), which attaches to the calcaneus. *Innervation*: Branches of the tibial portion of the sciatic nerve.

INSPECTION AND PALPATION. The gastrocnemius is largely responsible for the characteristic contour of the human calf. It is seen contracting in rising on tiptoes, walking, running, and jumping. In athletic individuals, particularly in males, the muscle bellies of the gastrocnemius when contracting are short and bulky, and the tendinous portions are comparatively long.

Soleus

The *soleus* (L. *soles*, sole, sandal), like the gastrocnemius, belongs to the posterior group of the leg. These two muscles together are also called the *triceps surae*, or three-headed muscle of the calf. *Proximal attachment*: Popliteal line of the tibia and the upper one third of the posterior surface of the fibula. *Distal attachment*: By means of a

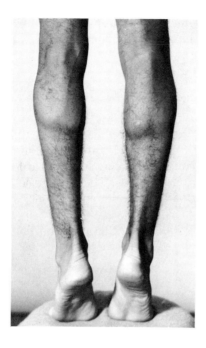

FIGURE 10-2. Both soleus and gastrocnemius muscles contract in rising on tiptoes. Note that the medial head of the gastrocnemius descends somewhat farther than the lateral head. Note the combined inversion of the heels.

tendinous aponeurosis covering the posterior surface of the muscle, which narrows distally and unites with the tendon of the gastrocnemius to form the *tendo-calcaneus*. *Innervation*: Tibial portion of sciatic nerve.

INSEPCTION AND PALPATION. The soleus is covered largely by the gastrocnemius, but in the lower portion of the calf it protrudes on both sides of the gastrocnemius so that it may here be observed and palpated. When the subject rises on tiptoes, both gastrocnemius and soleus contract strongly (see Fig. 10-2). A comparatively isolated contraction of the soleus may be seen if the subject lies prone with knee flexed and plantar-flexes the ankle against slight resistance (Fig. 10-3). The foot should be stabilized on the dorsal side so that the subject may press lightly against the examiner's hand.

Tibialis Posterior

The *tibialis posterior* is the most deeply situated muscle of the calf. It lies close to the interosseous membrane between the tibia and the fibula, covered by the soleus and the gastrocnemius. *Proximal attachment*: Posterior surface of the interosseous membrane and adjacent portions of the tibia and the fibula. In the upper calf, it occupies a central position between the flexor digitorum longus medially and the flexor hallucis longus laterally. In the lower calf, it takes a more medial course. Its tendon lies in a groove on the medial malleolus and is held down by a broad ligament. It then continues to the sole of the foot. *Distal attachments*: The tuberosity of the navicular bone and, by

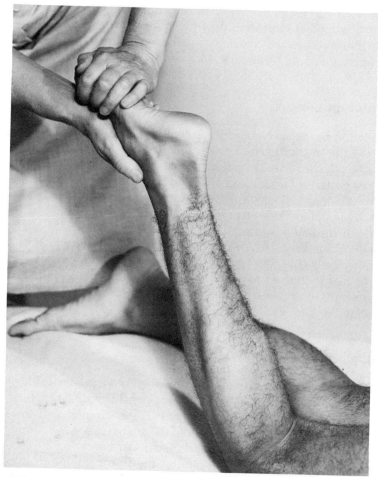

FIGURE 10-3. A comparatively isolated contraction of the soleus is obtained when plantar flexion is performed while the knee is flexed.

means of fibrous expansions, to adjacent tarsal bones and to the bases of the metatarsals. The spreading out of its attachments provides a tendo-muscular support on the plantar side of the foot.

INSPECTION AND PALPATION. The tendon of the tibialis posterior is observable and well palpable both above and below the medial malleolus. It is particularly easy to identify just proximal to the tuberosity of the navicular bone where it lies superficially. Above the malleolus, its tendon lies close to those of the flexor digitorum longus and the flexor hallucis longus. These tendons may be identified by inversion of the ankle (which brings out the toe flexors). For palpation of these tendons, have the subject seated on a chair, the limb to be tested being crossed over the other one so that the foot is relaxed and plantar-flexed. Notice that the tendon of the tibialis posterior lies closer to the medial malleolus than the other two tendons. The relationships among these three tendons just above the medial malleolus are expressed by the *Tom, Dick, and Harry rule*: Tom for tibialis, Dick for digitorum, and Harry for hallucis.

Flexor Digitorum Longus

The *flexor digitorum longus* is a deep muscle, lying medially in the calf, covered by the soleus and the medial head of the gastrocnemius. *Proximal attachment*: Tibia, below the distal attachment of the popliteus, and the intermuscular septum between it and the tibialis posterior. In the lower leg, it crosses over the tibialis posterior so that at the malleolus it comes to lie behind the tendon of the tibialis posterior. *Distal attachment*: The tendon enters the sole of the foot near the sustentaculum tali, crosses the tendon of the flexor hallucis longus, and divides into four parts that attach into the bases of the distal phalanges of the second to fifth toes. On the way to its attachment, each tendon perforates the corresponding tendon of the short toe flexor, this arrangement being similar to that of the hand. *Innervation*: Tibial nerve. *Palpation*: The tendon of the flexor digitorum longus can be palpated on the medial aspect of the medial malleolus when the toes are flexed.

Flexor Hallucis Longus

The *flexor hallucis longus* is located under the soleus on the lateral side of the calf. It is a rather strong muscle, its cross section being considerably larger than that of the flexor digitorum longus. *Proximal attachment*: Posterior surface of the fibular and intermuscular septa. Its tendon passes behind the medial malleolus, through a groove in the talus, and then under the sustentaculum tali. After entering the sole of the foot, it crosses to the medial side of the tendon of the flexor digitorum longus. At the metatarso-phalangeal joint, it passes between the two sesamoid bones in the tendon of the flexor hallucis brevis. *Distal attachment*: Base of the distal phalanx of the great toe. *Innervation*: Tibial nerve. *Palpation* of its tendon may be done above the medial malleolus, as previously described, and in the region of the sustentaculum talus, by alternating flexion and extension of the great toe. Since the average individual is unable to flex the great toe without simultaneously flexing the lesser toes, its tendon is difficult to distinguish from that of the flexor digitorum longus. Isolated contractions of the flexor hallucis longus and flexor digitorum longus are best observed with flexion of the distal interphalangeal joints of the toes.

Lateral Group of Muscles

This group is located on the lateral side of the shank, anterior to the calf group, occupying a comparatively small area and being separated from the anterior and posterior groups by intermuscular septa. There are two muscles in this group: the peroneus longus and peroneus brevis.

Peroneus Longus

In its location, the *peroneus longus* (Gr. *perone*, brooch, fibula) appears as a direct continuation of the biceps femoris. *Proximal attachment:* The principal attachment is to the head of the fibula near the distal attachment of the biceps femoris. The peroneus longus, however, has additional proximal attachments, including the neighboring area of the tibia, the shaft of the fibula, and intermuscular septa. The muscle fibers converge to form a tendon that passes in a groove behind the lateral malleolus and then to the cuboid bone where it enters the sole of the foot. There, the tendon follows a groove of the cuboid bone; the groove has an oblique direction coursing forward and medially. *Distal attachment:* Plantar surface of first cuneiform bone and base of first metatarsal.

Peroneus Brevis

The *peroneus brevis*, as its name indicates, is shorter than the peroneus longus. *Proximal attachment:* Fibula, lower than the longus, and intermuscular septa. Its tendon passes behind the lateral malleolus, then across the calcaneus and the cuboid. *Distal attachment:* The dorsal surface of the tuberosity of the fifth metatarsal bone.

The two peronei muscles are *innervated* by the superficial branch of the common peroneal nerve. (The common peroneal nerve is the lateral division of the sciatic nerve and it winds around the head of the fibula before dividing into a deep and a superficial branch.)

INSPECTION AND PALPATION OF THE TWO PERONEI MUSCLES. The muscular portion of the peroneus longus is identified just below the head of the fibula and may be followed down the lateral side of the leg. From halfway down the leg to the ankle, the two peronei muscles lie close together. Nearly all the brevis is covered by the longus, but in the lower part of the leg it can be felt separately from the longus.

When eversion is resisted, as illustrated in Figure 10-4, both muscles contract. The tendon of the peroneus brevis stands out more than the tendon of the peroneus longus and can be followed to its attachment on the fifth metatarsal bone. At the malleolus, the tendons of the peronei muscles appear as if they might slip over to the front side, but they are anchored firmly by retinacula. Above the malleolus, the tendon of the peroneus longus lies slightly posterior to that of the brevis, and, at least in some individuals, it is easily palpated. Below the malleolus, the tendon of the peroneus longus is held down close to the bone. It lies on the plantar side of the tendon of the peroneus brevis, but is rather difficult to identify (see also Fig. 10-10, B).

Note that when eversion of the foot is resisted in the sitting position, as in Figure 10-4, external rotation of the leg with respect to the thigh occurs simultaneously; the prominent tendon of the biceps femoris is seen at the knee.

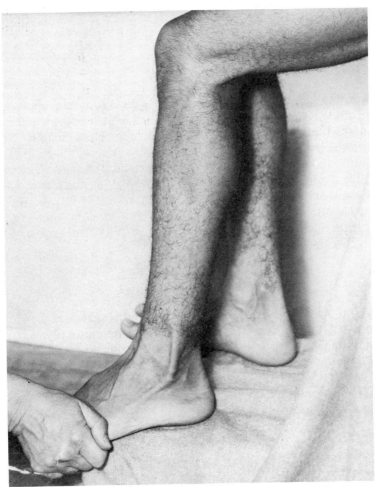

FIGURE 10-4. The tendons of the peroneus longus and peroneus brevis both pass posterior to the lateral malleolus. The tendon of the brevis may be followed to its attachment on the fifth metatarsal bone. Note also the tendon of the biceps femoris at the knee.

Anterior Group of Muscles

The anterior group is located on the lateral side of the anterior margin of the tibia, the sharp bony ridge palpable from the tuberosity of the tibia all the way down to the ankle. It is separated from the lateral group by an intermuscular septa but appears, on palpation, to be continuous with it. The muscles of the anterior group are the tibialis anterior, extensor hallucis longus, extensor digitorum longus, and peroneus tertius.

Anterior Tibialis

The *anterior tibialis* is responsible for the roundness of the shank anteriorly. When this muscle is paralyzed, a flatness or even slight concavity of this region results, so that the anterior margin of the tibia becomes even more prominent than normal. *Proximal attachment:* Lateral condyle and proximal half of the shaft of tibia, interosseous membrane, and fascia of leg. The muscle becomes tendinous well above the ankle, and its tendon passes over the dorsum of the ankle, held down by the transverse and cruciate ligaments. *Distal attachment:* Medial aspect of the medial cuneiform bone and base of the first metatarsal bone. *Innervation:* A branch from the common peroneal nerve and a branch from the deep peroneal nerve.

INSPECTION AND PALPATION. Because the muscle is superficial throughout its course, it may be observed and palpated all the way from proximal attachment to distal attachment. The muscular portion is palpated proximally, on the lateral side of the anterior margin of the tibia when the foot is dorsiflexed. Its tendon is observed and palpated as it passes over the ankle where it rises considerably when the foot is dorsiflexed (Fig. 10-5). In the illustration, the subject flexes the toes so that the tendon of the extensor hallucis longus, which lies just lateral to that of the anterior tibialis, will not be seen. If one wishes to observe both tendons simultaneously, the ankle should be held dorsiflexed and the great toe should be flexed and extended.

Extensor Hallucis Longus

In its upper portion the *extensor hallucis longus* is covered by the anterior tibialis and by the extensor digitorum longus. *Proximal attachment:* Middle portion of shaft of the fibula and interosseous membrane. Its tendon passes on the dorsum of the ankle, lateral to the tendon of the tibialis anterior, and is held down by ligaments. *Distal attachment:* Base of distal phalanx of great toes. *Innervation:* A branch from the deep peroneal nerve.

INSPECTION AND PALPATION. By resisting dorsiflexion of the great toe, as seen in Figure 10-6, the course of the tendon of extensor hallucis longus over the dorsum of the foot may be observed. The muscular portion is palpated in the lower half of the leg, but since it is almost entirely covered by the anterior tibialis and the extensor digitorum longus, it cannot be easily distinguished from these muscles.

Extensor Digitorum Longus

The *extensor digitorum longus* and *peroneus tertius* muscles are described together because they usually are not well differentiated in their upper portions. The peroneus tertius is the most lateral part of the extensor digitorum longus but is sometimes described as a separate muscle. The extensor digitorum longus is superficial, bordering laterally to the peronei muscles, medially to the anterior tibialis. *Proximal attachment:* The extensor digitorum longus to the upper portion of the tibia and fibula, interosseous membrane, intermuscular septa and fascia; the peroneus tertius to the distal portion of the fibula and to the interosseous membrane. The common tendon passes on the dorsum of the ankle, and, like the other tendon in this region, it is held down by the transverse and cruciate ligaments. The tendon divides into five slips, the most lateral one being the tendon of the peroneus tertius. *Distal attachment:* Four

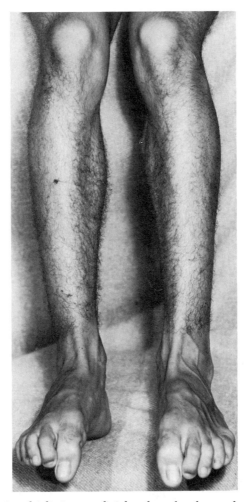

FIGURE 10-5. The anterior tibialis is superficial and can be observed all the way from proximal attachment to distal attachment. Its tendon is strong and prominent as it passes the ankle joint.

tendons go to the bases of the middle and distal phalanges of the four lesser toes; the tendon of the peroneus tertius goes to the dorsum of the fifth metatarsal bone. *Innervation:* A branch from the deep peroneal nerve.

INSPECTION AND PALPATION. To bring out the tendons of the toe extensors without simultaneous contraction of the anterior tibialis, the subject sits on a chair and lifts the toes off the floor while maintaining the sole on the floor. If resistance is given to the four lesser toes, the individual tendons stand out better (Fig. 10-7). The tendon of the peroneus tertius, when present and observable, is seen lateral to the tendon going to the fifth toe. The distal attachment of this tendon is variable, and the muscle may be missing altogether.

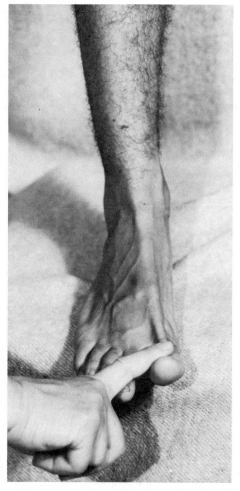

FIGURE 10-6. The tendon of the extensor hallucis longus is observed when the great toe is dorsiflexed against resistance. It lies just lateral to the tendon of anterior tibialis at the ankle.

The extensor digitorum longus also acts on the ankle joint, an action that can best be observed if dorsiflexion of the foot is resisted by pressure on the dorsum of the toes, as seen in Figure 10-7.

Muscles Originating Below the Ankle Joints

These muscles are comparable to the intrinsic muscles of the hand inasmuch as they are short muscles acting on the digits. Some of these muscles are almost identical with corresponding muscles of the hand, whereas others differ considerably.

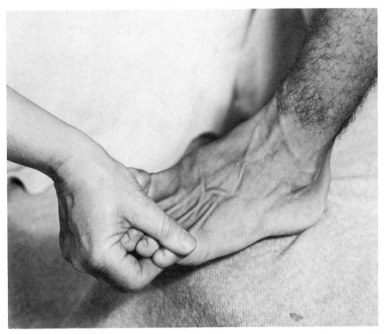

FIGURE 10-7. The tendons of the extensor digitorum longus are seen as they pass the ankle and proceed toward the four lesser toes. Examiner resists on the dorsum of the toes. In this subject, the tendon of the peroneus brevis, which passes lateral to the other tendons, could not be found.

Extensor Digitorum Brevis

The *extensor digitorum brevis* has its proximal attachment on the anterolateral side of the foot just below the sinus tarsi. Its muscular portion consists of four parts that lie largely beneath the tendons of the long extensor. Of the four tendon slips, the most medial one attaches to the base of the proximal phalanx of the great toe; the other three slips join the lateral side of those tendons of the extensor digitorum longus that serve the second to fourth toes. The muscle portion serving the great toe is the largest of the four and is sometimes described as a separate muscle, the *extensor hallucis brevis*. *Innervation:* Branch of the deep peroneal nerve.

INSPECTION AND PALPATION. The extensor digitorum brevis is variable in size. In some subjects, it is rather flat and hardly palpable; in others, a round firm muscle belly may be seen and palpated on the lateral side of the foot. It is seen in Figure 10-8 anterior to the lateral malleolus.

Since the tendons of the extensor digitorum brevis attach on the lateral side of the tendons of the longus, the tendons of the brevis compensate for the oblique direction of the longus. When the two muscles contract together, as they tend to do, the toes are extended without deviation.

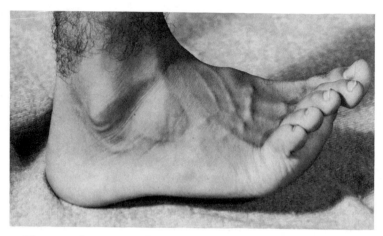

FIGURE 10-8. The muscular portion of the extensor digitorum brevis is seen on the lateral side of the dorsum of the foot. The tendons of distal attachment of this short muscle are hidden under those of the long toe extensors.

Muscles of the Sole of the Foot

The muscles of the sole of the foot should be studied in an atlas of anatomy, giving specific attention to the following:

Flexor digitorum brevis is comparable to the flexor digitorum superficialis in the hand, except that it is a short muscle.

Abductor hallucis is comparable to the abductor pollicis brevis. The abductor pollicis longus has no counterpart in the foot.

Quadratus plantae (flexor accessorius) attaches to the tendon of the flexor digitorum longus and has no counterpart in the hand.

The *lumbricals* have a similar location to those in the hand.

The *interossei* are much like those in the hand, except that with respect to abduction and adduction, they are oriented to the second instead of the third digit.

FUNCTION OF MUSCLES ACTING AT ANKLE JOINTS

Plantar Flexion of the Ankle (Talo-crural Joint)

Plantar flexion of the ankle is performed mainly, and almost exclusively, by the *triceps surae*. These muscles have both a large cross-sectional area (43 sq cm as compared with 33 sq cm for all the other muscles of the ankle combined; see Appendix A) and excellent leverage for plantar flexion. The perpendicular distance from the tendo-calcaneus to the ankle joint axis is approximately 5 cm (2 inches). Measurement of the maximum forces and torques that can be produced by the plantar flexors is difficult because of the large stabilizing forces that are imposed on the equipment, soft tissues, or intervening joints. Forces measured or calculated at the metatarso-phalangeal area during maximum isometric plantar flexion range from 225 to 400 lb (1000 to 1780 N or 102 to 182 kg) in adult men (Reys, 1915; Cureton, 1941; Haxton, 1944; Backlund and Nordgren, 1968; Tornvall, 1963; and Beasley, 1958 and 1961). Beasley measured plantar flexion force in the sitting position in more than 3000 normal subjects ranging in age from 5 to 70 years. He reported the mean value as 2.4 times body weight. After 30 years of age, the value decreases gradually, becoming about 1.7 times body weight at 70 years. Average values for young adult men were approximately 390 lb and those for women were 280 lb. Even greater forces would be expected if the knee were extended so that the gastrocnemius would have a more favorable length-tension relationship. This increase is demonstrated in two studies using young adult female subjects: with subjects in the sitting position and knees flexed to 90 degrees, Bernard (1979) recorded a mean of 98 ft-lb of torque. When the subjects were in the long sitting position with the knee extended, Belnap (1978) recorded a mean of 122 ft-lb of torque. When the sitting values were converted to force (dividing the torque by the length of the forefoot lever arm), they were similar to the force values recorded by Beasley (1958).

There are other muscles whose tendons pass posterior to the axis of motion of the talo-crural joint, but they have poor leverage and are quite *ineffective* as plantar flexors. These muscles do not act on the calcaneus but attach to more distal parts of the foot and have specific actions at other joints. The tendons of the posterior tibialis and the peronei muscles lie so close to the malleoli that they barely pass posterior to the axis. The tendon of the flexor digitorum longus lies only slightly further back. The flexor hallucis longus has somewhat better leverage, but its action as a plantar-flexor of the ankle still is insignificant compared with that of the triceps surae.

DIFFERENTIATION BETWEEN THE GASTROCNEMIUS AND THE SOLEUS IN PLANTAR FLEXION OF THE ANKLE

Because the two heads of the gastrocnemius attach above the axis of the knee, this muscle is most effective as a plantar flexor when the knee is extended. The soleus, attaching below the axis, is uninfluenced by the position of the knee. When the ankle is plantar-flexed while the knee is in a flexed position, the soleus is likely to be more active than the gastrocnemius. This is the case when the heel is being pushed off the floor in the sitting position and when the subject lies prone with the knee flexed and plantar-flexes the ankle (see Fig. 10-3). In both instances, palpation can verify that the soleus acts in a relatively isolated fashion. However, if, in the positions just mentioned, great force is required, both muscles may be felt contracting simultaneously.

Functions of the gastrocnemius and soleus muscles were investigated in six normal subjects (Herman and Bragin, 1967). Subjects were tested in a prone position with knees extended, and tension and electromyographic activity were recorded with respect to muscle length, and degree and rate of tension development in graded voluntary isometric contraction. Gastrocnemius activity was observed to be greatest when the ankle was plantar-flexed, when contractions were maximal and when tension developed rapidly. The soleus was most active in positions of ankle dorsiflexion and when contractions were minimal.

FUNCTION OF THE SOLEUS IN ERECT STANDING

Basler (1942) found that the force requirements of the plantar flexors at the ankle for maintaining equilibrium in normal erect standing never exceeded one seventh of the total strength of this muscle group. (When a load was carried, the tension would rise to one fifth or more of the total strength.) It would seem that either the soleus or the gastrocnemius, unaided by the other, would be capable of producing sufficient tension for normal equilibrium. Since the force needed is comparatively small, it is difficult to ascertain by palpation the extent to which one or the other muscle is involved.

The soleus has been found to contain a higher proportion of slow-twitch muscle fibers than the gastrocnemius, which possesses predominantly fast-twitch muscle fibers (Denny-Brown, 1929; Edgerton, Smith, and Simpson, 1975; see also Chapter 3). This would indicate that the soleus is concerned more with stabilization at the ankle and control of postural sway than is the gastrocnemius. Being composed of slow-twitch, fatigue-resistant motor units, the soleus operates economically, that is, with less fatigue for sustained contraction than the gastrocnemius, which contains predominantly fast-twitch and fast-fatiguing motor units.

The importance of the soleus as a postural muscle has been confirmed by electromyography. Joseph (1960), in studying the activity of various muscles in the "standing-at-ease" position, found continuous electric activity in the soleus in all the 12 subjects investigated; activity in the gastrocnemius could be detected in only 7 of the 12 subjects.

TRICEPS SURAE IN RISING ON TIPTOES, WALKING, RUNNING, AND JUMPING

The gastrocnemius and the soleus are both involved in activities requiring forceful plantar flexion of the ankle. In rising on tiptoes, both muscles are seen to contract simultaneously (see Fig. 10-2), and their state of contraction may be ascertained by palpation. In running and jumping, the action of the gastrocnemius is indispensable since its fibers possess the quality of producing a rapid rise in tension. (The function of the triceps surae in walking is discussed in Chapter 12.)

PARALYSIS OF THE PLANTAR FLEXORS OF THE ANKLE

When the gastrocnemius-soleus group is paralyzed, the patient cannot rise on tiptoes, and the gait is severely affected (see Chapter 12). The act of climbing stairs is awkward and slow, and activities such as running and jumping are all but impossible. The deep calf muscles and the peroneals, although passing posterior to the axis of the upper ankle joint, are incapable of substituting for the triceps surae.

The effect of paralysis of the triceps surae may be observed in patients with spina bifida (congenital defect in the vertebrae) who have lost innervation to the triceps surae but retain innervation to the posterior tibialis and the peroneals, and in postpoliomyelitic patients in whom the deep calf muscles have been spared. If these patients are children (whose feet are pliable), a calcaneo-caval deformity tends to develop (Fig. 10-9). It is obvious that the tibialis posterior, the flexor hallucis longus, and the flexor digitorum longus (although their tendons pass posterior to the joint axis) are incapable of plantar-flexing the ankle. These muscles have poor leverage at the upper ankle joint and, furthermore, do not attach to the calcaneus. Their tendons pass to the sole of the foot, and when the muscles contract, they affect more distal joints rather than the talo-crural joint. The tendons of the flexor digitorum longus and flexor hallucis longus have a shortening effect on the foot in a front-to-back direction, and the calcaneus, having lost the counterbalancing effect of the triceps surae, assumes a dorsiflexed position. These elements all contribute to the development of a calcaneo-caval deformity.

TIBIAL NERVE SEVERANCE. Clinically, the ineffectiveness of the peronei muscles as plantar flexors of the ankle was observed in a patient who had a complete paralysis of all the calf muscles as the result of a gunshot injury to the tibial portion of the sciatic nerve, an injury which left the common peroneal nerve intact. To induce the patient to perform plantar flexion, this movement was first carried out passively several times (Fig. 10-10, A), then the patient was asked to repeat the movement. No plantar flexion resulted, but the foot swung out in marked eversion (Fig. 10-10, B). Note in the illustration the sharp outline of the tendons of the peroneus longus above, and the peroneus brevis below, the lateral malleolus. The long lever arm of the triceps surae as

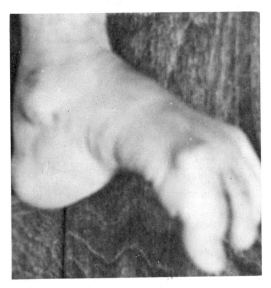

FIGURE 10-9. Postpoliomyelitic paralysis of the triceps surae. The long toe flexors, although passing posterior to the axis of the talo-crural joint, are incapable of plantar-flexing the ankle. With the triceps surae out of action, the long toe flexors are instrumental in the development of a calcaneo-caval deformity.

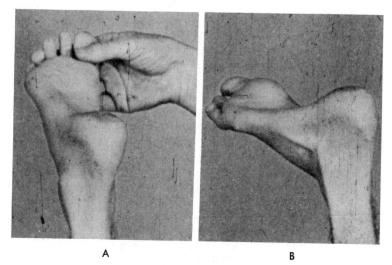

A   B

FIGURE 10-10. Severance of tibial portion of sciatic nerve with the common peroneal nerve preserved. *(A)* Patient prone, knee flexed. Passive plantar flexion is performed. *(B)* When patient attempts to plantar-flex the foot actively, the foot swings out in marked eversion. The tendons of the peroneus longus and brevis (plainly visible) course so close to the axis of the talocrural joint that their action in plantar flexion is practically nil. (Frames from a motion picture.)

compared with the short leverage of the peronei muscles can be well appreciated in this illustration.

Dorsiflexion of the Ankle (Talo-crural Joint)

This movement is performed by the anterior tibialis, the extensor hallucis longus, the extensor digitorum longus, and the peroneus tertius. Of these muscles, the tibialis anterior is by far the most important dorsiflexor—it has a straight line of pull for dorsiflexion, a comparatively large cross section, and favorable leverage. This muscle also has the advantage of acting exclusively over the talo-crural joint while the toe extensors tend to extend the toes first, thus losing effectiveness at the ankle.

ISOLATED PARALYSIS OF THE ANTERIOR TIBIALIS

When the anterior tibialis is paralyzed and the toe extensors are intact, dorsiflexion of limited range can be performed. The extensor hallucis longus is then seen contracting strongly, with the result that the great toe extends full range but comparatively little dorsiflexion of the ankle occurs. Extensor digitorum longus also participates in dorsiflexion and, if acting in an isolated fashion, will simultaneously produce strong eversion of the subtalar joint. Such eversion can be prevented by concurrent contraction of the tibialis posterior.

Inversion of the Ankle

Inversion is performed by the posterior tibialis, the gastrocnemius-soleus combination, and the long toe flexors. The tendons of each of these muscles course on the inversion side of the axis of the subtalar joint. The tibialis posterior is the inverter *par excellence*, while the others can invert in limited range only. The tibialis posterior, as previously stated, has extremely poor leverage as a plantar flexor, although its leverage for inversion is excellent. It controls this movement regardless of whether the ankle is dorsiflexed or plantar-flexed, and this can be readily ascertained by palpation. The inversion influence of the gastrocnemius-soleus combination is seen occurring simultaneously with ankle plantar flexion in Figure 10-2.

In many textbooks, the tibialis anterior is also identified with inversion. However, the point of distal attachment of this muscle is directly in line with the axis of the subtalar joint so that it is neutral with respect to inversion-eversion. Clinically, the inability of the anterior tibialis to invert the ankle was demonstrated by the patient (in Fig. 10-10) whose posterior tibialis was paralyzed. When asked to turn the foot out and in alternately, the patient everted the foot full range, then returned it to a neutral position. Thus, the anterior tibialis is capable of inversion from the fully everted position to the neutral position, but not beyond this point. (The anterior tibialis is also capable of everting the foot from the fully inverted position to the neutral position.)

Eversion of the Ankle

The movement of eversion is performed by the peroneus longus and brevis, the extensor digitorum longus, and the peroneus tertius. The tendon of the extensor hallucis longus, although slightly on the eversion side of the foot, courses so close to the axis of inversion-eversion that it has little effect on eversion. The peronei muscles are the main everters, and they act in this capacity regardless of the position of the talo-crural joint, whether this joint is dorsiflexed or plantar-flexed. The tendons of the peronei muscles may be palpated behind or below the lateral malleolus in all eversion movements. Figure 10-10 illustrates the strong eversion action of these muscles. In walking, the peroneals are important for foot placement and control of the leg on the planted foot.

Pronation-Supination

During standing (weight is carried on the foot) and particularly during walking (the body weight shifts from heel to toe), the longitudinal arch is depressed (pronated). This motion occurs at the subtalar, transverse tarsal, and other tarsal joints, and can be measured as a distance of the tuberosity of the navicular from the floor. In young adults, the change in this distance between non-weight-bearing and weight-bearing may range from 1 to 10 mm. The rigid arches show little movement, whereas those with obvious pronation will have higher values. When the body weight shifts forward to the ball of the foot, the *plantar aponeurosis*, which attaches to the calcaneus and crosses all the tarsals and metatarsals to attach distally into the phalanges, acts as a bowstring and is instrumental in raising the arch (Hicks, 1954). The tightness of the plantar aponeurosis may be palpated on passive dorsiflexion of the toes, whether performed in a non-weight-bearing position or in weight-bearing, as in rising on tiptoes. In walking and standing on the toes, the intrinsic muscles on the plantar surface of the foot contract strongly to supplement the plantar aponeurosis. These forces, along with the action of the triceps surae, cause an elevation of the arch and a supination of the calcaneus (see Fig. 10-2). The intertarsal joints become rigid and form a solid support structure.

A moderate amount of pronation-supination is characteristic of normal walking. In some individuals, the arch becomes almost obliterated during weight-bearing, but this must not be considered a "flat foot" as long as the condition reverses itself toward the end of the stance phase. The amplitude of the pronation-supination movement, which varies considerably in individuals, appears to depend mainly on the condition of the ligamentous apparatus of the foot rather than on the condition of the muscles. For example, a ballet dancer was seen in the clinic because she was worrying about getting flat feet. All of the muscles passing from leg to foot and the muscles in the sole of the foot were tested and found to be strong and under excellent control. Yet, in the standing position and on each step in walking, her feet pronated markedly. In this patient, the ligaments ordinarily responsible for arresting the motion probably had been excessively stretched during ballet practice. The muscles, although capable of preventing excessive pronation when attention was focused on the foot, did not do so automatically.

In the past, it was thought that the posterior tibialis, the peroneus longus, and the intrinsic muscles on the plantar surface of the foot maintained the longitudinal arch during standing. Electromyographic studies have shown this concept to be erroneous, in that normally there is no activity in these muscles during static standing (Basmajian, 1957). The normal arch is maintained by its osseous and ligamentous structures. The muscles do, however, become a secondary line of support to the arch when it is stressed. Gray (1969) found that in subjects with flat feet the anterior and posterior tibialis and the peroneus longus muscles were active during standing. In the normal foot that was statically loaded with up to 400 lb, Basmajian (1978) reports finding electromyographic activity in these muscles as well as in the intrinsic muscles of the foot. It has been suggested that in the presence of excessive pronation, these muscles may be subject to overuse and pain, particularly as a result of running on hard surfaces. In support of this theory, De Lacerda (1980) measured the amount of depression of the tuberosity of the navicular bone with weight-bearing. He found that those who later developed shin splints (pain to palpation, muscle testing, and weight-bearing of the anterior or posterior tibialis muscles) had an average depression of the navicular of 8.9 mm, whereas those who did not develop problems had a depression averaging 5.6 mm.

Flexion and Extension of Metatarso-phalangeal Joints

If the metatarso-phalangeal joints are compared with their counterparts in the hand, it will be seen that range in flexion predominates in the hand, while the range in extension is freer in the foot, corresponding to the grasping function of the hand and the weight-bearing function of the foot.

When, in walking, the body weight is transferred from heel to toe and the forefoot propels the weight of the body through space before the load is supported by the other foot, a considerable range in extension of the metatarso-phalangeal joints is required. This extension movement is caused by the superimposed body weight, but excessive movement is checked by the toe flexors. Since these muscles are being passively stretched, they are physiologically well prepared to produce tension, as they are first engaged in a lengthening contraction and then in a shortening contraction, the latter contributing to the "push-off," a particularly important action in running.

Abduction and Adduction of Metatarso-phalangeal Joints

These movements, like those in the hand, are performed by the interossei muscles, supplemented by the special abductors of the great and little toes. Infants move their toes freely in abduction and adduction, whereas adults have more difficulty. The first and the fifth toes are usually the easiest ones to move, but sometimes the ability of controlling the toes in these movements is lost through lack of use.

Movements at Interphalangeal Joints

Flexion and extension of these joints tend to occur as mass movements, it being difficult to move one toe without the others.

Use of Toes for Skilled Activities

With one exception, movements performed by the human hand can potentially be performed by the foot. Opposition of the thumb is not represented in the foot. The possibilities of developing the feet for grasping objects and performing skilled sensori-motor tasks have been amply demonstrated by children with congenital amputations of the upper extremities, particularly if the entire limbs are missing. These children learn to use their feet in an extraordinarily skilled manner and are capable of doing practically everything with their feet that normal children do with their hands.

CHAPTER **11**

HEAD, NECK, AND TRUNK

The vertebrae, ribs, and jaw have multiple purposes that frequently must be carried out simultaneously: protecting organs (spinal cord and viscera); providing vital functions of breathing, chewing, and swallowing; supporting head, arms, and trunk (HAT) against the force of gravity; transmitting forces between upper and lower extremities; and providing stability and mobility for hand function, locomotion, and other activities. The anterior portion of the vertebral column (bodies and disks) provides for weight-bearing, shock absorption, and mobility in all directions. The posterior portion of the column provides for protection of the spinal cord, guidance and limitation of motion, and elongated processes to increase the leverage of muscles of the trunk and extremities. Multiple motions can occur between the vertebrae: flexion, extension, lateral flexion, rotation, compression, and distraction, as well as horizontal and lateral shear. Although each motion may be as little as 1 degree, the additive effect over the multiple segments (up to 24) can produce a considerable amount of trunk motion. These small motions of the vertebral joints are complex, for each vertebra has more articulating surfaces than almost any other bone. The lumbar and cervical vertebrae have six articulations, whereas thoracic vertebrae may have up to 12 articulating surfaces (costo-vertebral joints). Injury, inflammation, hypomobility, or hypermobility of these structures can lead to pain and dysfunction and cause abnormal compensatory movement at other joints.

Nonpalpable Structures

Since the vertebral column is imbedded in muscles posteriorly and laterally and not available for palpation anteriorly, its general structure and the characteristics of its indi-

337

vidual parts should be studied using a disarticulated bone set and an anatomic atlas. *An anatomic orientation must precede clinical palpation.* It is suggested that the preliminary study include the following: (1) The *physiologic curves* of the vertebral column: cervical, thoracic, lumbar, and sacro-coccygeal. (2) The *general structure of a vertebra:* body and arch, enclosing the vertebral foramen; laminae; transverse, articular, and spinous processes; *specific characteristics* of the 7 cervical, 12 thoracic, and 5 lumbar vertebrae; the intervertebral disks. (3) *Ligaments* that bind the vertebrae together: anterior and posterior longitudinal ligaments, extending the entire length of the column; ligamenta flava (L. *flavus,* yellow), between the laminae of adjacent vertebrae; ligamenta intertransversaria, interspinalia, and supraspinalia; and ligamentum nuchae.

On the skull, the following structures should be identified: the *inferior nuchal line of the occipital bone,* which is almost parallel with the superior nuchal line but is hidden from palpation by muscles; the *occipital condyles,* one on each side, which go into the formation of the atlanto-occipital joints; the *jugular processes* of the occipital bone, which are located lateral to the occipital condyles and serve as attachment to one of the short posterior neck muscles (rectus capitis lateralis); and the *foramen magnum* of the occipital bone, which transmits the medulla oblongata.

On the anterior side of the foramen magnum is the *basilar part of the occipital bone.* This portion of the bone lies on the anterior side of the axis of motion of the atlanto-occipital joints and serves as attachment for the deep flexor muscles of the head (longus capitis, rectus capitis anterior).

On the mandible (lower jaw), the following parts should be identified: the *body, ramus,* convex *condyles,* and the *coronoid process* for attachment of the temporalis muscle. At rest, the condyles of the mandible lie in the glenoid fossa of the *temporalis* bone. When the mouth is opened, the condyles move down and forward to lie beneath the *articular tubercle* on the *zygomatic* process of the temporal bone.

Palpable Structures

If the fingers are placed behind the ear lobes, the mastoid portion of the temporal bone can be palpated, its lowest part being the *mastoid process* (Gr. *mastos,* breast, and *eidos,* resemblance). In the erect position, this process is best felt if the head is bent forward slightly so that the sternocleidomastoid muscle, which attaches to it, is relaxed. When the head is tipped backward, the muscle tightens, and only part of the process may be reached for palpation.

By moving the fingers in a posterior direction from the mastoid process, the *occipital bone* with its *superior nuchal line* is reached. The lateral portion of this ridge serves, in part, as a site for attachments of the sternocleidomastoid muscle, and its medial portion, in part, as a site for attachment of the trapezius.

At the point where the two superior nuchal lines of the right and the left sides meet in the median line is a small eminence, the *external occipital protuberance;* the external occipital crest extends from the protuberance to the foramen magnum, also in the median line. These bony eminences, which are not too well palpable, serve as sites for attachment of the *ligamentum nuchae*, a strong ligamentous band extending from the seventh cervical vertebra to the skull. This ligament is attached to the trapezius muscle and to a number of posterior neck muscles. It is best palpated when it is slack—when the head is tilted backward.

Just anterior to the external auditory canals, the *condyles of the mandible* can be palpated. When the subject opens the mouth or deviates the jaw, the condyles can be felt to move on the glenoid fossa and tubercle of temporal bones. The mandibular condyles also can be felt by placing the finger in the ear canal and pressing anteriorly.

For clinical orientation, the following *landmarks* may be used to determine the height of specific vertebrae: *C3*—level with the hyoid bone, which can be palpated anteriorly just below the mandible; *C4* and *C5*—level with the thyroid cartilage; *C6*—level with the arch of the cricoid cartilage; *body of T4*—height of junction of the manubrium and the body of the sternum; *body of T10*—level with the tip of the xiphoid process; *spinous process of L4*—level with highest portion of crest of ilium; *S2*—height of posterior superior iliac spines.

FIRST AND SECOND CERVICAL VERTEBRAE

The first cervical vertebra, the *atlas*, has a *transverse process* that protrudes more laterally than do those of the other vertebrae in this region. This process may be palpated and is found just below the tip of the mastoid process. This region is rather sensitive to pressure, and it is suggested that the student identify it on oneself before doing so on another person. The *posterior tubercle of the atlas* (its rudimentary spinous process) lies deep but may be found in its relation to the second cervical vertebra. The *spinous process of the axis*, the second cervical vertebra, is strong and prominent and is therefore easy to identify.

THIRD TO SIXTH CERVICAL VERTEBRAE

The lateral portions of these vertebrae present a number of processes and tubercles that are best palpated with the subject supine to relax the muscles of the neck. These vertebrae have short and perforated transverse processes, and their articular processes protrude laterally; therefore, the palpable areas of these vertebrae feel very uneven. Their short, bifid spinous processes may be felt in the median line though they are covered by ligamentum nuchae.

VERTEBRA PROMINENS (C7)

Because of the prominence of its spinous process, which is longer and sturdier than those of the other cervical vertebrae and not bifid, the vertebra prominens can be identified easily in most individuals. Often, however, the spinous process of the first thoracic vertebra is equally prominent. If the subject bends the head forward, identification of these processes is facilitated. If two processes in this region seem to be equal in size, they are identified as those of C7 and T1.

THORACIC AND LUMBAR VERTEBRAE

When the subject bends forward, flexing the entire spine, the spinous processes of the vertebral column become somewhat separated from each other and may be palpated throughout the thoracic and lumbar regions. The vertebra prominens is used as a starting point for counting the vertebrae, which can be done accurately in most subjects, particularly if the subject is told to "make the back round." Vertebral columns, however, present a great deal of individual variations. One or the other spinous process may be less developed and more difficult to locate, and minor lateral deviations of the processes are also common.

In the thoracic region, the spinous processes are directed downward and overlap each other, so that the spinous process of one vertebra is located approximately at the height of the body of the next lower one. In the lumbar region, the spinous processes are large and directed horizontally, so that the height of the spinous process more nearly represents the height of its body. The change from one type to another is a gradual one. The two lowest thoracic vertebrae resemble the lumbar ones, having rather horizontally directed spinous processes that are approximately at the height of the intervertebral disk between its own body and the body of the next lower vertebra.

SACRUM AND COCCYX

The exterior surface of the sacrum is palpated as a direct continuation of the lumbar spine. The *medial sacral crest* represents the rudimentary spinous processes of the sacral vertebrae, the processes being fused with the rest of the bone. On both sides of the crest are rough areas serving as sites for attachment of ligaments, fascia, and muscles. The approximate boundaries of the sacrum may be determined by following the crests of the ilia in a posterior direction, where the sacrum is interposed between the two ilia. The "dimples" medial to the posterior superior spines of the ilia indicate the posterior approach to the sacroiliac joints.

Caudally, the sacrum is continuous with the coccyx, and the two bones form a marked posterior convexity so that the tip of the coccyx has a deep location between the two gluteal eminences. If a subject sits on the front portion of a hard chair and then leans against the back of the chair, the coccyx may be felt contacting the chair.

THORAX, OR RIB CAGE

This consists of the 12 thoracic vertebrae in back, the sternum in front, and the 12 ribs. Most of the external surfaces of the thorax may be palpated. Some difficulty arises in palpating the upper ribs, which are hidden by structures of the neck and by the clavicle. In obese individuals, palpation of the last two, or "floating," ribs may be difficult also. Those portions of the ribs that lie close to the vertebral column are covered by muscles, but, beginning at their angles, the ribs may be palpated in their lateral, forward, and downward courses. It should be recalled that the first to seventh ribs attach to the sternum, the eighth to tenth ribs join with each other by means of cartilage, and the eleventh and twelfth ribs have free ends.

When the ribs on the left side are being palpated, it is suggested that the subject place the left hand on top of the head and stretch the left side so that the ribs become somewhat separated from each other. In stretching the side of the thorax, the distance between the lowest part of the rib cage laterally and the crest of the ilium increases, permitting the floating ribs to be more or less easily located. In the ordinary erect position, this distance is very short. In pathologic conditions, as in advanced states of lateral curvature of the spine, the ribs may actually come to rest on the ilium and nerves may become pinched, causing pain.

STERNUM

The sternum may be palpated from the xiphoid process below, to the manubrium and the sternoclavicular joints above.

JOINTS

Atlanto-occipital Joints

TYPE OF JOINTS

The atlanto-occipital joints have two degrees of freedom of motion. The two joints work in unison to provide movements between the head and the vertebral column. The shallow concave joint surfaces on the atlas, one on each side of the vertebral canal, support the two convex condyles of the occipital bone. The problem of supporting the head from below without interfering with the passage of the medulla oblongata into the vertebral canal, yet provide needed mobility of the head, has thus been solved excellently.

AXIS OF MOTION

The movement of the head at the atlanto-occipital joints is mainly a nodding movement in the sagittal plane, about a transverse axis through the two condyles. The approximate location of this axis is demonstrated by placing the tips of the two index fingers pointing toward each other on the mastoid processes. Small lateral bending movements are also permitted, but these are quite limited. Approximately 50 percent of the flexion-extension movement that occurs in the cervical spine occurs at the atlanto-occipital joints.

Atlanto-axial Joints

The two upper vertebrae articulate with each other by means of one centrally located joint and the two facet joints, which are formed by the inferior articular processes of the atlas and the superior articular processes of the axis. Centrally, the *dens of the axis* (odontoid process) fits into a ring formed by the arch of the atlas anteriorly and its transverse ligament posteriorly, so that a pivoting movement of the atlas around the dens can take place. Laterally, the nearly horizontal facet joints are slightly convex on both articular surfaces.

AXIS OF MOTION

The axis of motion for the centrally located joint is a vertical one, through the dens. The movement that takes place around the dens, however, is also determined by the shape of the joint surfaces of the lateral joints. Because of the convex shape of the joint surfaces of the facet joints, the *rotary movement* is not strictly in a horizontal plane, but a screwlike movement takes place. The atlanto-axial joint, therefore, is sometimes referred to as a "screw joint." The atlanto-axial joint contributes approximately 50 percent of the rotation that occurs in the cervical spine.

Intervertebral Joints From C2 to S1

The vertebral bodies from C2 to S1 are separated and flexibly bound together by intervertebral disks that allow small motions in all directions. The direction and amount of the motions in the various regions of the vertebral column are determined largely by the direction of the joint surfaces of the articular processes of the bilateral facet joints. This is similar to the way that railroad tracks control the direction of movement of a train.

INTERVERTEBRAL DISKS

Each disk (Fig. 11-1) is composed of three parts: the *annulus fibrosus*, a mesh of fibroelastic cartilaginous rings that enclose the *nucleus pulposus*, a gel with an 80 percent or more water content; and two hyaline *cartilaginous plates*, which separate the nucleus and the annulus from the vertebral bodies. The annulus is further reinforced by the anterior and posterior longitudinal ligaments (however, in the lumbar area, the posterior longitudinal ligament narrows to cover less than one half of the posterior aspect of the disk). The size of the disks basically corresponds to the bodies of the vertebrae, but becomes higher in the lumbar area. In total, the intervertebral disks account for approximately 25 percent of the length of the vertebral column.

With weight-bearing, forces are transmitted from the bodies of the vertebrae to the disk. The fluid nucleus is normally confined and therefore transmits the forces to the elastic annulus, which bulges (stretches) to absorb the weight forces and limit motion. If the force is central on the body (pure compression), the annulus will bulge in all directions. In most movements, the forces occur anteriorly, posteriorly, or laterally on the body of the vertebrae, causing the nucleus to exert pressure in the opposite direction. For example, lumbar flexion deforms the nucleus to cause an increase of posterior pressure. The annulus fibrosus becomes narrowed anteriorly and stretched posteriorly.

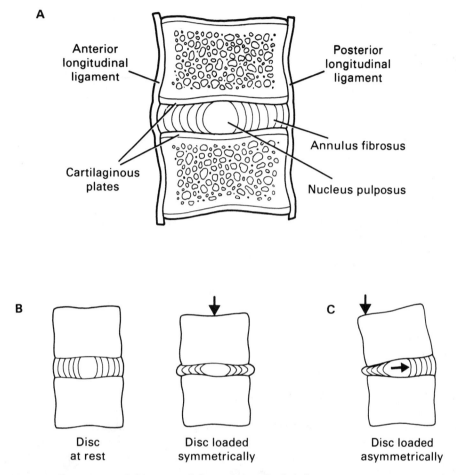

FIGURE 11-1. Structure and function of the intervertebral disk.

The nucleus pulposus is largely composed of water and is hydrophilic (loves water). Compression forces produced by standing and walking during the day cause the nucleus to lose small quantities of water, which are restored during sleep and recumbency when pressures inside the nucleus are reduced. Thus, changes in standing height of an individual may amount to as much as 2 cm between morning and evening. The supply of blood vessels to the disk disappears in the second decade of life (Cailliet, 1981), and the ability of the nucleus to restore lost water begins to decrease. Repeated microtrauma from lifting heavy objects, as well as the aging process, causes an increase in fibrous elements of the annulus and a decrease in the relative number of resilient elastic elements. The aging process causes mature adults (30 to 50 years) to become prone to injuries of the annulus and herniation of the nucleus onto the nerve roots. Older adults (50 to 90 years) may lose trunk height and be prone to develop thoracic *kyphosis* (Gr. *kyphos*, a hump), a prominent convex curvature of the spine.

CERVICAL REGION

In the upper cervical region, the articular surfaces of the facet joints are nearly horizontal, permitting mainly *rotation*. Caudally, these surfaces change their direction and become oblique, approaching the frontal plane. Some lateral bending is therefore permitted, together with a small amount of flexion and extension.

THORACIC REGION

The articular surfaces are somewhat oblique throughout, but may be said to be directed generally in the frontal plane so that *lateral flexion* can take place. This movement, however, is restricted considerably by the 10 upper ribs, and, consequently, only a small amount of motion can take place between adjacent segments. In the lowest thoracic region and at the thoracolumbar junction, however, there is more freedom of motion. Here the articular surfaces have a more oblique direction, approaching the sagittal plane, and a considerable amount of movement in all directions is permitted.

LUMBAR REGION

The articular surfaces are directed in a nearly sagittal plane throughout the lumbar region, and this permits mainly movements of *flexion and extension*.

LATERAL FLEXION AND ROTATION

Lateral flexion and rotation of the spine occur together. Lateral bend is always accompanied by some rotation, and rotation is accompanied by some lateral bend (Rasch and Burke, 1978; MacConaill and Basmajian, 1969; Kent, 1974). Although disagreement exists about the causes, the usual explanations refer to soft tissue tensions and to a mechanical principle that says, "If a flexible rod is bent first in one plane and then, while it is in this bent position, it is bent again in a plane at right angles to the first, it always rotates on its longitudinal axis at the same time" (MacConaill and Basmajian, 1969). Applying this principle to movements in the vertebral column, the "rod" (the spine) is normally "bent"—with an anterior concavity in the thoracic region and a posterior concavity in the lumbar region, causing compression on the concave side and soft tissue tension on the convex side. Thus, the "spinal column is already bent by its normal curves and lateral bending approaches a right angle to these curves" (Kent, 1974). The direction of vertebral rotation as lateral bending occurs is regulated by tension put on the ligaments and by the direction of the normal physiologic curves in combination with the direction of the lateral bend. The concave side of the normal curve turns to the convex side of the lateral curve (MacConaill and Basmajian, 1969). A lateral bend to the left would cause rotation of the thoracic vertebral bodies to the right. Lumbar bodies would tend to rotate left, but since the articular surfaces in this region are directed in a nearly sagittal plane, rotation here is limited. The effects of combined lateral flexion and rotation are particularly evident in pathologic curves of the spine.

Lumbosacral Junction

The angulation of the vertebral column at the lumbosacral junction that is marked in standing (see Fig. 8-11) indicates that the joint is subjected to a great deal of shearing stress by the superimposed body weight. Its ligamentous apparatus is comparable to that of other vertebral joints and is further reinforced by the strong *ilio-lumbar* and *sacro-lumbar ligaments*. Anatomic variations that weaken the joint and an unfavorable postural alignment may cause the fifth lumbar vertebra to slide forward on the sacrum, a pathology known as *spondylolisthesis* (Gr. *spondylos*, vertebra, and *olisthesis*, a slipping or falling).

Sacro-iliac Joint

The sacrum is firmly joined to the ilia at the two sacro-iliac joints. Reinforcing ligaments that should be noted are the *anterior and posterior sacro-iliac*, the *interosseous, sacro-tuberous*, and *sacro-spinous ligaments*. Small motions called *nutation* (nodding) occur between the sacrum and the ilia. Nutation is an anterior movement of the sacral promontory and increases the size of the pelvic outlet. Counternutation is a posterior movement of the promontory and increases the size of the pelvic inlet. A description of the motions of the sacro-iliac joints in walking and in childbirth can be found in Kapandji (1974).

Costal Joints

The ribs form two *costo-vertebral joints*. The head of the rib articulates with the bodies of two vertebrae and the intervening disk (ribs 1, 10, 11, and 12 articulate with one vertebral body). The tubercle of the rib articulates with the transverse process of the vertebra (except 11 and 12). Anteriorly, the cartilages of the ribs form synovial joints with the sternum (the first rib is cartilaginous only).

Normal Curves of the Vertebral Column

In posterior view, the normal spine is vertical. The linear alignment remains when the subject flexes the trunk. Laterally, the normal spine exhibits anterior and posterior physiologic curves that increase the resistance of the vertebral column to axial compression (Kapandji, 1974). At birth, the vertebral column is a single curve that is convex posteriorly. As the infant raises the head from the prone position and develops the ability to sit, the cervical vertebrae become convex anteriorly. As the child achieves standing and walking, the lumbar vertebrae develop an anterior convexity largely due to the tension of the psoas muscles (Cailliet, 1981). At about 10 years of age, the physiologic curves are similar to those found in the adult (Kapandji, 1974) with three curvatures: cervical (concave posteriorly), thoracic (convex posteriorly), and lumbar (concave posteriorly). The center of gravity of the head and subsequent superimposed segments falls on the concave side of all three curves (see Fig. 12-1). The inclined plane of the sacrum in the upright position is approximately 30 degrees from the horizontal (Kapandji, 1974). Alteration of the angle of the sacral base, which occurs with sitting or anterior pelvic tilt, causes in turn an alteration in the physiologic curves of the spine (see Chapter 8, pelvic balance).

When the normal subject is standing and slowly flexes the head, neck, and trunk, a lateral view of the spinous processes should reveal an unfolding of a posterior convexity without flattened areas or angulations. Lateral flexion to each side (viewed posteriorly) should also produce symmetric curves of the spinous processes. Lack of symmetry, straight areas, or angulations indicate hypomobility or hypermobility of joints or muscles. Although these deviations are considered abnormal, they may or may not be accompanied by back pain and dysfunction.

Pathologic Curves of the Vertebral Column

KYPHOSIS

A marked increase in the posterior convexity of the thoracic curve is referred to as a *kyphosis* (Gr. *kyphosis*, a humpback). In the strict sense of the word, it signifies a structural curvature of pathologic origin, as in paralysis of the erector spinae muscles in a high spinal cord injury, ankylosing arthritis, or vertebral epiphysitis. *Postural* or *functional* curves are flexible and are best referred to as "round back," "poor posture," or the like. *Senile kyphosis* refers to the rigid round back of old age, associated with collapse of the intervertebral disks, owing to desiccation of the nucleus pulposus.

LORDOSIS

Excessive increase in one of the forward convexities of the normal vertebral column is known as *lumbar lordosis* or *cervical lordosis*. Frequently, a lumbar lordosis may be attributed to faulty posture in general, but the determining factor may also be a hip flexion contracture, or various pathologies of the osseous or neuromuscular systems may be responsible.

SCOLIOSIS

Scoliosis (Gr. *skoliosis*, a curvature) is a lateral deviation of the spine and may be *functional* or *structural*. A functional curve is flexible and tends to disappear when, in standing, the subject bends forward. When the curve is structural, the vertebrae deviate laterally from the midline of the body and, at the same time, are rotated about a longitudinal axis. In the thoracic region, the ribs rotate with the vertebrae so that when the patient bends forward, a protuberance of the ribs on the side of the convexity of the curve is observed. For example, if there is a right thoracic curve (convexity to the right), the ribs protrude posteriorly on the right side. Deformities of the entire rib cage accompany such curves.

MUSCLES MOVING THE HEAD, NECK, AND TRUNK

Flexors of the Head and Neck

These muscles exert their action anterior to the axis of motion of the atlanto-occipital and the intervertebral joints. Some of these flexor muscles lie close to the anterior surface of the bodies of the cervical vertebrae, others lie further to the front.

The deepest of these muscles are the short *rectus capitis anterior*, acting on the atlanto-occipital joint only, and the *longus capitis*, acting both on head and the cervical spine. The *longus colli* acts on the neck only. Though the main action of these muscles is flexion of the head and neck, they may also have effect on lateral bending and on rotation because of their somewhat lateral location and oblique direction. In general, they aid in balancing the head and the cervical spine. The longus muscles cover portions of the anterior convexity of the cervical curve of the vertebral column and, therefore, may aid in preventing an undue increase of this curve because of the vertical pressure of the head on the spinal column. These muscles lie too deeply to be palpated or to be investigated by the electromyographic method, so objective evidence of their function is lacking. It may be assumed, however, that they are important postural muscles that aid in the maintenance of proper alignment of the cervical spine.

Scalene Muscles

The *scalene muscles* (Gr. *skalenos*, uneven; triangle with uneven sides) have *proximal attachments* on the transverse processes of the cervical vertebrae and *distal attachments* on the upper ribs. Acting bilaterally, they flex the neck on the thorax or elevate the upper ribs. Because of their antero-lateral location, when acting on one side, they bend the neck laterally. In the erect position, they contribute to the balance of the neck both anteriorly and laterally. With the cervical spine stabilized, they aid in elevation of the upper ribs, an action that is called upon in breathing.

PALPATION. The *scalenus anterior* and *scalenus medius* attach to the first rib and may be palpated during forced inspiration by placing the fingertips above the clavicle and behind the sternocleidomastoid muscle. They are also felt when, in the erect position, the head is tilted backward and when, in the supine position, the head and the neck are flexed on the thorax.

Sternocleidomastoid Muscles

The *sternocleidomastoid muscles,* one on each side, are the most superficial of the anterior neck muscles. *Proximal attachment:* By two heads: one head from the upper border of the manubrium sterni, partly covering the sternoclavicular joint, and the other from the upper border of the clavicle. *Distal attachment:* Mastoid process of the temporal bone and superior nuchal line of the occipital bone. *Innervation:* Spinal accessory nerve.

INSPECTION AND PALPATION. The two muscles may be observed in simultaneous action when the head is raised while the subject is in the supine position. One-sided action of the sternocleidomastoid is brought out if the subject's head is rotated toward one side, and resistance to lateral flexion toward the opposite side is given (Fig. 11-2). The left sternocleidomastoid is also seen in Figure 7-11, and both muscles in Figure 7-7.

There are a number of other muscles located in the anterior neck region that may participate to a certain extent in head and neck flexion. These muscles belong to the suprahyoid and infrahyoid groups, but since their main use is for purposes other than neck flexion, that is, swallowing, they will not be discussed.

Extensors of the Head and Neck

Numerous muscles are concerned with extension of the head and the neck. Some muscles are deep; others are more superficial. The posterior muscles as a group have considerably more bulk than the anterior ones, indicating that greater strength is needed in extension than in flexion.

Among the deepest extensor muscles is a group of short muscles, the *suboccipital muscles,* which connect the upper two cervical vertebrae with the occipital bone and with each other. Some of these muscles are concerned mainly with extension; others are concerned with rotation.

The *longissimus capitis,* the *transversospinalis capitis* (semispinalis capitis), and the *transversospinalis cervicis* (semispinalis cervicis) are also deep muscles of the neck, acting on the head and neck. The muscles are covered by the *splenius muscle,* which in turn is covered, in part, by the trapezius and by the upper portion of the sternocleidomastoid muscle.

PALPATION. Many of the neck extensors are too small and lie too deeply to be palpated; others can be palpated only as a group. Palpation of this group, with the subject in the erect position, should be done both with the head inclined backward (the muscles are relaxed) and with the head bent forward (the muscles become tense). If the head is inclined backward and then rotated left and right, some of the deeper muscles can be felt acting in their rotary capacity.

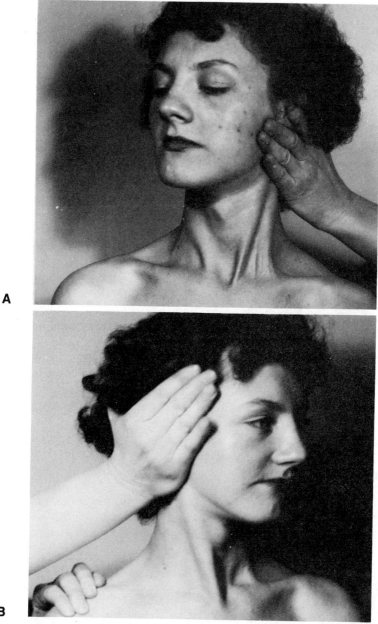

A

B

FIGURE 11-2. Testing the sternocleidomastoid muscle unilaterally. *(A)* For strong activation of the left sternocleidomastoid muscle, the head is rotated to the right, and resistance is given to lateral flexion of the head to the left. Both sternal and clavicular portions are seen. *(B)* In this patient, the clavicular portion of the right sternocleidomastoid muscle is missing. The sternal portion is seen contracting. Patient also has paralysis of the right trapezius, as seen in Figure 7-16.

Anterior and Lateral Trunk Muscles

The anterior and lateral trunk muscles, in addition to their function as supporters of the abdominal viscera and breathing, are concerned with movements of the trunk—flexion, lateral bending, and rotation. They consist of large sheaths of muscles in several layers. The fibers of the various layers run in different directions, a factor that contributes to the strength of the combined layers. A similar arrangement of fibers is seen in the thoracic region where the external and internal intercostals represent two layers corresponding to the external and internal oblique abdominal muscles.

The *linea alba* is a fibrous band in the median line of the abdominal region, extending from the xiphoid process above to the pubis below. This line unites the aponeuroses of the muscles of the right and left sides.

Rectus Abdominis

The *rectus abdominis* is a superficial muscle and consists of two parts, one on each side of the linea alba. *Proximal attachment:* Xiphoid process of the sternum and adjacent costal cartilages. *Distal attachment:* Pubic bones, near the pubic symphysis. The longitudinally arranged muscle fibers are interrupted by three *tendinous inscriptions* (L., a mark or line), the lowest one at, or slightly below, the level of umbilicus. *Innervation:* Ventral portions of the fifth through the twelfth intercostal nerves.

INSPECTION AND PALPATION. In well-developed subjects, the rectus abdominis may be observed and palpated throughout its length in flexion of the trunk (Fig. 11-3). The tendinous inscriptions and the muscular portions between them are well recognized. In the subject shown, the lowest inscription is well below the level of the umbilicus, and three "muscle hills" above this inscription can be seen. (See also Figure 11-4.) The widest portion of the linea alba (it is unusually wide in this subject) is found above the umbilicus. The lowest portion of the rectus is usually uninterrupted by inscriptions; in the illustration, however, the lowest portion of the rectus is hidden by the subject's shorts.

In obese individuals, the tendinous inscriptions and the boundaries of the muscle cannot be recognized very well but, when the subject raises the head while in the supine position, the tension in the muscle can always be palpated.

Obliquus Externus Abdominis

The *obliquus externus abdominis* (external oblique abdominal muscle) constitutes the superficial layer of the abdominal wall. It is located lateral to the rectus abdominis and covers the anterior and lateral regions of the abdomen. *Proximal attachment:* Anterolateral portions of the ribs, where it interdigitates with the serratus anterior and, at its lowest point of origin, with slips from the latissimus dorsi. *Distal attachment:* The upper fibers have a downward-forward direction and attach into an aponeurosis by which they are connected to the linea alba; the lower fibers are attached to the crest of the ilium. *Innervation:* Lower intercostal nerves.

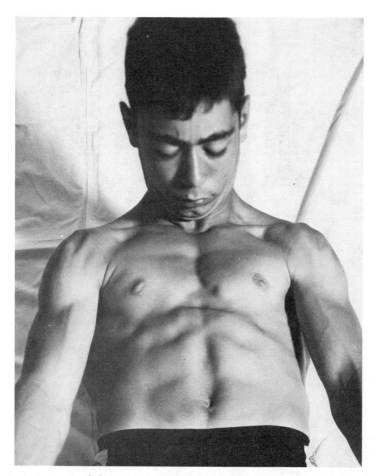

FIGURE 11-3. Activation of the rectus abdominis. In the supine position, the head and the shoulders are raised so that the spine flexes. The three tendinous inscriptions across the muscle are seen, the lowest one slightly below the umbilicus.

INSPECTION AND PALPATION. Because of the oblique direction of the fibers of the externus, flexion of the trunk combined with rotation brings out a strong contraction of this muscle, particularly if the movement is opposed by the weight of the upper part of the body (Fig. 11-4). To activate the muscle on the right side, the trunk is rotated to the left; the muscle on the left side contracts in trunk rotation to the right. Bilateral action helps to produce flexion of the trunk without rotation. The muscles are also active bilaterally when "straining."

Obliquus Internus Abdominis

The *obliquus internus abdominis* (internal oblique abdominal muscle), being covered by the external oblique, belongs to the second layer of the abdominal wall. The muscle

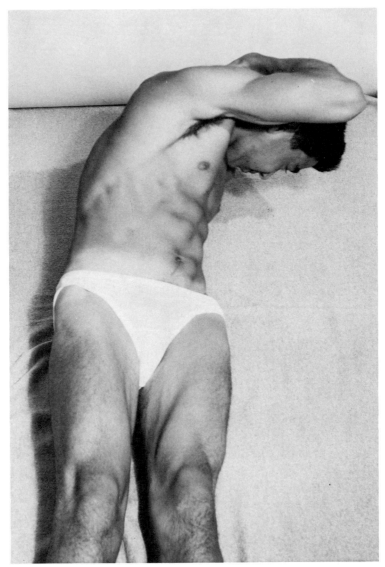

FIGURE 11-4. Activation of the right external oblique abdominal muscle. In the supine position, head and shoulders are raised and the trunk rotated to the left. The interdigitations of the right external oblique with the latissimus dorsi and serratus anterior are seen. The rectus abdominis is also contracting.

extends essentially over the same area as the externus, but its fibers cross those of the externus. *Proximal attachment:* Inguinal ligament and crest of ilium. From this region, the fibers fan out to *distal attachments* on the pubic bone, on an aponeurosis connecting with the linea alba, and on several ribs where the direction of the fibers is continuous with those of the internal intercostals. *Innervation:* Lower intercostal nerves and branches from the iliohypogastric nerve.

INSPECTION AND PALPATION. In palpation, the internal oblique cannot be well differentiated from the other layers of the abdominal wall. However, the tension of the abdominal wall (seen and felt on the left side of the abdomen when the trunk is rotated to the left, as in Fig. 11-4) is due, at least in part, to the internal oblique. In this movement, the line of action of the external oblique on the right side and the internal oblique on the left side is a continuous one, both muscles contributing to the rotation.

Transversus Abdominis

The *transversus abdominis* composes the innermost layer of the abdominal wall. This muscle has been named the "corset muscle" because it encloses the abdominal cavity like a corset. The direction of its fibers is transverse. *Proximal attachment:* Lower ribs, thoracolumbar fascia, crest of ilium, inguinal ligament. *Distal attachment:* By means of an aponeurosis, partly fused with those of the other abdominal muscles, into the linea alba. *Innervation:* Lower intercostal nerves, iliohypogastric, and ilioinguinal nerves.

PALPATION. In forced expiration, a tightening of the abdominal wall is felt anterolaterally between the lower ribs and the crest of the ilium. The transversus is partly responsible for this tension, which involves all the layers of the abdominal wall.

Quadratus Lumborum

The *quadratus lumborum* is a muscle of the posterior abdominal wall, having a close relation to the psoas major. *Proximal attachment:* Crest of ilium (posterior portion), transverse processes of lower lumbar vertebrae, iliolumbar ligament, and thoracolumbar fascia. *Distal attachment:* Transverse processes of upper lumbar vertebrae, 12th rib, and lumbar fascia. *Innervation:* Branches from the upper lumbar nerves.

Palpation is best accomplished with the subject in a supine position. The examiner palpates posteriorly at the waist lateral to the vertebral column. The subject then hikes the hip (pulls the pelvis on that side up toward the ribs, which involves shortening of the muscle). The muscular contraction felt in this region when hiking the hip is not of the quadratus lumborum alone, but involves other lateral abdominal muscles and some of the muscles belonging to the erector spinae group.

External and Internal Intercoastals

The *external and internal intercostal muscles*, as their names indicate, are located between the ribs. They may be looked upon as the thoracic continuation of the external and internal oblique abdominal muscles. Each intercostal muscle extends between two adjacent ribs, but all of them together compose a two-layered muscle sheath enclosing the thoracic cavity. *Innervation:* Intercostal nerves.

PALPATION. If an attempt is made to insert the tip of a finger between two ribs, the intercostals offer resistance. The muscles may also be felt in movements of the trunk involving a widening or narrowing of the intercostal spaces. For example, in sitting or standing, the subject reaches overhead with the left arm; then flexes the trunk to the right while spreading the ribs apart on the left side; the subject then returns the trunk to the upright position. The intercostals on the left side may be felt in both parts of this movement as they oppose the action of gravity, and in particular during the return movement.

Posterior Trunk Muscles

The posterior trunk muscles, or simply back muscles, are concerned with extension, lateral flexion, and rotation of the trunk, and, in general, with balance of the vertebral column. Anatomically and functionally, they have much in common with the posterior neck muscles with which they are continuous.

The entire extensor group is referred to as the *erector spinae* muscle. It is a large muscle mass that fills the space between the transverse and the spinous processes of the vertebrae and extends laterally beyond the transverse processes, partly covering the posterior portion of the thorax.

The many muscles which comprise the erector spinae group have proximal and distal attachments at various levels and are named in accordance with their attachments, their shape, or their action. It is suggested that the student consult an atlas of anatomy to become familiar with the following muscles: *iliocostales*, *longissimus*, *spinales*, *transversospinales* (including semispinalis, multifidus, and rotatores), *interspinales*, and *intertransversarii*. Most of these muscles are represented in all regions of the vertebral column, and their specific locations are indicated by adding *lumborum*, *thoracis*, *cervicis*, or *capitis* to their respective names, such as iliocostalis lumborum, semispinalis thoracis, semispinalis cervicis, semispinalis capitis. *Innervation:* Numerous branches of the spinal nerves from cervical, thoracic, and lumbar regions.

INSPECTION AND PALPATION. The action of the erector spinae as a group may be observed best in the lumbar and lower thoracic regions when the subject, in the prone position, raises the upper part of the body off the floor (Fig. 11-5). These muscles should also be palpated in erect standing, and the effect of swaying the upper part of the body forward and backward should be observed (during forward sway, the muscles become tense; during backward sway, the muscles are relaxed). These muscles are active also in lateral bending and in rotation of the trunk; the muscles should be palpated in these movements and their action analyzed. In walking, the erector spinae group in the lumbar region may be felt contracting on each step (see also Chapter 12).

FUNCTION OF HEAD, NECK, AND TRUNK MUSCLES

Balancing of Vertebral Column and Head

The muscles that surround the vertebral column and that are located close to it provide a flexible support for the upright column, and they act to stabilize its parts in

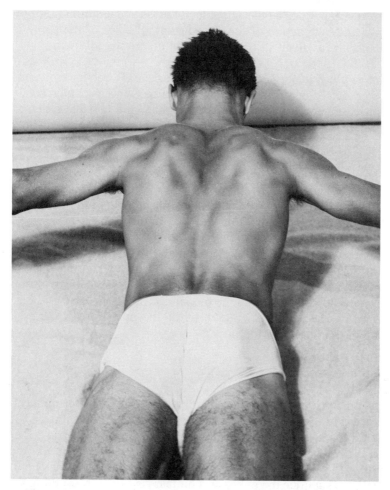

FIGURE 11-5. The erector spinae group is best observed in the lumbar region. In the thoracic region, this group is covered by the rhomboids and the trapezius. The latter muscle is seen contracting strongly.

relation to each other and in balancing the trunk as a whole in relation to the pelvis. In this action, they are aided by the abdominal and intercostal muscles, which act indirectly on the vertebral column.

Many of these muscles have a function that may be compared to that of guy-ropes supporting an upright pole. As long as the pole is vertical, little or no tension in the guy-ropes is required, but as soon as there is a slight inclination of the pole, the guy-ropes opposite the side toward which the pole is inclined become tense to prevent the pole from falling over.

The "guy-ropes" of the vertebral column are capable of producing tension at various lengths and, therefore, can allow deviations of the trunk or its segments in various directions while maintaining their stabilizing functions. Since some of these muscles are short (bridging two or three vertebrae only) and others are long, their actions may be adjusted to affect small or large segments of the vertebral column. For proper stabilization, a give-and-take action of the muscles on all sides of the spine is required. Among the muscles involved in such equilibration are the following:

1. *Anteriorly:* psoas major, longus colli, longus capitis, rectus capitis anterior, scalenes, sternocleidomastoid, anterior abdominal muscles, intercostals.
2. *Posteriorly:* erector spinae in lumbar, thoracic, and cervical regions.
3. *Laterally:* psoas major, quadratus lumborum, scalenes, sternocleidomastoid, erector spinae, lateral abdominal muscles, intercostals.

If one of the above groups of muscles is paralyzed, the body will assume a position that eliminates the necessity of action of this group. In accordance with this rule, the *vertebral column or the head will deviate toward the side of the paralyzed muscles,* which throws the muscles on the opposite side into action. This rule applies to the upright position and is illustrated by examples in the next paragraph.

If the back muscles are paralyzed or weakened, the trunk tends to be inclined backward so that the anterior muscles take over the balancing function. Paralysis of the abdominal muscles results in a forward flexion of the vertebral column. With the anterior neck muscles out of function, the subject tends to keep the head inclined slightly forward by the action of gravity, while the posterior neck muscles prevent further flexion of the head and the neck.

Stabilization

An important function of the trunk musculature is to fixate the thorax, pelvis, and vertebrae in order to stabilize the proximal attachments of the muscles of the neck, shoulders, and hips as the extremities are moved. In the supine position, head and neck flexions are synergistically accompanied by a strong isometric contraction of the rectus abdominis to stabilize the rib cage. During leg raising, all the abdominal muscles are activated to stabilize the pelvis and lumbar vertebrae. By varying the lever arm length of the lower extremity (flexing or extending the knees) and by using one or both extremities, a finely graduated exercise program for weak abdominal muscles can be developed. Manual resistance to shoulder motions such as extension-adduction (an action of the pectoralis major) will cause abdominal muscle activity, particularly of the external oblique on the same side and the internal oblique on the opposite side.

In the prone position, similar activation of the erector spinae occurs. Hip extension produces a synergistic contraction of the back extensors to stabilize the pelvis. If the arms are placed over head and then lifted, the back extensors automatically contract.

Functional Activities

Activities of lifting the body using the upper extremities, such as crutch-walking, pull-ups, or sitting pushups, activate the trunk muscles to prevent distraction of the intervertebral joints. Paraplegic patients, who must use their upper extremities to lift and move their bodies, have to lift their bodies higher to compensate for the loss of trunk musculature.

Surprisingly little activity of the neck and trunk musculature occurs in normal relaxed standing or in walking. There is very slight activity of the erector spinae and the internal abdominal obliques in standing. Activity in these muscles increases slightly in walking. Even in walking, the rectus abdominis is normally electromyographically silent. Activity of the back extensors increases in the standing position when the center of gravity of the trunk is moved anteriorly, as in swaying forward from the ankles, flexing at the hips, or flexing the vertebral column. While flexion of the spine (in either the sitting or standing position) is initially accompanied by increased activity of the erector spinae, their activity decreases and may be absent when the full range of flexion has been achieved. In this position, the vertebrae lose active muscle control, and their support is dependent upon passive ligamentous tensions. The extreme position of trunk flexion occurs in many daily activities such as leaning over to touch the toes or to pick up a piece of paper. Such apparently innocuous motions are common in the history of acute back injuries.

For specific electromyographic studies of the trunk muscles the reader is referred to the classic studies of Floyd and Silver (1950), Campbell (1952), Jones and associates (1953, 1957), Koepke and associates (1955), Partridge and Walters (1959), Morris and associates (1962), and Taylor (1960), as well as the summaries presented by Basmajian (1978).

Breathing and Coughing

The primary muscles used in inspiration are the diaphragm (which produces about two thirds of inspiratory capacity), the external intercostals, and the scaleni. Muscles of expiration are the abdominals and the internal intercostals. In normal quiet breathing, the only muscles that contract are those of inspiration. Expiration is accomplished by relaxation of these muscles and the passive recoil of the lung (elastic tissues and the surface tension produced by the fluid interface on the 3 million alveoli).

During exercise or when performing forceful breathing activities such as a vital capacity maneuver or in coughing, all the primary muscles of respiration are activated, along with accessory muscles and stabilizing muscles. Accessory muscles of inspiration are the sternocleidomastoids, the pectoralis minor, and the suprahyoid and infrahyoid muscles. The pectoralis major and the serratus anterior have also been found to be active in forced inspiration. During exercise or forced ventilation, expiration occurs by contraction of the abdominal muscles. The latissimus dorsi can assist with expiration when the arms are stabilized by placing the hands on the thighs or a table. During coughing, the latissimus dorsi can be seen to contract sharply.

The upper trapezius, erector spinae, and the quadratus lumborum are activated in forced breathing, probably more as stabilizers than as primary muscles of respiration. The erector spinae contract strongly in coughing to prevent trunk flexion that would occur with abdominal muscle contraction.

SUPPORT OF THE FLEXED SPINE
UNDER CONDITIONS OF STRAIN

The functions of the abdominals, the intercostals, and other trunk muscles in compressing the thoracic and abdominal cavities when weights are lifted or traction is applied against a firm resistance were investigated by Morris and associates (1961).

Electromyograms of the various muscle groups were recorded, and simultaneously the intra-thoracic and intra-abdominal pressures were measured in both dynamic and static loading of the spine. *Dynamic loading* consisted of bending forward and lifting weights of varying heaviness while (1) flexing hips and knees and (2) flexing hips and maintaining knees extended. *Static loading* involved pulling on a strain ring while the trunk was erect and at various degrees of hip flexion.

The hypothesis of Morris and associates (1961) is, in part, as follows: The thoracic cavity, filled with air, and the abdominal cavity, filled with liquid and semisolid material, under certain circumstances, are capable of giving substantial support to the flexed spine. The contraction of the trunk muscles converts these chambers into nearly rigid-walled cylinders that resist a part of the force generated in loading the trunk, and thereby relieves the load on the spine itself.

Calculations of forces acting on the lumbosacral disk when a 170-lb man lifts a 200-lb weight (the role of the trunk is omitted) disclose that this force would amount to more than 2000 lb, much more than this region could endure without structural failure. The research data revealed that, owing to the "inflatable support," the force in the lumbosacral region was reduced by 600 lb. Similarly, the force acting on the lower thoracic region was found to be reduced from 1568 to 791 lb.

An often-observed fact is that when a heavy weight is lifted, the person holds the breath and tightens the trunk muscles. This is an automatic compensatory action that helps to prevent strain and injury of the vertebral column.

Temporo-mandibular Joint

The temporo-mandibular (TM) joints are among the most frequently used joints in the body. In their functions of chewing, talking, yawning, swallowing, and sneezing, Hoppenfeld (1976) estimates that the TM joints may move 1500 to 2000 times per day. These joints provide jaw motions of opening, closing, protrusion, retrusion, and lateral deviation to each side. Normally, the jaw should open smoothly in a straight line without lateral deviations in the motion, and the subject should be able to place the width of three fingers between the teeth.

JOINT

Interposed between the condyle of the mandible and the glenoid fossa of the temporal bone is a movable meniscus (articular disk) that is attached anteriorly to the pterygoid lateralis muscle. Opening of the jaw begins with a hinge-type motion, which is rapidly followed by a gliding of the condyles *down and out of the glenoid fossa* to lie under the convex articular tubercle on the zygomatic process. This is a complex motion in which the condyle moves on the disk and the disk moves forward on the tubercle.

MUSCLES

Specific attachments of the muscles of mastication and their lines of pull should be studied using an anatomic textbook and a skull. The *lateral pterygoid* muscle is primarily responsible for opening the jaw and is supplemented by the *suprahyoid* and *infrahyoid* muscles. Closure and the forceful movements of chewing are performed by the *temporalis, masseter,* and *medial pterygoid* muscles, all of which have excellent leverage advantages. Slight activity in the temporalis muscle maintains jaw closure in the upright position (Basmajian, 1978). Protrusion is performed by the two pterygoid muscles, and retrusion by the temporalis. Lateral deviation is performed by the temporalis and masseter on the same side and the pterygoids on the opposite side.

The TM joints are subject to injury and dysfunction with injuries of the head or cervical spine, malocclusion, or poor dentition. Although the teeth can sustain great forces, the TM joints are not designed for weight-bearing, and they may be injured by cervical traction (see Fig. 2-4).

CHAPTER 12

STANDING AND WALKING

POSTURE

Posture is a general term that is defined as a *position or attitude of the body, the relative arrangement of body parts for a specific activity, or a characteristic manner of bearing one's body.* Postures are used to perform activities with the least amount of energy. Thus, posture and movement are intimately associated, for movement begins from a posture and may end in a posture—as when a person is in a sitting position and then moves to a standing position. Postural relationships of body parts can be altered and controlled voluntarily, but such control is short-lived for it requires concentration. In normal function, postural "sets" and adjustments are rapid and automatic (see Chapter 3).

STATIC OR STEADY POSTURES

The body can assume a multitude of postures that are comfortable for long periods, and there are many that accomplish the same purposes. In many cultures, for example, people do not sit in a chair to rest the body but rather use a variety of floor-sitting postures such as crossed legs, side sitting, or the deep squat. Normally, when discomfort occurs from joint compression, ligamentous tension, continuous muscle contraction, or circulatory occlusion, a new posture is sought. If a joint has been in one position for a long time, the able-bodied person will move and stretch the joint and muscles. Habitual postures without positional changes can lead to injury, limitation of motion, or deformity. Patients with sensory losses (e.g., peripheral nerve injuries, spinal cord transection) fail to perceive the discomfort of vascular occlusion. If this is not alleviated by relieving the pressure periodically, tissue destruction may occur,

361

leading to *decubitus ulcers* (bedsores). Patients with lower extremity amputations are especially prone to adaptive shortening *(contractures)* of the hip and knee flexors caused by resting the residual limb on a pillow and by prolonged sitting. If the joints of patients with muscle paralysis are not passively moved through their ranges of motion, the joint structures and muscles will adaptively shorten to the habitual position.

STANDING POSTURE

Asymmetric Standing

If erect standing must be maintained for any length of time, the posture of choice is to stand with the weight first on one and then on the other foot, the contralateral foot being on the ground but supporting very little weight. The hip posture is of the Trendelenburg type, in which the abductors are relieved of action and the ligaments are relied on. A vertical projection through the center of gravity passes slightly anterior to the knee axis so that the quadriceps muscle is not used and the knee is also supported by ligaments (see Chapters 2 and 9). This is an energy-saving posture because there is less metabolism in ligaments than in contracting muscles. Overstretching of the ligamentous apparatus is avoided by frequent shifting from one foot to the other. Another common standing position is on both feet with the hips and knees in extension (hyperextension) and with the hands clasped behind the back or arms folded on the chest. Some people when standing on one foot will place the opposite foot on the knee. This stance is not socially acceptable in this country, and adults are usually reluctant to admit this preference. The one-leg standing posture is called the nilotic stance (belonging to the Nile), and it is commonly practiced in Africa and among sheep herders.

Symmetric Standing

Evaluation of posture and body alignment requires a symmetric stance with the arms relaxed at the side of the body. Although this position is called "comfortable, relaxed standing," it is not comfortable for any length of time, and the individual will choose a posture that is less tiresome. Nevertheless, the standing position of humans is extremely efficient as compared to that of animals, which must stand on flexed extremities. In the human, the line of gravity falls very close to (or through) the joint axes (Fig. 12-1). Therefore, only minimal contraction of a few muscles such as the soleus, erector spinae, trapezius, and temporalis (jaw closure) are needed to maintain the erect posture. Some subjects may have slight contraction of the hamstrings and the iliopsoas. Discomfort in this position, therefore, cannot be caused by muscle contraction and excessive energy expenditure, but must rather be caused by vascular insufficiency of the structures that are under compression or tension. Another factor that may become pertinent is the need for intermittent contraction of muscles in the extremities to prevent pooling of venous blood. Tensing skeletal muscles compresses veins in the

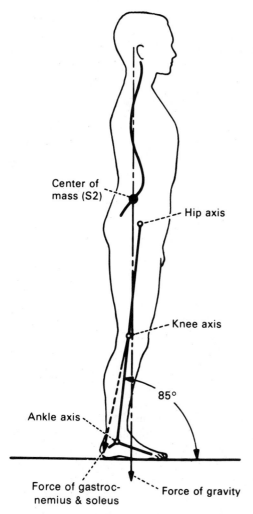

Center of mass (S2)

Hip axis

Knee axis

85°

Ankle axis

Force of gastroc-
nemius & soleus

Force of gravity

FIGURE 12-1. In the relaxed, standing posture, the gravitational force line through the center of mass falls behind the hip joint, in front of the knee joint, and in front of the ankle joint. In the lower limbs, active muscle contraction for balance is required, but only in the gastrocnemius-soleus muscles. (Redrawn from Rosse and Clawson, 1980.)

region and assists in returning venous blood to the right atrium of the heart so that cardiac output is maintained within the physiologic range. A person standing quietly in a fixed posture (particularly in a hot environment) can have excessive pooling of venous blood. The decline in venous return results in insufficient cardiac output to supply the needs of brain cells, thus producing an episode of fainting.

Balance at Ankle Joint

The vertical projection of the center of gravity of the body mass above the ankle joints falls anterior to the axis of the upper ankle joint. This is inevitably so because the center-of-gravity line of the entire body remains close to the center of the base of support, which lies well ahead of the ankle joints (see Figs. 2-13, 2-21). A rotary force is thus set up at the ankle that would cause the body to topple forward unless opposed by a muscular force. The calf muscles furnish this equilibrating force, thereby preventing dorsiflexion of the ankle (excessive forward inclination of the shank with respect to the foot). The soleus muscle, in particular, is thought to be responsible for this equilibration (Denny-Brown, 1929; Joseph, 1960). During postural sway, the body weight seldom, if ever, passes behind the axes of the ankle joints, and consequently the calf muscles remain continuously, although variably, active (Smith, 1957). When high-heeled shoes are worn, the vertical projection of the center of gravity moves forward between the feet, and activity of the soleus increases (Basmajian, 1978). The normal ankle and foot are supported by bony and ligamentous structures. No electromyographic activity is found in the other intrinsic or extrinsic muscles of the foot during bilateral stance.

EFFECT OF BILATERAL CALF MUSCLE PARALYSIS

If the calf muscles are paralyzed bilaterally, the subject is forced to keep the weight in vertical alignment with the axes of the upper ankle joints, or nearly so. If the body weight passes further to the rear, the dorsiflexors of the ankle spring into action, but the safe range of backward sway is extremely limited. A subject with calf muscle paralysis tends to keep the feet a certain distance apart or to hold on to a nearby object to provide stability.

Balance at Knee Joints

The body mass above the knee joints consists of the head, arms, trunk, and thighs. A vertical line through the center of gravity of this body mass falls slightly in front of the axis for flexion and extension of the knees (see Fig. 12-1). During postural sway, this vertical line may occasionally, though rarely, move behind the axis of the knee joints. Most of the time, therefore, a rotary force in the sense of extension is present at the knees. What, then, prevents the knees from being extended and hyperextended? Electromyographic studies usually show slight activity of either the hamstrings or the gastroctnemius muscles.

This question was investigated by Smith (1957), who found that the counterbalancing force had three components of variable size, depending on the knee angle. As an example, in a subject who stood with the knees 6 degrees short of full extension (knee angle 174 degrees), the proportion of the three components were 50 percent, passive resistance in extra-articular tissues; 30 percent, postural activity of the knee flexor muscles; and 20 percent, resistance by an articular mechanism.

FUNCTION OF THE QUADRICEPS IN STANDING

In most subjects, no electromyographic activity is detected in the quadriceps during bilateral standing (Basmajian, 1978). Continuous quadriceps action is required only in subjects who stand in such a manner that the center-of-gravity line of the supra-tibial mass falls posterior to the axis of the knee joint. But such subjects are exceptions. A short burst of quadriceps activity also appears if, during postural sway, the center-of-gravity line momentarily passes behind the knee axis. The above has been confirmed by statography (Åkerblom, 1948) and by electromyography (Åkerblom, 1948; Joseph and Nightingale, 1954).

Hyperextension increases knee stability, but it has a delaying effect in activity situations when quick flexion of the knee is required. The "readiness position" in athletics, therefore, avoids complete knee extension. The failure of some individuals to make a quick start is due, to a great extent, to the knees being somewhat hyperextended, and "being caught flat-footed" depends as much on knee alignment as on ankle position.

STABILITY VERSUS MOBILITY

Clinically, in the rehabilitation of the disabled, the individual's requirements with respect to stability and mobility must be carefully evaluated. If *stability* is the prime requirement, as may be the case in elderly persons with amputations, the prosthetic knee must have a large margin of safety. But a young active person with an amputation, whose skill in controlling the prosthetic knee may develop to a remarkable extent, will prefer *mobility*, which requires a readiness position of the prosthetic knee for quick starting and for ease and grace in walking.

BILATERAL QUADRICEPS PARALYSIS

Because of the stabilizing effect of gravity on the knee joints, an individual with bilateral paralysis of the quadriceps muscle is capable of standing erect without braces, provided that there are no other complicating factors. In order to minimize the danger of collapse at the knee during postural sway, the individual will tend to keep the knees maximally extended, which might lead to hyperextension and *genu recurvatum*. The person may also choose to incline the trunk somewhat forward, which increases the stabilizing effect of gravity.

EFFECT OF CALF MUSCLE PARALYSIS ON KNEE STABILITY

A prerequisite for stabilization of the knee by gravity is that the body weight be kept forward as in normal erect posture, which is possible only if the calf muscles are functioning. Indirectly, therefore, these muscles are responsible for knee stability. A subject with a combination of calf muscle and quadriceps paralysis benefits from wearing a foot-ankle orthosis with dorsiflexion limited at 90 degrees because this materially improves knee stability. Similarly, a blocking of dorsiflexion of the prosthetic foot in the above-knee artificial limb improves knee stability, whereas allowing dorsiflexion beyond 90 degrees causes the knee to become unstable.

Balance at Hip Joints

As previously stated, the center of gravity of head, arms, and trunk (HAT) is located inside the thorax, approximately at the height of the xiphoid process. A vertical line through this center may fall directly through, in front of, or in back of the common hip axis, depending on how the individual stands. Muscle action will vary accordingly.

There has been much controversy with respect to the location of the center-of-gravity line of HAT in relation to the common hip axis in standing. In the latter half of the 19th century, anatomists (Meyer, 1853; Braune and Fischer, 1889; Fick, 1911) differed considerably in their opinions. Schede (1941), in his analysis of common ways of standing, shows that the center-of-gravity line may fall on either side of the common hip axis, or directly through it. He stresses that *incomplete extension of the hip is essential if the knees are to be stabilized by gravity*, for when the hip is completely extended, a backward sway of the center of gravity of HAT can no longer be absorbed at the hip and, therefore, will result in flexion of the knees.

Åkerblom (1948) reported that 22 subjects (out of 25 studied) stood with incomplete extension at the hip, varying from 2 to 15 degrees. His subjects stood "comfortably," with the feet slightly apart and the arms hanging relaxed. Variations of the center-of-gravity line with respect to the hip axis from one measurement to the other were found, indicating postural sway at the hip as well as at the ankle. He concluded that in *comfortable symmetric standing, the upper body is usually balanced over the hip joint in unstable equilibrium*. Basmajian (1978) registered slight electric activity in the iliacus in standing at ease, thus substantiating Åkerblom's findings of incomplete hip extension.

HIP POSTURE WHEN KNEE CONTROL IS LACKING

It is of particular importance for individuals who have lost their ability to control the knee actively (such as patients with above-knee amputations and patients with paralysis of certain muscles, e.g., the quadriceps) to stand with the hips short of full extension so that some postural sway can be absorbed at the hip. As pointed out by Schede (1941), when an above-knee prosthesis is worn, equilibration at the hip is mandatory for knee stability. These patients tend to have some increase in the lumbar curve, but a backward tilt of the pelvis for the purpose of decreasing the lumbar curve is contraindicated, because it would cause the artificial knee to buckle.

HIP POSTURE OF PARAPLEGIC PATIENTS

The paraplegic patient, having lost control of the muscles of the ankles, knees, and hips, needs bracing to stand erect. Bracing at ankles and knees is essential to maintain the knees in extension and to provide stability at the ankle, but the hips may be left free. Such a patient assumes a characteristic posture with the upper part of the body inclined backward so that the center-of-gravity line of HAT comes to fall well behind the hip axis (Fig. 12-2). The upright posture of the patient standing in bilateral knee-ankle-foot orthoses (KAFO) is supported at the hips by the ilio-femoral (Y) ligaments.

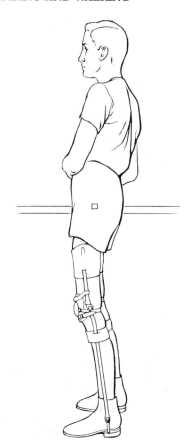

FIGURE 12-2. Characteristic posture of a paraplegic patient standing in knee-ankle-foot orthoses that stabilize the knees and ankles but leave the hips free. Center-of-gravity line of the upper part of the body falls well behind the common hip axis. The square on the shorts is positioned over the greater trochanter, which represents the approximate location of the center of the hip joint.

If the ligaments have been permitted to shorten, or if there is hip flexor spasticity, the hips will be in flexion. The patient will demonstrate lordosis as the patient attempts to maintain the erect position. The patient will not be able to bring the center of gravity of HAT posterior to the hip axis and will require constant support for HAT from the upper extremities. Crutch-walking will be laborious and impractical.

If the paraplegic patient wishes to lean forward, as when picking up an object from the floor, the patient must brace self on a firm object with one hand while picking up the object with the other hand. Otherwise, the patient will collapse at the hip as soon as the center of gravity of HAT moves in front of the hip axis.

Balance of the Trunk and Head

In the erect position, slight electromyographic activity is recorded from the erector spinae muscles. The rectus abdominus is inactive, and in some subjects slight activity may be recorded from the internal abdominal oblique muscles (Basmajian, 1978).

The center of gravity of the head is located about 1 inch (2 to 3 cm) above the transverse axis of the atlanto-occipital joints so that the head is in unstable equilibrium, much like that of a seesaw. When the head is erect, a perpendicular line through the center of gravity of the head falls somewhat anterior to the transverse axis for flexion and extension (Fig. 12-3, A). Therefore, in ordinary standing and sitting, the posterior neck muscles are moderately active to prevent the head from dropping forward. When the head is inclined forward, as in reading, writing, and sewing, the demands on these muscles increase (Fig. 12-3, B). But when the head is allowed to drop all the way forward, the ligamentum nuchae becomes tense and muscular activity is no longer needed. If the head is tipped backward, the center-of-gravity line falls posterior to the transverse axis (Fig. 12-3, C), and the head will tip all the way back unless the flexors of the head spring into action. By palpating the anterior neck muscles (sternocleidomastoid, scalenus anterior), the point at which the center of gravity passes behind the transverse axis can be ascertained.

Perpendicular Posture

The perpendicular posture is assumed when one is standing at attention or when one is told to "stand up straight." The weight is shifted posteriorly until a plumb line through the center of gravity of the body falls directly through the axes of the talocrural, knee, and hip joints as well as through the tips of the shoulder and ear. Maintenance of this unnatural posture requires conscious effort and a marked increase in muscle activity (as compared with relaxed standing).

Unfortunately, perpendicular posture has been equated with good or desirable posture. This has come about because of an error in translation and a misinterpretation of the work of Braune and Fischer (1889). This position was used by the authors to facilitate measurements of body points in the coordinate system. The position was referred to as "Normalstellung" (reference upright) but not as normal posture. Comfortable relaxed standing was called "Bequeme Haltung" (comfortable hold).

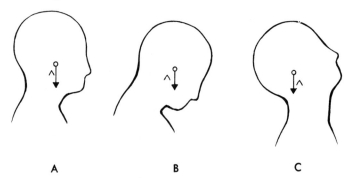

A   B   C

FIGURE 12-3. Relation of center-of-gravity line of head to axis of atlanto-occipital joints in different head positions. (A) Head erect, center of gravity slightly anterior to axis, posterior neck muscles moderately active. (B) Head forward, increased activity of posterior neck muscles. (C) Head backward, center of gravity posterior to axis, anterior neck muscles active.

AMBULATION (WALKING)

Ambulation can be defined in a broad sense as a type of locomotion (L. *locus*, place, plus *movere*, to move; in this case, moving from one place to another). Other types of locomotion include crawling or the use of a wheelchair. In the human, a bipedal (L. *bi*, two, plus *pes*, foot) pattern of ambulation is acquired during infancy. With practice (training), the sensory-motor system becomes very adept at automatically generating a repeating set of motor control commands to permit an individual to walk without conscious effort. Disease or injury of the nervous system or of the musculoskeletal system can disrupt the normal pattern of ambulation. A variety of compensatory mechanisms may be called into action in an effort to maintain functional ambulation. These compensations manifest themselves as abnormal patterns of walking and are invariably less efficient and more costly in terms of energy expenditure than the normal mechanisms.

Historical Notes on the Study of Locomotion

Humans have long appreciated the more apparent distinctions between activities such as walking and running, but analysis of their fundamental mechanics was not possible before the development of the science of physics. With so many other important problems awaiting physical analysis, locomotion received only sporadic attention from pioneers such as Borelli (1679) and the Weber brothers (1836). More adequate records of the sequence of changes in position were produced by Marey, the eminent French physiologist, by methods that led to the development of motion pictures (1873, 1885, 1887, 1894). The real founder of the scientific study of locomotion was Otto Fischer, a German mathematician, who was the first person to calculate the forces involved in walking (1895–1904). His work on muscles was restricted to the free swing of the leg but was a remarkable advance over previous studies. The next important step was the introduction of the force plate by Elftman (1938, 1939a), allowing the direct recording of the ground reaction forces (see page 379), and, with this as a starting point, the computation of all the muscle moments from motion picture records. Since that time, the use of force plates of increasingly accurate design, combined with various ingenious methods of photographic recording of body positions, has been the standard method of analysis of human locomotion (see Chapter 1). Especially active in the accumulation of data has been a group of workers, headed by Eberhart and Inman, at the University of California, Berkeley. A summary of the results of this work is found in *Human Walking* by Inman, Ralston, and Todd (1981). Sophisticated instrumentation available today makes possible a multifactorial computer analysis of gait. This method, now gaining acceptance, was first introduced by Basmajian and associates (1974).

Locomotion has also been studied from the standpoint of metabolic cost by measuring the amount of oxygen consumed during walking. Studies of this nature were undertaken by Benedict and Murschhauser (1915), Studer (1926), Atzler and Herbst (1927), Margaria (1976), and others.

The results achieved by these early investigators have since been added to by others, notably by Murray and associates at the Kinesiology Research Laboratory, Veterans Administration Center, Wood, Wisconsin; by Basmajian and associates at Queen's University, Kingston, Ontario, Canada, and later at Emory University in Atlanta, Georgia; and by Perry and associates at Rancho Los Amigos Hospital in Downey, California.

PATTERNS OF WALKING

Gait Cycle

Gait is defined as the manner or style of walking. One of the attributes of normal walking, as compared with most pathologic gait patterns, is the wide latitude of safe and comfortable walking speeds available. Thus, a description of the gait pattern of an individual ordinarily includes the *speed of locomotion* (m per sec) and the number of *steps* completed per unit of time (steps per min; this is also called *cadence*), as well as other characteristics of the gait pattern (Larsson et al, 1980).

During a walking cycle, a given foot is either in contact with the ground (*stance phase* of the gait cycle) or in the air (*swing phase*). The duration of the gait cycle for any one limb extends from the time the heel contacts the ground (called *heel-strike* or *heel-on*) until the same heel contacts the ground again as illustrated in Figure 12-4. The stance phase begins with initial contact of the foot (usually heel-strike, but in some pathologic conditions, other parts of the foot may contact the ground first) and ends with the foot (usually the ball of the foot and the toes) leaving the ground (called *toe-off* or *ball-off*). The swing phase begins with toe-off and ends with heel-strike. At ordinary walking speeds, the stance phase occupies approximately 60 percent and the swing phase 40 percent of a single gait cycle. Figure 12-4 depicts a full gait cycle for the left and right legs along the same time axis. A typical cycle can be expected to last 1 to 2 sec, depending on walking speed. Figure 12-4 shows that a period of double support exists when both limbs are in a stance phase. The duration of double support varies inversely with the speed of walking. In slow walking, this period is comparatively long in relation to the swing phase; but as the speed increases, the period becomes shorter and shorter. In running, double support is no longer present. In fact, for a brief time, both feet may be off the ground simultaneously.

Each of the two primary phases of the gait cycle can be subdivided into various stages called the *subphases* of gait. For example, the stance phase is comprised of heel-strike, foot-flat, heel-off, and toe-off subphases. Perry (1974) has suggested terminology to improve the precision of communication among scientists and clinicians who analyze gait patterns. In that classification system, the stance phase includes *initial contact, loading response, midstance, terminal stance,* and *preswing* subphases. The swing phase is comprised of *initial swing, midswing,* and *terminal swing* subphases.

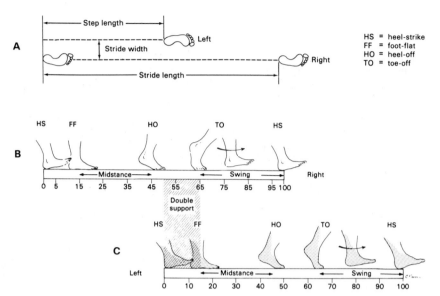

FIGURE 12-4. The phases of the gait cycle shown on the same time axis for left and right legs. *(A)* Representation of the stride dimensions as viewed from above or beneath the subject. *(B)* Side view of one complete cycle of the right leg. *(C)* Side view of one complete cycle of the left leg. The time axes indicate the percentage of the gait cycle completed, starting and ending with heel-strike (HS). Note that two steps occur during each stride. (Adapted from Rosse and Clawson, 1980.)

RECORDING OF THE WALKING CYCLE

A record of the duration of sole contact with the ground in walking was first accomplished by a pneumatic method (Marey, 1873); electric contacts attached to the sole of the shoe are now commonly used. Scherb (1927), Mülli (1940), and Scherb and Arienti (1945) had their subjects wear a sandal into which was incorporated three electric contacts so that separate signals were obtained from the heel, ball of great toe, and ball of little toe. Murray and associates (1964) used a method of interrupted-light photography (like that shown in Fig. 1-15) with a mirror mounted over the walkway, so that overhead projections as well as sagittal projections of targets on the subject were recorded. Targets of a reflective fabric were fixed to reference points on both shoes. The duration of the walking cycle and its phases (stance, swing, and double-limb support), stride length and foot positions, and angles were measured. Andriacchi and associates (1977) in their study used pressure-sensitive transducer foot pads placed inside the subjects' shoes for recording.

Variation of Walking Speed

It is customary to speak of *slow, medium* (or ordinary), and *fast* walking speeds. In the Berkeley study, cadences of 70, 95, and 120 steps per min were chosen to represent slow, medium, and fast speeds (see Klopsteg and Wilson, 1968). Murray and associates (1964, 1966) refer to "free" and "fast" walking speeds. They found that free cadence selected by individuals varied widely; in order to assure meaningful comparisons of subjects, they put them all through a pretrial pacing at 112 steps per min (this figure from Drillis, 1958) before conducting investigations. For "fast" walking, their subjects were instructed to "walk as fast as you can comfortably walk" (Murray et al, 1966, p 9). Andriacchi and associates (1977) studied normal subjects and subjects with knee pathologies whom they had asked to walk a prescribed distance at "normal, fast, and slow" speeds. The natural way to increase walking speed is to increase the cadence or walking rate (number of steps taken per min) and to lengthen the stride simultaneously. The studies of Murray and Clarkson (1966a, 1966b) and Andriacchi and associates (1977) confirmed this observation.

Increased speed results in diminished duration of all the component phases of the walking cycle (stance, swing, double support). Swing phase time decreases less than other phases, apparently because "the swinging extremity moves forward through a greater distance in a shorter time to achieve the longer and more rapid step length needed for faster walking. This appears to be a major factor in accomplishing the faster walking speed" (Murray et al, 1966, p 21).

The cadence used at different speeds of walking varies in individual subjects, being related to such factors as the length of limbs and the weight distribution of body segments. For example, an individual with short limbs usually takes shorter strides and more steps per min than an individual with long limbs for a particular walking speed. When heavy boots are worn, the length of the stride tends to increase as compared with when light shoes are worn.

KINEMATICS OF LOCOMOTION

The kinematics, or "geometry," of locomotion may be studied objectively by recording movements of points on the body, such as the summit of the head or the crest of the ilium, or surface landmarks representing the centers of joints or the long axes of bones. If the movement paths of these landmarks are projected on the sagittal, frontal, and horizontal planes, a three-dimensional record is obtained.

Chronophotography

The chronophotographic method developed by Marey (1885, 1887, 1894) consisted of making a series of exposures of a walking subject on a photographic plate. By means of a rotating shutter, exposures were made at intervals of 0.1 sec. Since superimposition of several pictures on one another gave a confused record, "geometric chronophotography" was subsequently employed. The subject was dressed in black, and brilliant metal buttons and shining bands were attached to the clothing to represent joints and bony segments. The subject, strongly illuminated by the sun, was photographed as he or she walked in front of a black screen. Dots and lines thus appeared on the photographic plate since the rest of the body did not show against the black background. The principles of this method of recording have since been used extensively by subsequent investigators.

Displacements in the Plane of Progression

Angular and linear displacements of body parts have been measured in all three reference planes, but the greatest displacements occur in the plane of progression (the sagittal plane).

Vertical oscillations of the head or center of gravity of the body occur twice in the gait cycle (see Fig. 1-15)—at midstance for each foot.

Murray and associates (1964) used a method of interrupted-light photography (see Fig. 1-15) to analyze movements of the pelvis, hip, knee, and ankle. Figure 12-5 shows a summary of their findings in which the mean patterns of sagittal rotation of the main joints of the lower extremity are plotted with respect to the percent of completion of the gait cycle. Pelvic tipping anteriorly and posteriorly was minimal. The *pelvis* remains relatively level and shows a mean excursion of only 3 degrees. The *hip*, which is flexed when the heel strikes the ground, extends gradually as the trunk moves forward over the supporting limb. Studies showed that when the contralateral heel strikes the ground, the ipsilateral hip has extended to an average of 10 degrees more than it did in a standing posture. At the beginning of the swing phase, the ipsilateral hip starts to flex, and it continues to do so and to remain flexed until the end of the cycle. The knee is extended at heel-strike and flexes about 15 degrees in early stance phase, then extends in late stance phase, and flexes to a peak of about 70 degrees at midswing. The ankle plantar-flexes in early stance phase to permit contact of the entire foot with the floor. With the body weight on the foot shifting forward, the tibia moves forward and the ankle is in dorsiflexion. Following this, the heel rises, and the ankle plantar-flexes strongly. During the swing phase of the pattern, the ankle dorsiflexes to neutral so that the toes and foot may clear the floor. Note that more dorsiflexion motion is used in the stance phase than in the swing phase.

Recording of Transverse Rotations

For accurate recordings of transverse rotations of bony segments, Eberhart and associates (1947) attached targets directly to the bones. This was done under local anesthesia by drilling stainless steel pins into the ilium, the femur, and the tibia at suitable locations. The targets, which consisted of small spheres mounted on light wooden rods, protruded laterally, and this magnified the excursions of the segments. A camera operating above the subject recorded the top view. This study yielded information concerning the rotation of each bony segment in space, as well as concerning the rotation of one segment with respect to another.

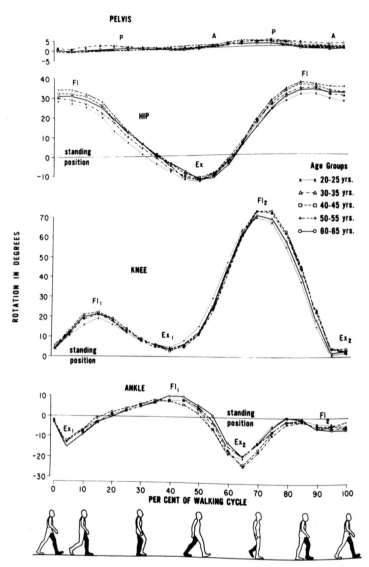

FIGURE 12-5. Mean patterns of sagittal rotation for the five age groups, twelve men in each group, two trials for each man. The zero reference positions for the hip, knee, and ankle excursions are the angular positions of the joints in the standing posture. Flexion (*Fl*) in these three curves is always represented by an upward deflection; extension (*Ex*), by a downward deflection. The reference position for pelvic tipping is the angle formed by the pelvic target and the horizontal at the time of the preceding heel-strike. *P* is the upward and backward movement of the anterior aspect of the pelvis; *A* is the downward and forward movement of the anterior aspect of the pelvis. Note that the hip has one wave of flexion-extension, while the knee and ankle have two each. (From Murray et al, 1964, with permission.)

The magnitudes of the transverse rotations of the three segments (pelvis, femur, and tibia) varied considerably in the subjects investigated. The composite curves for all subjects (Fig. 12-6) indicate that, in general:

1. Pelvic rotation is comparatively slight; the femur rotates more than the pelvis; and the tibia rotates more than the femur.
2. All three segments rotate inward during the swing phase, and this inward rotation continues through the first portion of the stance phase. A sudden change from inward to outward rotation takes place at midstance, and outward rotation continues until the toe-off position is assumed.

The data in Figure 12-6 were used to plot the curves seen in Figure 12-7, which illustrates rotations of femur with respect to pelvis and rotation of tibia with respect to femur.

Murray and associates (1964) using a mirror mounted over the walkway, studied overhead projections of transverse rotations of the thorax and the pelvis simultaneously with the sagittal displacements. The thoracic target was a rod secured to the sternum with elastic webbing and projecting forward. The pelvic target, a similar rod strapped to the sacrum, projected backward. These projections magnified the excursions. Pelvic and thoracic rotation excursions (Fig. 12-8) were more variable in the group of normal men subjects than any of the other patterns studied. The investigators suggest that these ''excursions are influenced more by an individual's attitude of locomotion than by mechanical demands'' and that ''these patterns may be optional movements, available in particular circumstances of movements'' (Murray et al, 1964, p 358). The magnitudes and directions of pelvic rotation were similar to those reported in the Berkeley study in that the pelvis moved forward on the side of the forward-

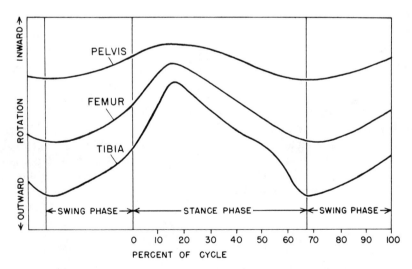

FIGURE 12-6. Transverse rotations of bony segments of lower extremity during walking cycle. (Composite curves for all subjects; redrawn from Eberhart et al, 1947.)

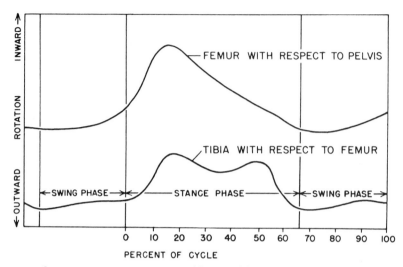

FIGURE 12-7. Relative transverse rotations of hip and knee joints for all subjects. (Redrawn from Eberhart et al, 1947.)

swinging limb. Thorax rotation was less and in a direction opposite that of the pelvis. The amount of rotation between thorax and pelvis increased with increased walking speed, probably related, according to the investigators (Murray et al, 1966), to the more vigorous arm swing of the faster gait.

Displacements in the Frontal Plane

Two displacements in the frontal plane are important for adjustment of the body to the line of weight-bearing and to maintenance of body balance. Although the motions are minimal, the loss of their control results in pronounced abnormalities of gait. The first is a lateral shift of the center of gravity of the body to the weight-bearing side that occurs as body weight is transferred from one leg to the other. "The total magnitude of this lateral displacement is approximately two inches" (Eberhart et al, 1968, p 458).

The other factor is a downward tilting of the pelvis on the swing side. The upward thrust on the hip of the stance side together with the weight of HAT and the swing leg tends to cause this tilt. The tendency is opposed by contraction of the hip abductors on the stance side (see Fig. 8-9, B), but some drop of the pelvis on the unsupported side does occur. "The amount of this rotary displacement is approximately eight degrees" (Eberhart et al, 1968, p 460).

Gait Determinants

"Determinants in normal gait" is a phrase used by Saunders, Inman, and Eberhart in their interpretive article on locomotion (1953). They discuss, particularly, the dis-

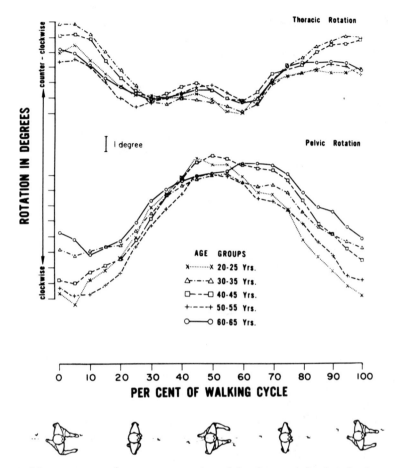

FIGURE 12-8. Mean patterns of transverse rotation of the thorax and pelvis for five age groups, twelve men in each age group, and two trials for each man. (From Murray et al, 1964, with permission.)

placement of the body's center of gravity during locomotion and describe its slowly undulating movement approximately 2 inches (5 cm) vertically and 2 inches horizontally during forward progression. They assert that abrupt changes in the direction of the locomotive movement compel a high expenditure of energy and that translating the center of gravity forward through this undulating pathway conserves energy. Certain gait determinants, they say, smooth out the pathway and limit the vertical and lateral displacements to an excursion of only 2 inches.

The first determinant described is *transverse pelvic rotation*. The pelvis on the ipsilateral side moves forward with the swing leg to the extent that the rotation lessens the hip flexion-extension movements and thereby *elevates the low points* of the arc of the center-of-gravity pathway. The second and third determinants serve to *depress the summit* of the center-of-gravity pathway, one by *downward tilt of the pelvis on the unsupported side*, the other by *knee flexion* that occurs in the stance phase. Fourth and fifth determinants concern foot, ankle, and knee mechanisms and the intimate relationships of their angular displacements throughout the period of stance phase to decrease abrupt changes in acceleration or deceleration of the center of gravity, thus producing a smooth sinusoidal curve. The sixth determinant of gait reduces the lateral oscillations of the center of gravity. This determinant is the adducted position of the shaft of the femur (neck-shaft angle approximately 125 degrees; see Fig. 8-2) and the tibio-femoral angle, which permits body weight to be placed over the supporting foot without large lateral shifts of the center of gravity.

Kinematic aspects of the classic study by Eberhart and associates have been re-examined and, in general, have been substantiated by later investigators. New material and certain details of gait previously not sufficiently studied have been given special attention, notably by Murray and associates, Kinesiology Research Laboratory, Veterans Administration Center, Wood, Wisconsin (1964, 1966a, 1966b, 1967, 1969, 1970, 1971). They studied the influence of age, height, sex, and walking speed on walking patterns of normal persons. Their studies showed that configurations of the patterns of motion were similar for all but that amplitudes of the patterns were quite different, with women showing smaller excursions of motions than men. Walking speeds of women were slower, resulting from their shorter stride lengths, but their cadence was slightly more rapid. Women showed less arm swing and less vertical and lateral motion of the head. In walking, the mass of the center of the body must be shifted to a position over the base of support; which part of the body shifts seems "to be an optional and attitudinal characteristic of gait" (Murray et al, 1970, p 647). Men showed greater lateral shifting of head and thorax; women showed greater lateral shifting of the pelvis. The investigations of women's walking patterns showed differences with changes in heel heights. Women's slower walking speed was more pronounced with high heels. Higher heels had little effect on cadence, so the slower speed resulted from shorter stride lengths. Women in high heels showed increased knee flexion early in the stance phase and a rapid movement to lower the whole forefoot to the floor, seemingly to enlarge the base of support quickly to receive the oncoming body weight.

Older men walked with slower speed, shorter and wider steps, more toe-out, and less pelvic rotation, especially for fast-speed walking. In general, their gaits, though surprisingly rhythmic, seemed "guarded" or "restrained" in an attempt to obtain maximum stability and security. Men beyond age 65 spent a longer time in the stance phase and a shorter time in the swing phase, attributable perhaps to their instability during periods of single limb support or to their shorter steps. They showed decreases in the excursions of the lower limbs in the swing phase, except that toe clearance was actually slightly greater than that of the younger men, perhaps to guard against toe-scuffing. Arm swing for the older men was less, especially elbow extension on the back swing and shoulder flexion on the forward swing, and their general posture tended toward one of shoulder hyperextension and elbow flexion (Murray et al, 1969).

KINETICS OF AMBULATION

Importance of Understanding the Physical Principles of Kinetics

For an analysis of the contribution of muscles to movement, a more extensive knowledge of physics than that usually included in the background requirements for students of physical therapy and occupational therapy is required. The present chapter, therefore, does not attempt such an analysis, but some of the general features are described so that the reader may become somewhat familiar with methods used in the study of locomotion, and may become aware of the difficulties that arise if the student is to go beyond an evaluation of muscles *in static conditions* to an understanding of how they control the body in motion.

When the body is stationary, the torque produced by the muscles about each joint must balance the torque produced by gravity, and the contribution of each muscle fiber is determined by the length-tension relationship, by the angle of pull, and by the lever arm relationships. When the body is in motion, these factors are still present, but more difficult ones are added. The tension produced by each muscle fiber decreases with its speed of shortening and increases more the faster it is stretched (see Chapter 4). The torque exerted by the muscle does not move the body directly but changes its acceleration. The change in acceleration changes its velocity, which finally results in displacement. To gauge the participation of muscles in movement, one must be able to visualize the movement in terms of its acceleration, a characteristic not readily appreciated.

Ground Reaction Forces

The force platform (or plate) described both by Hellebrandt and by Elftman in 1938 is still widely used (with technologic improvements, of course) to record postural sway of a stationary subject and the ground reaction forces transmitted through the foot of a walking subject. The typical force platform is comprised of a metal plate approximately one 1 sq m resting on four short pillars that support the plate midway along the length of each side. Strain gauges bonded to each pillar detect changes in the load supported by that pillar. When a load (mass) is placed anywhere on the force platform, the strain gauges generate voltage signals in proportion to the load being supported by each pillar. By amplifying and recording the output signals of the strain gauges, the magnitude and direction of the forces being transmitted to the supporting surface, called the ground reaction forces, can be determined.

Three components of the ground reaction to the stance phase of a single step are illustrated in Figure 12-9. The components shown are (1) the vertical component (Z), which reflects the total force pressing down at a right angle to the surface of the plate; (2) a horizontal, anterior-posterior component (X), which reflects the total force acting to push the plate forward or backward; and (3) a horizontal, lateral component (Y),

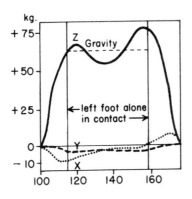

FIGURE 12-9. Vertical and horizontal components of ground reaction on the foot, as obtained from force plate studies. (Redrawn from Elftman, 1939a.)

which reflects the total force acting to push the plate to one side or the other. The curve for the vertical component Z rises rapidly after heel contact and exhibits two peaks (maxima). The first peak occurs as the supporting limb receives the full impact of the body weight. The second peak occurs near the end of the stance phase when the foot begins to "push-off" and accelerate the body mass. During both of these peaks, the vertical force exceeds the subject's body weight of 63 kg (horizontal dotted line), while in midstance the vertical force is slightly less than the body weight. These fluctuations in vertical force on the plate are the result of adding or subtracting the influence of momentum on the body. The curve showing anterior-posterior forces (X) has negative values (arbitrary designation for a force in the walking direction) after heel contact and positive values during push-off. The Y component is directed laterally at a right angle to the walking direction and remains small unless the subject veers to the right or left of the original walking direction.

Figure 12-10 shows the path of the point of application of the ground reaction to the sole of the foot, from heel contact to toe-off position (Elftman, 1939a). The subject weighed 63 kg and walked at a medium-fast speed. Following heel contact, the path moved toward the midline of the foot and remained in the midline until the heel began to rise, then deviated medially toward the great toe. Center-of-pressure data of this kind are variable among normal subjects, and in pathologic conditions, marked changes are observed.

Muscle Activity

In later years, the method of choice for the study of muscle action has been electromyography. The onset, duration, and peaks of contraction of muscles are seen on the electromyogram, but quantitative values in terms of tension are not obtainable. Needle electrodes have been used to record the action of individual muscles during walking (Scherb and Arienti, 1945), or surface electrodes for recording muscle group action (Eberhart et al, 1947). Current research on the activity of deep muscles often uses fine wire electrodes (Basmajian, 1978).

Electric activities of muscle groups were recorded as the subjects walked on level ground or ascended and descended slopes and stairs (Eberhart et al, 1947). The main

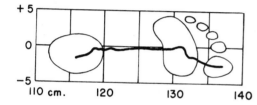

FIGURE 12-10. Path of the point of application of the ground reaction on the foot, as obtained from force plate studies. (Redrawn from Elftman, 1939a.)

muscle groups of the lower limb, with the exception of the hip flexors, were included in the study. The electromyographic signal as recorded by an oscillograph gave certain information about the activities of the muscle groups, but the wave had a complicated shape and interpretation proved difficult. A so-called integrator, a device that rectifies and filters the wave, was therefore introduced in the circuit, yielding an "integrated electromyogram." The records of integrated electromyogram shows the total amount of electric activity "seen" by the recording electrodes at each instant of time.

For each muscle group studied, records of integrated electromyograms of 10 normal adult male subjects (representative strides being picked out) were superimposed upon each other, such superimposition leading to "summary curves." From the summary curves, the "idealized" curves presented in Figure 12-11 were constructed to indicate the patterns of activity of the various muscle groups during the walking cycle.

Inspection of the various curves (see Fig. 12-11) shows that muscular activity is marked at the beginning of stance, while in midstance there is little or no activity of the various muscle groups. In late stance, activity again increases. During the swing phase, these records show only minor activity of the groups investigated. The sharp rise and fall of the electromyographic curves indicate a burst of activity followed by periods of inactivity. The alternation between short periods of activity and relatively long periods of recovery accounts in part, for our ability to walk comparatively long distances without experiencing fatigue. Most of the muscles activated in walking perform eccentric contractions, at which time they resist a stretching force (gravity, momentum); then they may contract isometrically or reverse to a brief shortening contraction. Such a scheme, as has been discussed previously (Chapter 4), is most economical from the standpoint of expenditure of energy.

With the electromyographic records as a basis, functions of main muscle groups of the lower extremity during the gait cycle will now be discussed.

DORSIFLEXORS OF ANKLE

The dorsiflexors of the ankle show slight activity during the swing phase, at which time these muscles prevent the front part of the foot from dropping. Because the weight of the foot is comparatively small, only slight to moderate activity is needed. But following heel contact, a marked activation of the dorsiflexors is required, or the impact of the body weight on the heel would cause the foot to slap vigorously on the ground. Owing to the action of these muscles, the sole of the foot is lowered to the ground in a gradual and controlled fashion.

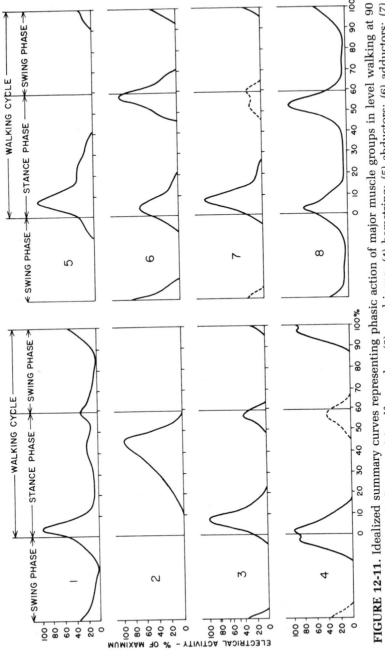

FIGURE 12-11. Idealized summary curves representing phasic action of major muscle groups in level walking at 90 steps per min. (1) Pretibial group; (2) calf muscles; (3) quadriceps; (4) hamstring; (5) abductors; (6) adductors; (7) gluteus maximus; (8) erector spinae. The amount of electric activity recorded from the muscle group is expressed as a percentage of the maximum electric activity recorded from that group *while walking*. It is not the maximum amount of activity that the particular muscle group is capable of producing with a maximum contraction. (Redrawn from Eberhart et al, 1947.)

CALF GROUP

The activity of the calf group (triceps surae) occurs in the stance phase only, the curve rising to a maximum during the last third of stance, to control the forward movement of the tibia on the ankle. Its peak contraction is synchronous with the maximum ground reaction on the ball of the foot, indicating that this group is importantly involved in the push-off.

If the proximal joints of the limb were to remain extended, plantar flexion of the ankle would exert a direct forward and upward force on the trunk. But the records show that the knee flexes rapidly as the ankle plantar-flexes and that, simultaneously, the hip is also in the process of flexing, so that the action of the calf muscles on the trunk becomes debatable. The calf muscles, however, have another important function to fulfill in late stance.

Francillion (1941a, 1941b) pointed out that when the triceps surae contracts late in the stance phase, after heel rise—the soleus is said to be particularly active at this time—this contraction causes not only plantar flexion of the ankle, but also flexion of the knee, a flexion that is needed during the swing phase. Eberhart and associates (1947) state, "during the period of double support at the end of stance, ankle extension forces will go into driving the thigh forward and flexing the knee." The importance of the calf muscles for the initiation of swing has been particularly stressed by Elftman (1955): "The impulse which they (the calf muscles) provide is usually referred to as the push-off. This indeed it is, but the pushing is exerted on the limb which is preparing for its free swing and not on the trunk, as is frequently supposed."

That muscles may transmit their actions also to distant segments is exemplified by the calf muscles. When the entire sole has reached the ground in the stance phase, the ankle angle becomes acute (see Fig. 12-5), and the calf muscles are being stretched by the momentum of the body. By resisting this stretching force, the calf muscles are instrumental in slowing down the forward motion of the body and, acting through the pelvic link, in decelerating the forward swing of the opposite limb (Elftman, 1955).

QUADRICEPS GROUP

The peak of contraction of the quadriceps group occurs after heel contact, and this peak coincides with weight-bearing on a somewhat flexed knee during "double knee action." At this moment, the center-of-gravity line of the body falls behind the axis of the knee joint, and quadriceps action is required or the knee will buckle. Note that in midstance, when the center of gravity of the body has moved in front of the axis of the knee joint, no quadriceps action is registered. The height and shape of the second quadriceps peak varies considerably among different individuals.

HAMSTRINGS

The peak of activity of the hamstring group occurs earlier than that of the quadriceps group. As the limb swings forward, these muscles are being stretched over hip and knee simultaneously, and at this time their tension builds up. It may be assumed that their function is to decelerate the forward swing of the limb and to prevent, first, excessive hip flexion, and, second, an abrupt extension of the knee due to inertia. After the heel has contacted the ground and the foot is receiving the body weight, the hamstrings continue to exhibit a high level of activity. With the foot secured on the ground by the body weight and the quadriceps acting at the knee, the hamstrings can now transfer their action to the hip. Note that at this time the quadriceps and the hamstrings act as synergists in their task to control the knee and to extend the hip, respectively.

GLUTEUS MAXIMUS

The gluteus maximus shows peak activity in early stance as the body weight is being transferred to the forward foot. It acts synchronously with the quadriceps group and partly with the hamstrings. Scherb and Arienti (1945), recording action potentials from various portions of the gluteus maximus, verified what had been observed earlier by palpation, namely, that the posterior fibers of the gluteus maximus start contracting first and that the contraction then moves forward in a wavelike fashion. This "fan symptom" was also found to be present in the gluteus medius.

In addition to furnishing hip control on the side of the stance limb, the gluteus maximus may also, through the pelvic link, aid in the forward swing of the contralateral limb (Elftman, 1955).

HIP FLEXORS

The Weber brothers (1836) postulated that the forward swing of the leg in walking was a pendulum motion requiring little or no muscular effort. This theory was challenged by Fischer (1895–1904) who proved that a muscular force was needed, a subject that has been further elucidated by the energy studies of Elftman (1955). This still leaves unanswered the question: Which muscles are responsible for the forward swing of the limb? The calf muscles on the side of the limb that is to begin its forward swing and the hip extensors on the opposite side may supply a portion of this force, but it may be assumed also that the hip flexors become active.

During the late stance and early swing phases of gait, electric activity has been recorded from the tensor fasciae latae by Altenburger (1933) and from the sartorius by Scherb and Arienti (1945). In using the "myokinesiographic method"—recording muscle action by palpation—the group headed by Scherb noted activity in the gracilis, sartorius, adductor longus, and a portion of the adductor magnus (but found no activity in the rectus femoris). More refined methods—dual wire electrodes in the muscle—reveal that only scant electric activity may be derived from the iliopsoas during the above period. In fact, during level walking, the muscle was found to be virtually silent in many subjects (Close, 1964). This would indicate that the superficial hip flexors are mainly responsible for the initiation of the swing phase. However, in cases when other hip flexors are weak, the iliopsoas may become quite active prior to toe-off and during early swing phase (Close, 1964).

Abductor Group

The *abductor group*, to fulfill its function as a lateral stabilizer of the pelvis, rapidly intensifies its action after heel contact, its activity curve rising steeply to a maximum in early stance at a time when the impact of the body weight must be prevented from lowering the pelvis on the opposite side. The activity is maintained at a lower intensity during single stance, and it fades out as double stance begins. Note that the peak of contraction of the gluteus medius is synchronous with those of the quadriceps and the gluteus maximus (Fig. 12-11). The gluteus medius, like the maximus, shows a wave-like contraction that starts posteriorly and proceeds anteriorly (Scherb and Arienti, 1945).

Adductor Group

The *adductor group* has two peaks of activity that occur in early and in late stance. The early peak is the smaller of the two and is almost synchronous with the peaks of the quadriceps, the hamstrings, the gluteus maximus, and the abductor group. The adductors thus join the numerous muscle groups that show high activity just after heel contact. The second peak is seen at or just before toe-off.

If an attempt is made to interpret the function of the adductor group, several things must be kept in mind: first, that the adductor group is located partly anterior and partly posterior to the axis of flexion and extension of the hip and that, therefore, one portion may aid in flexion, another in extension; second, that the adductors are mechanically capable of performing transverse rotations; and third, that muscle groups such as the abductors and adductors (which are anatomic antagonists) often act synergically when firm stabilization of a joint is required. The muscles of the adductor group, it may be assumed, do not limit their activities to the control of lateral oscillations of the body but may be significantly involved in the control of numerous other movements.

ERECTOR SPINAE GROUP

Two periods of activity are registered, one in early stance, the other one in late stance. Following heel contact on the *right* side, the right erector spinae has its first peak of activity, and following heel contact on the *left* side, the right erector spinae has its second (higher) peak. Because the erector spinae on the left side acts in the same manner as the one on the right, the muscles on both sides support the vertebral column after heel contact when, owing to inertia, excessive forward motion of the trunk must be prevented. A stabilizing effect of the erector spinae muscles on the vertebral column in a lateral direction may also be inferred from the anatomic position of these muscles.

ABDOMINAL MUSCLES

Sheffield (1962) reported *inactivity of the abdominal muscles* in slow, level walking at 60 steps per min. By means of fine needle electrodes, the upper and lower portions of the rectus abdominis were investigated; activity of the lateral abdominal muscles was sampled at two different points at the height of the crest of the ilium, medially and laterally, but no effort was made to differentiate between the layers of the lateral abdominal muscles. None of the areas sampled yielded records of electric activity in the muscles under the conditions tested.

MUSCLES OF THE FOOT AND TOES

An electromyographic study of six of the intrinsic muscles of the foot by Mann and Inman (1964) revealed that during the swing phase of level walking, these muscles remained inactive. But all six muscles showed electric activity in the last half of the stance phase. In subjects with flat feet, the activity of the intrinsic muscles was of longer duration. For example, the abductor hallucis was found to be active during the entire stance phase. A study of six leg and foot muscles (tibialis anterior, tibialis posterior, flexor hallucis longus, peroneus longus, abductor hallucis, flexor digitorum brevis) by Gray and Basmajian (1968) throws further light on the function of individual muscles in walking. Most of the muscles studied were definitely more active in flatfooted persons than in subjects with normal arches. None of the muscles contracted continuously during both stance and swing phases. "Contingent arch support by muscles rather than continuous support is the rule, muscles being recruited to compensate for lax ligaments and special stresses during the walking cycle" (Gray and Basmajian, 1968).

ARM MUSCLES

Electromyographic studies of the arms of normal subjects during gait show activity in the posterior and middle deltoid slightly before the arm starts its backward swing, and this continues throughout the backward swing. During forward swing the main shoulder flexors were silent and activity was noted only in some of the medial rotators (subscapularis, latissimus dorsi, teres major) (MacConaill and Basmajian, 1969). In studying 12 shoulder and arm muscles, Hogue (1969) found greatest activity in the posterior deltoid. He interpreted this as activity that decelerated the forward-swinging arm and extended the backward-swinging arm. Posterior deltoid activity, as well as that in the middle deltoid and teres major, increased with increased cadence but did not show any appreciable increase as subjects ascended an incline.

Potential for Reprogramming Control of Muscle Action After Surgical Transfer of Its Tendon of Attachment

When the ability to perform a motion or to stabilize a joint has been lost because of permanent paralysis of the muscles primarily responsible for the action, the tendon of another muscle that is still capable of voluntary contraction may sometimes be surgically detached and then re-attached at a new location that provides a line of pull suitable for causing the desired action. *Tendon transfer* has been successfully used in selected instances to restore muscle balance at a joint, to restore lost motion, and to increase the active tension developed during joint motion. An expendable muscle of suitable strength and excursion must be available for transfer across a joint with a suitable range of motion. The vascular and neural supply to the muscle must, of course, be preserved. Muscles from synergistic groups provide the best candidates for transfer since the central nervous system is already "programmed" to activate the muscle when attempting the desired motion. However, antagonists have also been used to restore lost function. For example, Bunnel (1951) reported restoring elbow flexion to patients by passing the distal tendon of the triceps brachii through a lateral subcutaneous tunnel to the front side of the humerus where the tendon of the triceps was attached to that of the biceps. Transfer of the pectoralis major tendon has also been used to restore active flexion of the elbow (Brooks and Seddon, 1959; de Bruijn, 1980).

In the lower extremity, retraining a muscle to become active during a different portion of the gait cycle has generally been less successful. However, with the more widespread use of electromyographic biofeedback techniques (Basmajian, 1979) to improve muscle re-education, a few investigators have reported that muscles such as the peroneus brevis (a plantar-flexor) can be retrained to produce functional dorsiflexion (Takebe and Hirohata, 1980).

Energy Cost in Walking

Muscles affect the rate of energy expenditure of the body during movement partially by doing work on the body to increase the speed of motion or to lift portions or all of the body against gravity. An equally important role of muscles is to decelerate different parts, to stabilize joints so that they do not move, and to lower the weight of the body. The details of these processes can be studied only by elaborate laboratory methods, but the overall metaboic cost can be assessed by measuring oxygen consumption and converting the results to energy units (Calories or METS; see Chapter 3).

The influence of speed and rate of walking on oxygen consumption was investigated by Studer (1926) and by Atzler and Herbst (1927). As would be expected, oxygen consumption per unit of time was found to rise as walking speed increased (Studer, 1926). But when interest was centered on the oxygen consumption per "walking unit" (transportation of 1 kg of body weight a distance of 1 m on level surface), the picture became more complicated.

The energy cost per distance traveled when a subject walked at different speeds and with prescribed cadences of 50, 75, 100, 130, and 150 steps per min was investigated by Atzler and Herbst (1927). At each of the five cadences, the subject increased speed by lengthening the stride. In Figure 12-12, the energy cost (Calories per meter) is plotted against length of stride for the various cadences. With the exception of the lowest cadence, energy cost remains comparatively low at stride lengths between 45 and 75 cm. In Figure 12-13, Calorie cost per meter is plotted against rate of walking for stride lengths of 45, 60, 75, and 90 cm. The lowest portions of the curves are found at

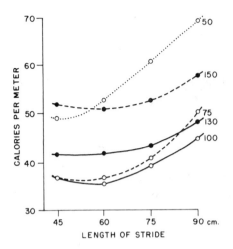

FIGURE 12-12. Calorie consumption as related to length of stride and cadence of walking. Steps per min are indicated at the right-hand end of each curve. (Redrawn from Atzler and Herbst, 1927.)

walking rates between 75 and 100 steps per min. Energy cost per distance traveled depends, then, on the length of the stride as well as on the rate of walking, and individuals sometimes choose the most efficient combination of stride length and cadence. Elftman (1966) emphasizes the "profound" effect of stride length and suggests that "the usual custom of reporting only velocity in metabolism measurement results in an inadequate experiment" (Elftman, 1966, p 375).

Studies of energy cost of walking have "produced surprisingly similar data" in the past half century (Corcoran, 1971). Results are reported with respect to walking speed (i.e., steps per min, miles or km per hour, and so on). Work is greater at very slow walking speeds than at ordinary speeds. Calorie cost of walking a given distance is lowest at a walking speed of about 3 miles (4.8 km) per hour. The energy requirement increases at very high walking speeds and changes considerably in walking up an incline, doubling on a 10 to 12 percent grade and tripling on a 20 to 25 percent grade (Corcoran, 1971).

Energy Cost in Walking of the Handicapped

Of special interest to rehabilitation personnel are studies of energy consumption of patients with amputations and of hemiplegic and paraplegic subjects. Original studies by Ralston (1958) and more recently by Corcoran and Brengelmann (1970) on able-bodied individuals helped establish bases for comparison. Bard and Ralston (1959) found that a person with an above-knee amputation wearing a well-fitted suction socket prosthesis and walking at "comfortable" speed used only slightly more energy than control subjects walking at the same speed. When a pylon without a knee joint was used, the energy cost was higher, and rose still higher when the subject walked without a prosthesis, using elbow crutches. Waters and associates (1976) compared the energy cost of walking of patients with amputations to study the influence of the level of amputation. The subjects' performance was significantly better, the lower the

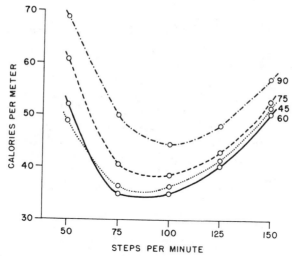

FIGURE 12-13. Calorie consumption as related to rate of walking and stride length. Stride length in centimeters is indicated at the right-hand end of each curve. (Redrawn from Atzler and Herbst, 1927.)

level of amputation. Most of the subjects kept energy expenditure within normal limits by adjusting their gait velocity; it was this somewhat slower walking speed that reflected the loss of efficiency.

The walking efficiency of hemiplegic patients was found to be rather low, and the more severe the spasticity, the less the efficiency. However, the metabolic cost to these patients when they walk at a comfortable speed is not so high as to make walking hazardous if no complications are present (Bard, 1963). The energy-saving effect of wearing an ankle brace was demonstrated in the case of a moderately spastic subject (Bard and Ralston, 1959). When the subject walked with a cane but without a brace, the energy expenditure was 41 percent greater than when the subject walked with a cane and wore a brace; the speed was identical in both test runs. Corcoran and associates (1970) found higher than normal (51 to 67 percent) energy expenditures when they investigated maximum and comfortable walking speeds and the energy cost of walking at these speeds. They also observed lower energy costs when patients used ankle-foot orthoses.

Gordon and Vanderwalde (1956) investigated energy requirements of ambulation when both legs are paralyzed and found that metabolic work was at least three times the basal rate, and sometimes five to eight times higher. The magnitude of this energy cost reflected the degree of motor loss. Energy cost for persons with paraplegia who ambulate with crutches is two to four times greater than that of a normal person walking. In fact, wheelchair locomotion may be the desirable and realistic method of locomotion for those with paraplegia in terms of energy expenditure, since it has been shown that wheelchair use on a smooth surface requires the same or slightly less energy than normal walking (Corcoran, 1971).

The addition of extra weight, clothing, and braces during walking causes a linear increase in energy cost of walking. Lehneis and associates (1976) measured differences in consumed oxygen between patients wearing advanced-design lower limb orthoses and the same patients wearing conventional braces. The new designs, developed at the Institute of Rehabilitation Medicine, New York City, were found to result in a reduction of oxygen consumption of 9 to 16 percent.

The energy used for walking with canes and with crutches was determined by McBeath and associates (1974). All forms of assisted ambulation tested required more energy than normal walking. The swing-through and the three-point non-weight-bearing gait required about 78 percent more energy; the use of canes or the use of crutches with two-point-alternating and three-point partial-weight-bearing gaits required about 33 percent more. Use of either type of crutches, Lofstrand or axillary, required about the same expenditure of energy.

APPENDIX **A**

TABLES 1 THROUGH 13

TABLE 1. Leverage Factors for Individual Muscles Flexing the Elbow. Figures Show Force Moments per Unit Cross Section of Each Muscle (1 sq cm) and per Unit of Muscle Force (1 kg). Muscle Force Is Assumed to Be Constant Throughout Range.

Flexion degrees	Pronator teres	Ext. carpi rad. long.	Brachialis	Biceps, long head	Biceps, short head	Brachioradialis
0	4.9	−5.7	11.0	11.5	12.2	9.7
10	5.7	−0.5	12.5	13.7	13.8	13.5
20	6.3	+4.5	13.8	16.8	16.4	20.5
30	6.8	8.6	15.3	21.4	20.7	30.5
40	7.3	12.3	17.0	27.0	26.3	39.8
50	8.1	16.0	19.6	32.4	31.9	48.4
60	9.3	19.5	23.0	37.4	36.9	56.4
70	10.5	22.9	26.6	40.7	40.2	64.0
80	11.4	26.4	30.0	43.5	43.0	70.3
90	12.3	29.3	33.5	45.4	45.5	75.2
100	12.9	31.4	36.5	45.5	46.1	79.8
110	12.8	32.5	35.9	42.8	43.8	81.4
120	11.8	31.9	33.4	39.2	41.0	79.9
130	10.2	28.6	31.4	35.9	37.5	72.7

Adapted from R. Fick, 1911, pp 318, 319.

TABLE 2. Maximal Work Capacities of Flexors of Elbow, From Extension (0 Degrees) to Flexion (145 Degrees)

Name of Muscle	Shortening (in meters)	Cross Section (in sq cm)	Work Capacity (in kg m)
FOREARM IN SUPINATION			
Brachialis	0.060	6.4	3.84
Biceps, long head	0.073	3.33	2.43
Biceps, short head	0.073	3.22	2.42
Brachioradialis	0.102	1.86	1.90
Pronator teres	0.039	3.24	1.26
Extensor carpi radialis longus	0.039	3.14	1.22
Flexor carpi radialis	0.022	2.16	0.47
Extensor carpi radialis brevis	0.015	2.22	0.33
Palmaris longus	0.010	0.93	0.09
			13.96
FOREARM IN MIDPOSITION			
Brachialis	0.060	6.4	3.84
Biceps, long head	0.070	3.33	2.33
Biceps, short head	0.070	3.22	2.25
Brachioradialis	0.119	1.86	2.21
Extensor carpi radialis longus	0.047	3.14	1.47
Pronator teres	0.043	3.24	1.39
Flexor carpi radialis	0.024	2.16	0.52
Extensor carpi radialis brevis	0.015	2.22	0.33
Palmaris longus	0.011	0.93	0.10
			14.44
FOREARM IN PRONATION			
Brachialis	0.060	6.4	3.84
Biceps, long head	0.069	3.33	2.30
Brachioradialis	0.130	1.86	2.25
Biceps, short head	0.069	3.22	2.22
Pronator teres	0.024	2.16	1.52
Extensor carpi radialis longus	0.048	3.14	1.51
Flexor carpi radialis	0.047	3.24	0.52
Extensor carpi radialis brevis	0.017	2.22	0.38
Palmaris longus	0.013	0.93	0.12
			14.66

Adapted from R. Fick, 1911, p 320.

TABLE 3. Maximal Work Capacities of Extensors of Elbow, From 35 Degrees (Elbow Flexed) to 180 Degrees (Elbow Extended)

Name of Muscle	Shortening (in meters)	Cross Section (in sq cm)	Work Capacity (in kg m)
Triceps, lateral head	0.050	6.78	3.39
Triceps, medial head	0.047	5.66	2.66
Triceps, long head	0.051	4.75	2.42
Anconeus	0.026	3.18	0.83
			9.30

Adapted from R. Fick, 1911, p 131.

TABLE 4. Maximal Work Capacities of Supinators of Forearm, From Complete Pronation (0 Degrees) to Complete Supination (120 Degrees)

Name of Muscle	Shortening (in meters)	Cross Section (in sq cm)	Work Capacity (in kg m)
ELBOW IN EXTENSION			
Biceps brachii, short head	0.011	3.22	0.36
Supinator	0.015	2.20	0.33
Biceps, long head	0.008	3.33	0.26
Brachioradialis	0.014	1.86	0.16
Extensor carpi radialis longus	0.005	3.14	0.16
Abductor pollicis longus	0.004	1.84	0.07
Extensor pollicis brevis	0.004	1.84	0.07
Extensor pollicis longus	0.003	0.56	0.02
Extensor indicis proprius	0.003	0.37	0.01
			1.44
ELBOW AT 90 DEGREES			
Biceps brachii, short head	0.019	3.22	0.61
Biceps brachii, long head	0.016	3.33	0.53
Supinator	0.015	2.20	0.33
Abductor pollicis longus	0.004	1.84	0.07
Extensor pollicis brevis	0.004	1.84	0.07
Brachioradialis*	0.002	1.86	0.04
Extensor pollicis longus	0.003	0.56	0.02
Extensor indicis proprius	0.003	0.37	0.01
			1.68
ELBOW IN COMPLETE FLEXION			
Biceps brachii, short head	0.019	3.22	0.61
Biceps brachii, long head	0.016	3.33	0.53
Supinator	0.015	2.20	0.33
Abductor pollicis longus	0.004	1.84	0.07
Extensor pollicis brevis	0.004	1.84	0.07
Extensor pollicis longus	0.003	0.56	0.02
Extensor indicis proprius	0.003	0.37	0.01
			1.64

*To 20 degrees, starting from complete pronation.

Adapted from R. Fick, 1911, pp 348, 349.

TABLE 5. Maximal Work Capacities of Pronators of Forearm From Complete Supination (0 Degrees) to Complete Pronation (120 Degrees)

Name of Muscle	Shortening (in meters)	Cross Section (in sq cm)	Work Capacity (in kg m)
ELBOW IN EXTENSION			
Pronator teres	0.010	3.24	0.32
Flexor carpi radialis	0.013	2.16	0.28
Pronator quadratus	0.008	2.22	0.18
Palmaris longus	0.012	0.93	0.11
			0.89
ELBOW AT 90 DEGREES			
Pronator teres	0.019	3.6	0.68
Flexor carpi radialis	0.011	2.16	0.24
Brachioradialis*	0.012	1.86	0.22
Pronator quadratus	0.008	2.22	0.18
Extensor carpi radialis longus	0.005	3.14	0.16
Palmaris longus	0.011	0.93	0.10
			1.58
ELBOW IN COMPLETE FLEXION			
Pronator teres	0.015	3.24	0.49
Brachioradialis	0.015	1.86	0.28
Flexor carpi radialis	0.010	2.16	0.22
Pronator quadratus	0.008	2.22	0.18
Extensor carpi radialis longus	0.005	3.14	0.16
Palmaris longus	0.008	0.93	0.07
			1.40

*To 105 degrees, starting from complete supination.

Adapted from R. Fick, 1911, p 351.

TABLE 6. Maximal Work Capacities of Muscles in Flexion, Extension, Ulnar Abduction, and Radial Abduction of Wrist, Complete Range of Motion

Name of Muscle	Shortening (in meters)	Cross Section (in sq cm)	Work Capacity (in kg m)
FLEXORS OF WRIST			
Flexor digitorum superficialis	0.045	10.7	4.815
Flexor digitorum profundus	0.042	10.8	4.536
Flexor carpi ulnaris	0.039	5.0	1.950
Flexor pollicis longus	0.041	2.9	1.189
Flexor carpi radialis	0.038	2.16	0.821
Abductor pollicis longus	0.005	1.84	0.092
All flexors:		33.40	13.403
EXTENSORS OF WRIST			
Extensor digitorum communis	0.040	4.30	1.720
Extensor carpi ulnaris	0.021	5.30	1.113
Extensor carpi radialis longus	0.034	3.14	1.068
Extensor carpi radialis brevis	0.040	2.22	0.888
Extensor indicis proprius	0.038	1.20	0.456
Extensor pollicis longus	0.025	0.56	0.140
All extensors:		16.72	5.385
ULNAR ABDUCTORS OF WRIST			
Extensor carpi ulnaris	0.020	5.30	1.060
Flexor carpi ulnaris	0.014	5.00	0.700
All ulnar abductors:		10.30	1.760
RADIAL ABDUCTORS OF WRIST			
Extensor carpi radialis longus	0.036	3.14	1.130
Abductor pollicis longus	0.021	1.84	0.386
Extensor carpi radialis brevis	0.014	2.22	0.311
Extensor indicis proprius	0.007	1.20	0.084
Extensor pollicis longus	0.014	0.56	0.078
Flexor carpi radialis	0.003	2.16	0.065
All radial abductors:		11.12	2.054

Adapted from R. Fick, 1911, pp 396–398.

TABLE 7. Maximal Work Capacities of Muscles Acting on Glenohumeral Joint

Name of Muscle	Shortening (in meters)	Cross Section (in sq cm)	Work Capacity (in kg m)
IN FLEXION OF SHOULDER			
Subscapularis	0.011	25.2	2.77
Supraspinatus	0.031	7.7	2.39
Coracobrachialis	0.039	5.8	2.26
Infraspinatus and teres minor	0.014	16.5	2.21
Biceps, short head	0.048	3.2	1.54
Biceps, long head	0.030	3.3	0.99
			12.16
IN EXTENSION OF SHOULDER			
Teres major	0.101	9.8	9.90
Triceps, long head	0.054	4.7	2.54
			12.44
IN ADDUCTION OF THE SHOULDER			
Teres major	0.066	9.8	6.47
Coracobrachialis	0.052	5.8	3.01
Triceps, long head	0.041	4.7	1.92
Biceps, long head	0.019	3.2	0.61
			12.01
IN ABDUCTION OF THE SHOULDER			
Supraspinatus	0.033	7.7	2.54
Infraspinatus and teres minor	0.011	16.5	1.81
Subscapularis	0.004	25.2	1.01
Biceps, long head	0.012	3.3	0.40
			5.76
IN INWARD ROTATION OF SHOULDER			
Subscapularis	0.047	25.2	11.84
Teres major	0.023	9.8	2.25
Biceps, long head	0.021	3.3	0.69
Biceps, short head	0.003	3.2	0.10
			14.88
IN OUTWARD ROTATION OF SHOULDER			
Infraspinatus and teres minor	0.042	16.5	6.93
Coracobrachialis	0.003	5.8	0.17
			7.10

NOTE: The pectoralis major, latissimus dorsi, and deltoid are missing in this table. Cross section of middle deltoid is given elsewhere as 25.3 sq cm.

Adapted from R. Fick, 1911, pp 280, 281.

TABLE 8. Maximal Work Capacities of Flexors and Extensors of Knee

Name of Muscle	Shortening (in meters)	Cross Section (in sq cm)	Work Capacity (in kg m)
EXTENSORS			
Vasti	0.080	148.30	118.640
Rectus femoris	0.081*	28.89	23.400
Tensor fasciae latae	0.010	7.56	0.756
			142.796
FLEXORS			
Semimembranosus	0.064*	26.38	16.833
Semitendinosus	0.134	7.27	13.242
Biceps femoris	0.059	17.37	10.248
Gracilis	0.075	4.11	3.082
Sartorius	0.070	3.17	2.319
			45.774

*Muscle is "actively insufficient."

Adapted from R. Fick, 1911, p 585.

NOTE: These are the figures appearing in Fick's table, but errors in calculation seem to have crept in. Furthermore, the work capacities for biarticular muscles must be re-evaluated, since these muscles are actively insufficient in a portion of the joint range. S.B.

TABLE 9. Maximal Work Capacities of Rotators of Knee

Name of Muscle	Shortening* (in meters)	Cross Section (in sq cm)	Work Capacity (in kg m)
EXTERNAL ROTATORS			
Tibia with respect to femur			
Biceps femoris	0.0247	19.80	4.891
Tensor fasciae	0.0077	8.40	0.647
INTERNAL ROTATORS			
Tibia with respect to femur			
Semimembranosus	0.0133	26.39	3.400
Semitendinosus	0.0109	7.65	0.834
Sartorius	0.0156	3.75	0.585
Popliteus	0.0150	5.32	0.798
Gracilis	0.0127	3.30	0.419

*Shortening by a rotation of 37.5 degrees.

Adapted from R. Fick, 1911, p 586.

TABLE 10. Maximal Work Capacities of Muscles Acting on Talocrural Joint

Name of Muscle	Shortening (in meters)	Cross Section (in sq cm)	Work Capacity (in kg m)
DORSIFLEXORS OF ANKLE			
Tibialis anterior	0.033	7.7	2.54
Extensor digitorum longus	0.033	2.5	0.82
Peroneus tertius*	0.031	1.7	0.49
Extensor hallucis longus	0.029	1.3	0.42
			4.27
PLANTAR FLEXORS OF ANKLE			
Gastrocnemius	0.039	23.0	8.97
Soleus	0.037	20.0	7.40
Flexor hallucis longus	0.019	4.5	0.85
Peroneus longus	0.0103	4.3	0.44
Tibialis posterior	0.007	5.8	0.41
Flexor digitorum longus	0.013	2.8	0.36
Peroneus brevis	0.0065	3.8	0.25
			18.68

*In two out of four cadavers investigated, the peroneus tertius was unusually well developed, hence the cross section given (average of 4) is quite high.

Adapted from R. Fick, 1911, p 610.

TABLE 11. Maximal Work Capacities of Muscles Acting on Lower Ankle Joint

Name of Muscle	Shortening (in meters)	Cross Section (in sq cm)	Work Capacity (in kg m)
INVERTORS			
Gastrocnemius	0.011	23.0	2.53
Soleus	0.0116	20.0	2.32
Tibialis posterior	0.025	5.8	1.45
Flexor hallucis longus	0.015	4.5	0.67
Flexor digitorum longus	0.0205	2.8	0.57
Tibialis anterior	0.0041	7.7	0.32
		63.8	7.86
EVERTORS			
Peroneus longus	0.0245	4.3	1.05
Peroneus brevis	0.0227	3.8	0.86
Extensor digitorum longus	0.0194	2.5	0.48
Peroneus tertius	0.0226	1.7	0.38
Extensor hallucis longus	0.0090	1.35	0.12
Tibialis anterior	0.0043	7.7	0.33
		21.35	3.22

Adapted from R. Fick, 1911, p 629.

TABLE 12. Maximal Work Capacities of the Long Toe Flexors and Extensors

Name of Muscle	Shortening (in meters)	Cross Section (in sq cm)	Work Capacity (in kg m)
FLEXORS			
Flexor hallucis longus	0.0370	4.5	1.66
Flexor digitorum longus	0.0307	2.8	0.86
			2.52
EXTENSORS			
Extensor digitorum longus	0.0200	2.5	0.50
Extensor hallucis longus	0.0280	1.35	0.38
			0.88

Adapted from R. Fick, 1911, p 639.

TABLE 13. Maximal Work Capacities of Some of the Hip Muscles

Name of Muscle	Shortening (in meters)	Cross Section (in sq cm)	Work Capacity (in kg m)
FLEXORS (sagittal plane motion of 120 degrees)			
Rectus femoris	0.060	28.89	17.33
Tensor fasciae	0.154	8.40	12.94*
Sartorius	0.133	3.75	4.99
Gracilis to 40 degrees flexion	0.013	3.3	0.43
EXTENSORS (sagittal plane motion of 120 degrees)			
Semimembranosus	0.074	26.39	19.53*
Gluteus maximus, lower portion	0.0805	22.2	17.77
Biceps, long head	0.101	14.25	14.25*
Adductor magnus, upper portion	0.1052	11.65	12.26
Adductor magnus, middle portion	0.1008	11.65	11.74
Gluteus maximus, middle portion	0.0521	22.2	11.57
Adductor magnus, lower portion	0.0695	11.65	8.10
Semitendinosus	0.074	7.65	5.66
Gluteus maximus, upper portion	0.022	22.2	4.88
Gracilis from 40 to 120 degrees	0.041	3.3	1.35
ABDUCTORS (frontal plane motion of 37 degrees)			
Rectus femoris	0.0115	28.89	3.32
Tensor fasciae	0.0281	8.40	2.36
Sartorius	0.0152	3.75	0.57
ADDUCTORS (frontal plane motion of 37 degrees)			
Gracilis	0.0490	3.3	1.61
Biceps, long head	0.0105	14.25	1.50
Semimembranosus	0.0030	14.55	0.44
Semitendinosus	0.0030	7.65	0.23

*The work capacity given for this muscle must be considered too large because the muscle is actively insufficient owing to the shortness of its fibers.

Adapted from R. Fick, 1911, p 502.

SUMMARY: RANGES OF JOINT MOTION

Although many textbooks provide values for normal range of motion, standardized normal tables according to age, sex, body build, and type of motion (active or passive) have not been established. Thus, the most accurate measurement of normal motion is the patient's opposite extremity if it is present and unimpaired. The following goniometric values may be used as guidelines to the approximate normal joint range of motion in the adult. *The single value given below is a round number that is convenient to remember in estimating the amount of normal motion present.* The values in parentheses are the range of *average* normal motion reported in several sources (Daniels and Worthingham, 1972; Kendall, Kendall, and Wadsworth, 1971; Gerhardt and Russe, 1975; Kapandji, 1970a, 1970b; Department of the Army and Air Force, 1968; American Academy of Orthopaedic Surgeons, 1965). For details of positioning and landmarks for the measurements, the original references should be consulted.

SHOULDER flexion **0°** to **180°** (150° to 180°)
extension **0°**
hyperextension **0°** to **45°** (40° to 60°)
abduction **0°** to **180°** (150° to 180°)
internal rotation **0°** to **90°** (70° to 90°)
external rotation **0°** to **90°** (80° to 90°)

ELBOW flexion **0°** to **145°** (120° to 160°)
extension **0°**

FOREARM supination from midposition **0°** to **90°** (80° to 90°)
pronation from midposition **0°** to **80°** (70° to 80°)

403

WRIST   neutral when the midline between flexion and extension is 0° and when
            forearm and third metacarpal are in line
            flexion **0°** to **90°** (75° to 90°)
            extension **0°** to **70°** (65° to 70°)
            radial abduction **0°** to **20°** (15° to 25°)
            ulnar abduction **0°** to **30°** (25° to 40°)

FINGERS metacarpophalangeal flexion **0°** to **90°** (85° to 100°)
            metacarpophalangeal hyperextension **0°** to **20°** (0° to 45°)
            metacarpophalangeal abduction **0°** to **20°**
            metacarpophalangeal adduction **0°**
            proximal interphalangeal flexion **0°** to **120°** (90° to 120°)
            distal interphalangeal flexion **0°** to **90°** (80° to 90°)

THUMB   metacarpophalangeal flexion **0°** to **45°** (40° to 90°)
            metacarpophalangeal abduction and adduction NEGLIGIBLE
            interphalangeal flexion **0°** to **90°** (80° to 90°)

HIP   flexion **0°** to **120°** (110° to 125°)
            hyperextension **0°** to **10°** (0° to 15°)
            abduction **0°** to **45°** (40° to 55°)
            adduction **0°** (30° to 40° across midline)
            external rotation **0°** to **45°** (40° to 50°)
            internal rotation **0°** to **35°** (30° to 45°)

KNEE   flexion **0°** to **120°** (120° to 140°)
            extension **0°**

ANKLE   neutral with foot at a right angle to the leg and knee flexed
            plantar flexion **0°** to **45°** (40° to 50°)
            dorsiflexion **0°** to **15°** (10° to 20°)

Ranges of motion for other body parts, such as the neck, trunk, carpometacarpal
joint of the thumb, and temporomandibular joint, and for other motions, such as axial
rotation of the knee and inversion-eversion of the ankle, have not been included because of the variability of the methods used and the resulting *apparent* disparity of the
values. In the absence of accepted standardized techniques of measurements of these
areas, quantitative evaluation of these motions requires standardization by clinicians
in their local treatment settings.

APPENDIX C

SUGGESTED LABORATORY ACTIVITIES

The following suggested laboratory activities and review questions are to guide your study of material presented in this book. Your application of clinical kinesiology will vary according to your professional role. Many of you, as workers in the field of rehabilitation of physically handicapped persons, will need to use the basic knowledge and skills emphasized here. With practice you should be able to:

1. identify and palpate (i.e., examine by touch) anatomic structures in the living human.
2. develop some tactile sensitivity so that you can identify, through overlying skin, the anatomic structures you feel (i.e., bone, tendon, muscle).
3. analyze an isolated or a gross movement.
4. determine synergic muscle actions that will produce movement.

MATERIALS NEEDED

For laboratory study you will need the following:

1. a skeleton and disarticulated bones.
2. a comprehensive anatomy text.
3. "relatively" normal subjects (fellow classmates or others).
4. appropriate laboratory attire to permit exposure of body segments.
5. some additional equipment, instruments, materials, objects (to be identified within the units of study).

GENERAL PROCEDURE

Follow this procedure for studying all muscle action:

1. Identify bony landmarks on a skeleton. Identify the palpable bony landmarks on yourself and on a subject. Bony landmarks are firm and stable structures and provide a starting point for locating the mobile soft tissue structures like muscle bellies and tendons.
2. Study articulating joint surfaces and joint axes of movement. Locate on yourself and on a subject the palpable bony landmarks that will identify approximate joint axes.
3. Define, describe, observe, and perform joint motions.
4. Study muscle groups and individual muscles. Identify their:
   a. attachments
   b. lines of action
   c. relationship of action lines to joint axes.
   A knowledge of the joint axes and of muscle action lines and their relationships to these axes is the key to being able to analyze muscle function.
5. Palpate muscle groups and individual muscles and tendons.
6. Given a specific muscle name, state and demonstrate movements it will perform.
7. Given specific joint movements, state and identify muscles that will perform these movements.
8. Analyze an isolated or a gross movement and determine synergic muscle actions that will produce these movements.

PRINCIPLES

Always consider the kinesiologic principles. The following statements summarize the main mechanical and physiologic principles in this book. The chapter numbers following each statement identify the locations in the text of a reference to the principle.

1. A body is stable when the vertical projection of its center of gravity falls within the base of support (Chapters 2 and 12).
2. Body movements can be described, for convenience in communication, with reference to three anatomic planes: sagittal, frontal, and horizontal (Chapter 1).
3. Movements are most appropriately described by referring to the joints at which the movements occur rather than with reference to the moving segments (Chapters 1 and 4).
4. The concepts of rotary motion and degrees of freedom of motion form a basis for analyzing bodily movements (Chapter 1).
5. A combination of several joints uniting successive segments constitutes a kinematic chain or joint chain. In an open kinematic chain, the most common formed in the human body, the distal segment terminates free in space. Through summation of freedom of movement of successive joints, a high degree of freedom of

movement is allotted not only to the end of the segment but also to various segments in relation to each other (Chapter 1).

6. Vector quantities (i.e., forces that involve magnitude and direction) play a fundamental part in body motion (Chapter 2).

7. In body movement, the effectiveness with which a gravitational force or a muscular force produces rotation about a point (i.e., a joint axis) increases as the perpendicular distance from the action line of the force to that point (i.e., axis or fulcrum) increases (Chapter 2).

8. Muscle actions are best analyzed if their attachments and thus their action lines are visualized with respect to the joint axes that they cross. Any muscle action line that crosses any joint axis may produce some movement about that axis (Chapter 2).

9. A muscle tends to produce motion at the point of attachment having the least stability (Chapter 2).

10. A muscle having extensive attachments has the capacity to perform multiple actions (Chapter 2).

11. Effectiveness of a muscle force or gravitational pull in rotating a body segment increases as the angle of application of that force to the part approaches 90 degrees (Chapters 2 and 4).

12. The larger the physiologic cross section of a muscle, the more tension it can produce (Chapter 3).

13. Velocity of muscle shortening influences muscle tension as follows:
    a. Isometric contractions (i.e., velocity zero) have higher tension values than shortening contractions.
    b. As velocity of shortening increases, tension decreases.
    c. During a lengthening contraction, more tension can be produced than during isometric or shortening contractions.
    d. Up to a certain point, as velocity of stretch of the muscle increases, the tension rises (Chapter 4).

14. Muscle performance must be visualized with consideration of lengthening as well as shortening muscle contractions (Chapter 4).

15. Maximum contractile tension is obtained when the muscle is elongated slightly beyond its "resting length." For optimum effect, the muscle should be elongated before it is made to contract (Chapter 4).

16. A typical torque curve (maximal torque that a muscle or muscle group can produce at various joint positions) shows that maximal torque occurs at a joint position where the muscles are elongated and that curves, such as produced by the elbow flexors, are exceptions (Chapter 4).

17. Isokinetic exercise allows control of speed of muscular performance irrespective of the magnitude of the force generated by the participating muscles (Chapter 4).

UNIT 1—GENERAL CONCEPTS

1. Turn to Table 1, Appendix A. On a piece of graph paper, draw two perpendicular axes, placing the point of intersection in the lower left corner of the paper. On the

vertical axis, allow for values from −10 (below the point of intersection) to +80. On the horizontal axis, allow for values from 0 to +130. Label the vertical axis "force moments—leverage," and label the horizontal axis "joint angle." Plot the degrees of elbow flexion against the leverage factors shown in Table 1 for pronator teres, extensor carpi radialis longus, brachialis, biceps (long head), and brachioradialis. Draw the curves. Compare the results. In what way do the curves differ? How are they similar? Explain the meaning of the curves.

2. On a piece of graph paper, plot torque curves (force against joint angle) for pronator teres, brachialis, biceps (long head), and brachioradialis. To determine muscle force, multiply leverage factor (in Table 1) by the physiologic cross section (in Table 2, listed under "forearm in supination"). Joint angles are those listed in Table 1. Compare these curves with the previous ones you drew. In what ways are they the same or different? How do you interpret or explain the meaning of these curves?

3. Study torque curves in Figures 4-10 to 4-17. Note the peaks of the curves. Observe a classmate perform the various upper limb movements, and estimate the position in the range of motion where the torque is greatest for elbow flexion, elbow extension, shoulder extension, shoulder flexion, shoulder abduction, and shoulder adduction. Consider factors that influence the tension developed by a contracting muscle. Which factors seem to predominate in these six movements? Using appropriate laboratory equipment (i.e., dynamometers or tension-meters and goniometers) determine the maximal torque that various muscle groups can produce over a joint. Have a subject make maximal effort against a stationary resistance, the resistance being applied at a 90-degree angle to the bony lever at all positions of the joint. Read the magnitude of the resistance on a dynamometer or tension-meter. Read the joint angle on a goniometer. Be sure to provide stability to entire body and to prevent assistive movements of other body parts as subject exerts maximal effort. (See Williams and Stutzman, 1959, for details.)

4. Stand erect. Perform a movement (any joint, any body segment) in the sagittal plane. Observe a subject do the same. Perform movements in the frontal plane and in the horizontal plane. Observe a subject do the same. How many movements can you perform in the three planes? Name and describe them. Identify the direction of the axes about which these various movements occur. Compare movements in these planes with natural movements that occur in everyday activities (i.e., opening a door, putting on a coat, climbing stairs, reaching up to a cabinet, walking).

5. Estimate the location of the center of gravity in a variety of objects and then estimate their most stable positions for balance (i.e., a square box, a cone-shaped object, a telephone pole, a ball, a book, a yardstick, body segments, the human body). Under what conditions is an object or a body in stable equilibrium? (See Chapter 2.)

6. Describe how the center of gravity shifts with changes in body posture as you do the following:
   a. Rise from a seated position to standing.
   b. Stand with back and heels touching a wall and bend forward to reach the floor without moving your feet.

c. Face the edge of an open door with nose and abdomen touching the edge, feet straddling it; rise on tip toes.

Account for any difficulty you had in accomplishing these activities. Describe some sport or clinical activities that exemplify the importance of control and of shifting of the center of gravity of the total body.

UNIT 2—ELBOW AND FOREARM

1. On the skeleton, identify these bones and bony landmarks of the elbow:

Humerus	Ulna	Radius
shaft	shaft	head
capitulum	olecranon process	neck
coronoid fossa	coronoid process	shaft
trochlea	trochlear notch	tuberosity of radius
olecranon fossa	head	radio-ulnar
medial epicondyle	radial notch	articulation
lateral epicondyle	styloid process	Lister's tubercle

2. Which of these bony landmarks can you palpate? Locate these on yourself and then on a partner.
3. Identify and examine the skeleton joint surfaces where the movements of elbow flexion, elbow extension, pronation, and supination take place. Move the skeleton forearm by turning palm of the hand up (supinate) and then by turning it down (pronate). Note that when the palm turns up (supination), radius and ulna are parallel; when palm turns down (pronation), these bones are crossed, that is, the radius rotates and crosses over the ulna.
4. Perform elbow and forearm movements on yourself and then observe as a subject performs them:
    a. Flex and extend the elbow first with the forearm supinated, then with the forearm pronated.
    b. Pronate and supinate the forearm. As you do this, hold your upper arm against side of body, maintain wrist in one position, and maintain elbow flexed at a right angle. Note that isolated forearm movement occurs.
    c. Pronate both forearms as described. Now extend elbows, lift your arms to shoulder height, and continue to turn palms of hands in the direction of pronation as far as they will move. Note increased movement which results from shoulder rotation. With arms elevated to shoulder height this way, continue movements of pronation and supination. Now isolate the forearm movement by again flexing the elbow and holding the upper arm against the side of your body. Which forearm and shoulder movements occur synchronously?

5. On the skeleton, on yourself, and on a partner, identify and visualize the axes for elbow flexion and extension and for forearm pronation and supination. Identify and palpate bony landmarks to locate these axes.
6. Using anatomy text and skeleton determine points of attachment for:

biceps brachii	triceps brachii	anconeus
brachialis	pronator teres	pronator quadratus
brachioradialis	supinator	wrist extensors

Note particularly the action line of each muscle and the axes each one crosses; from these observations, determine the movements each can perform. A helpful method to facilitate such observations is to cut lengths of adhesive tape to reach from one attachment of the muscle to the other and then to tape these pieces on the skeleton from the point of proximal attachment to point of distal attachment.
7. Determine muscles that will:
   a. flex the elbow.
   b. extend the elbow.
   c. pronate the forearm.
   d. supinate the forearm.
8. Select a partner. Following the descriptions in Chapter 5, palpate the biceps brachii, brachialis, brachioradialis, pronator teres, triceps brachii, supinator, and anconeus. Identify these muscles and tendons first on yourself and then on your partner.

UNIT 3—WRIST AND HAND

1. On the skeleton, identify the following bones and bony landmarks of the wrist and hand. Determine which of these are palpable and palpate them on yourself and on a partner.

head of the ulna	carpal bones
styloid process of the ulna	shafts of metacarpal bones
styloid process of the radius	heads of metacarpal bones
dorsal radial tubercle	phalanges

2. On the skeleton, examine and identify the following joint surfaces:

radiocarpal	metacarpophalangeal
midcarpal	interphalangeal
carpometacarpal	carpometacarpal joint of the thumb

3. Analyze wrist and finger movements (excluding thumb) on yourself and on a partner. Identify and palpate bony landmarks that will locate axes of these movements.

4. Analyze all thumb movements (carpometacarpal, metacarpophalangeal, interphalangeal) on yourself and on a partner. Palpate in your own hand and in several subjects' hands the location of the "saddle" joint of the thumb.

5. On the skeleton, locate the points of attachment for these muscles:

extensor carpi radialis longus   flexor carpi ulnaris
extensor carpi radialis brevis   flexor carpi radialis
extensor carpi ulnaris   flexor digitorum profundus
extensor digitorum   flexor digitorum superficialis

flexor pollicis longus
abductor pollicis longus
extensor pollicis longus
extensor pollicis brevis

Analyze the:
a. joints these muscles cross.
b. distal attachments of these muscles.
c. innervation of these muscles.

6. Palpate muscle bellies of wrist and finger flexors and extensors, tracing their action line to their proximal bony attachments in the region of the elbow. Palpate tendons about the wrist and analyze their relationships so that you can identify them accurately irrespective of forearm or hand position. From the class select four students, two whose wrist tendons are prominent and easily identified and two whose tendons may be palpable although not easily observed. All students study these subjects and compare their observations. Compare with wrist tendons in the rest of the group. Determine muscles that will perform wrist flexion and extension and radial and ulnar abduction of the wrist.

7. Using skin pencils, sketch on your own hand the extrinsic tendons, including those of the thumb. Next add the "short" (i.e., intrinsic) muscles and analyze their relationships to the extrinsic muscles. Determine hand, finger, and thumb movements performed by the intrinsics. Analyze integrated action of intrinsic and extrinsic hand muscles.

8. Pick up or manipulate these objects: thumb tacks, straight pins, paper clips, cards, coins, keys, glass, weights, pencil or pen, briefcase, handbag, cup, doorknob, scissors, magazine, newspaper, screwdriver, book, ball. Analyze prehension patterns, noting particularly the wrist positions, the specific finger movements and the continuous transition from pattern to pattern. (See Figs. 6-27—power grip and precision grip, 6-32—palmar prehension, 6-33—lateral prehension, 6-31—tip prehension, 6-29—cylindric grasp, 6-30—spheric grasp, 6-28—hook grasp.)

9. With a hand dynamometer and a pinch meter, test strength of your grip, chuck pinch, and lateral pinch (Figs. A-1—grip, A-2—chuck pinch, A-3—lateral pinch). Test your major and your minor hand. Compile and compare results among all class members and determine average scores. Assure standardization of test pro-

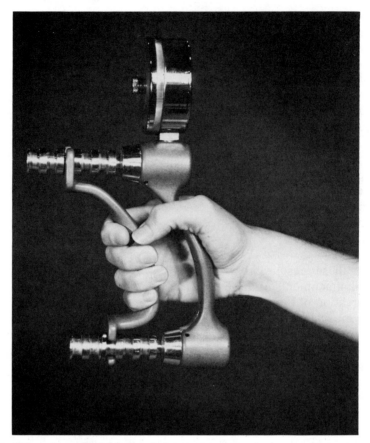

FIGURE A-1. Grip using adjustable hand dynamometer.

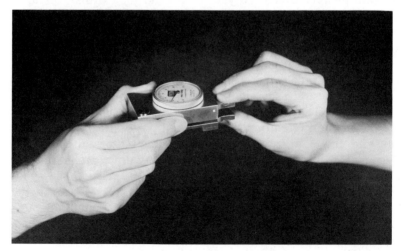

FIGURE A-2. Chuck pinch. Examiner (left) holds pinch meter. Subject (right) pinches the instrument.

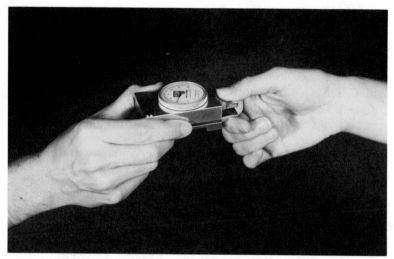

FIGURE A-3. Lateral pinch. Examiner (left) holds pinch meter. Subject (right) pinches the instrument.

cedure with respect to the number of repetitions and to the position and support (or nonsupport) of the forearm.

10. Analyze synergic muscle action of wrist and fingers for the following activities:
    a. Close the fist tightly. Open the fist and extend the fingers completely. Continue these movements, alternating quickly between the open and closed positions. What kinesiologic principle does this activity exemplify?
    b. With forearm and hand supported, perform thumb and little finger movements described in Chapter 6.
    c. Pick up and release objects of different sizes and shapes.
    d. Perform other activities relevant to your professional function such as the use of the hand to manipulate crutches and to support the body weight in the activity of crutch walking.
11. Predict dysfunction of elbow, wrist, and hand that could occur when:
    a. radial nerve is severed in the region of the spiral groove in the humerus.
    b. median nerve is cut at the wrist joint.
    c. ulnar nerve is crushed at the elbow between the medial epicondyle of the humerus and the olecranon process.
    d. the lateral cord of the brachial plexus is damaged.
    In your analysis, determine functions that will be lost, functions decreased, and functions remaining.

UNIT 4—SHOULDER REGION

1. On the skeleton, identify the following bones and bony landmarks. Determine which ones are palpable, and identify these on a partner. (Wear appropriate attire for this unit to permit exposure of the shoulder and shoulder girdle.)

Scapula	*Humerus*	*Sternum*	*Clavicle*
acromion process	head	manubrium	trapezoid line
spine	neck	body	conoid tubercle
coracoid process	greater tubercle	xiphoid process	
supraspinous fossa	lesser tubercle	jugular (sternal)	
infraspinous fossa	bicipital (inter-	notch	
glenoid cavity	tubercular) groove	facet for clavicle	
superior angle	deltoid tuberosity		
inferior angle			
medial border			
axillary border			
supraglenoid tubercle			
infraglenoid tubercle			

2. Locate the sternoclavicular, acromioclavicular, and glenohumeral joints on the skeleton, and perform all movements that are possible at these joints. Identify axes about which these movements occur. Analyze forearm movements that occur synchronously with internal and external shoulder rotation.

3. Palpate scapular bony landmarks on a subject and maintain your palpation as your subject abducts the shoulder. Analyze the scapular movements. Repeat the same as your subject flexes the shoulder. Note particularly the synchronous scapular rotation and elevation of the humerus (i.e., shoulder abduction and shoulder flexion). Analyze scapular movements as your subject elevates, depresses, protracts, and retracts the shoulder girdle.

4. On the skeleton, determine attachments for the muscles connecting:
   a. shoulder girdle with trunk.
   b. scapula and humerus.
   c. trunk and humerus.
   Note particularly the:
   a. lines of action.
   b. muscles with extensive proximal attachments and, hence, the multiple actions.
   c. movements these muscles can perform.

5. Determine muscles that will:
   a. flex the shoulder.
   b. extend the shoulder.
   c. abduct the shoulder.
   d. adduct the shoulder.
   e. internally and externally rotate the shoulder.
   f. elevate the shoulder girdle.
   g. depress the shoulder girdle.
   h. protract the shoulder girdle.
   i. retract the shoulder girdle.
   j. upwardly rotate the scapula.
   k. downwardly rotate the scapula.

6. Select a partner. Following the descriptions in Chapter 7, palpate muscles of the shoulder region:

Shoulder girdle to trunk	Scapula to humerus	Trunk to humerus
serratus anterior	deltoid	pectoralis major
trapezius	supraspinatus	latissimus dorsi
rhomboids	infraspinatus	
pectoralis minor	teres minor	
levator scapulae	subscapularis	
	teres major	
	biceps	
	triceps	
	coracobrachialis	

7. Analyze synergic muscle action for the following:
   a. Upward rotation of the scapula and humeral elevation (i.e., shoulder flexion or shoulder abduction).
   b. Shoulder girdle depression when body weight is supported on the upper limb.
   c. Other activities relevant to your professional functions, such as any shoulder region activity needed to position the upper limb for use of the hand.

UNIT 5—HIP AND PELVIC REGION

1. On the skeleton, identify these bony landmarks. Which are palpable? Locate them on yourself and on a subject:

Femur	Pelvis
head	iliac crest
greater trochanter	anterior superior iliac spine
lesser trochanter	anterior inferior iliac spine
neck	posterior inferior iliac spine
intertrochanteric crest (anterior)	posterior superior iliac spine
intertrochanteric line (posterior)	posterior gluteal line
trochanteric fossa	anterior gluteal line
gluteal tuberosity	inferior gluteal line
linea aspera	acetabulum
	sciatic notch (greater, lesser)
	tuberosity of ischium
	ramus of ischium
	ramus of pubis
	obturator foramen
	iliac fossa

2. Review, describe, perform, and observe all hip movements and their conventionally chosen axes. Describe the angulation of the femoral neck with the femoral
   shaft in the frontal and horizontal planes. Differentiate the anatomic and mechanical hip axes.
3. Locate the skeletal attachments of all muscles that cross the hip joint. Note particularly the action lines and the muscles with extensive origin. Determine muscles
   that will flex, extend, abduct, adduct, and internally and externally rotate the hip.
   Note how changes in hip position will alter hip muscle action lines. How will this
   change influence the movements the muscles may perform (e.g., adductors act as
   hip flexors or extensors)? Analyze iliopsoas action with special attention to its
   influence on the spine.
4. On a subject, measure with a goniometer and record the following hip and knee
   ranges of motion:
   a. Hip flexion with knee extended—your subject back-lying.
   b. Hip flexion allowing knee to flex—your subject back-lying.
   c. Knee flexion with hip extended—your subject prone.
   d. Knee flexion allowing hip to flex—your subject back-lying.
   Compare the measurements. Give reasons for similarities and differences you observe. What are some clinical implications? Compare similar range of motion measurements for ankle dorsiflexion with the knee extended and with the knee flexed.
5. On a subject, palpate the hip musculature as described in Chapter 8:

iliopsoas	tensor fasciae latae
gluteus maximus	rectus femoris
gluteus medius	adductors (as a group)
hamstrings (as a group)	six external rotators
sartorius	

6. Analyze hip muscle action in the weight-bearing position:
   a. Stand with weight on both feet, and incline your trunk forward and then back-
      ward. In each position, forward and back, explain the relationship of the weight
      line of the suprafemoral body mass to the hip axes. What muscle activity must
      counteract the effect of the gravitational force?
   b. Stand on one foot. Explain the effect on one-legged balance of the weight of the
      head, arms, trunk, and the unsupported limb. What muscle activity counteracts
      this effect? In this force system, identify the fulcrum, the weight and its lever
      arm, and the force and its lever arm.
   c. Assume you have a positive Trendelenburg sign. Shift the body weight to one
      side and lift the opposite foot off the ground. Allow the pelvis to sag on the side
      opposite the stance limb; then reverse the pelvic movement so the pelvis again
      becomes level. Repeat and describe hip movements and hip muscle actions that
      occur.

UNIT 6—KNEE REGION

1. On the skeleton, identify the following bones and bony landmarks and determine those that are palpable.

Femur

medial and lateral condyles
epicondyles
adductor tubercle
linea aspera
medial and lateral
   supracondylar lines
intercondylar notch
popliteal surface
patellar surface
distal articular surfaces

Tibia

medial and lateral condyles
tibial plateau
intercondylar eminence
tibial tuberosity
anterior border
interosseous border
proximal articular surfaces

Fibula

head, neck, shaft

Patella

anterior and posterior surfaces

2. While seated with the knee bent, palpate on yourself and then on a classmate the patella, anterior border of tibia, head of the fibula, tibial tuberosity, medial and lateral epicondyles of femur, and lateral condyle of tibia. Locate medially and laterally the joint space between the tibia and femur. With the knee extended, grasp your patella and move it passively from side to side and in an up and down movement from proximal to distal. Keep the quadriceps muscle completely relaxed to accomplish this maneuver. Repeat this same procedure on a subject.
3. Analyze knee movements on yourself and on a partner. Determine the extent of transverse rotation that can occur with knee flexed and with the knee extended. Analyze patellar excursion that accompanies knee motion. Palpate bony landmarks that will identify location of the approximate axis for knee flexion and extension.
4. On the skeleton, locate points of attachment of all muscles that cross the knee joint, noting particularly their action lines and their relationships to other joints of the lower limb.
5. Determine muscles that will:
   a. flex the knee.
   b. extend the knee.
   c. externally rotate tibia on femur when knee is flexed.
   d. internally rotate tibia on femur when knee is flexed.
   e. have influence on movements of joints other than knee joint. (Which joints? Which movements?)

6. Select a partner. Following the descriptions in Chapter 9, palpate knee muscles and tendons:

quadriceps femoris
biceps femoris
semimembranosus
semitendinosus
adductor gracilis
proximal attachments of gastrocnemius
distal attachments of sartorius and tensor fasciae latae

7. Observe the alignment of upper and lower segments of the legs of several standing subjects and evaluate the knee positions from an anterior and a lateral view. What is genu recurvatum? Genu valgum? Genu varum? Tibial torsion? Do any subjects show evidence of these misalignments?

8. Analyze (observe and palpate) on yourself and on a subject the knee movements and synergic muscle actions of knee joint musculature in a weight-bearing position:
   a. Stand, knees straight, and slowly shift body weight forward and back, then side to side.
   b. Stand, knees bent, and slowly shift body weight as above.
   Explain the relationship of the weight line of the supratibial body mass to the knee axis as you analyze these activities. What muscles counteract the gravitational forces as balance shifts?

UNIT 7—ANKLE AND FOOT

1. On the skeleton, identify the following bones and bony landmarks. Locate on yourself and on a subject those that are palpable:

tibia	cuboid
fibula	three cuneiform bones
medial and lateral malleoli	metatarsal bones
tuberosity of navicular	(heads, bases, shafts)
talus	phalanges
calcaneus	sustentaculum tali
	tuberosity of fifth metatarsal

2. Examine and identify the joint surfaces where ankle and foot movements occur. What are the movements? At which joints? Analyze these movements on yourself and on a subject in a non-weight-bearing position (tibia is stable; foot moves) and in a weight-bearing position (foot is stable on the floor; tibia moves).

3. Measure the amount of external rotation of the axis for ankle dorsiflexion and plantar flexion with respect to the axis of knee flexion and extension in the following way:
   a. Stand with weight evenly distributed on both feet, knee caps pointing straight forward (knee axes lie in frontal plane).
   b. Trace around one foot on a piece of paper, keeping back edge of paper parallel with knee axis.
   c. Mark vertical projections of the malleoli on the paper. Connect the two projections. This line represents the upper ankle (talocrural) axis.
   d. With a protractor, measure degrees of deviation of this upper ankle axis from the frontal plane. Record deviation from 0 degrees toward 180 degrees (i.e., 0 degrees to ____ degrees).

   Compare with measurements on the other leg. Compare measurements of several subjects. Compare with discussion on pages 314 to 315.

4. On the same traced outline of your foot, draw another line representing the lower ankle joint (subtalar) axis (see Fig. 10-1). Identify and palpate on yourself and on a subject the bony landmarks to locate these axes.

5. On the skeleton, locate the attachments of all muscles that cross the two ankle axes. Sketch their relationships to the axes on the tracing you have drawn. Identify muscles that dorsiflex, plantar-flex, invert, and evert the ankle.

6. Study intrinsic foot muscles in an anatomy text and compare these with the intrinsic hand muscles. Palpate extensor digitorum brevis in your own foot and on a subject.

7. On yourself and on a subject, palpate ankle muscles and tendons (follow descriptions for palpation in Chapter 10):

gastrocnemius	peroneus longus
soleus	peroneus brevis
tibialis posterior	anterior tibialis
flexor digitorum longus	extensor hallucis longus
flexor hallucis longus	extensor digitorum longus

8. Analyze (i.e., observe, palpate) the synergic ankle muscle action in a weight-bearing position:
   a. Stand, weight evenly distributed on both feet. Shift body weight backward, almost to the point of losing balance.
   b. Shift body weight forward.
   c. Stand and balance on one foot. Observe co-contraction of many ankle muscles and interplay of muscle contractions as balance is maintained.
   d. Walk forward slowly. Which muscles contract strongly at the point of heel contact? At the point of "push off" to propel the body forward?

   Explain the relationship of the weight-line of the suprapedal body mass to the ankle axes as you analyze these activities. What muscles counteract the gravitational forces as balance shifts?

UNIT 8—HEAD, NECK, AND TRUNK

1. On the skeleton, identify the following bones and bony landmarks, and on a subject identify those that are palpable:

Skull	*Vertebrae*	*Ribs*
temporal bone	atlas	head
mastoid process	axis	articulating facets
occipital bone	cervical	tubercle
foramen magnum	thoracic	shaft
occipital condyles	lumbar	
superior nuchal line	sacral	
mandible	transverse processes	
	spinous processes	

   Review and palpate landmarks of the pelvis and shoulder region. Identify landmarks that will determine the approximate height of the following vertebrae:

   first cervical
   body of the fourth thoracic
   body of the tenth thoracic
   spinous process of fourth lumbar
   second sacral

   Judge the symmetry or asymmetry of a subject's standing posture by identifying the following landmarks:
   a. height of anterior superior iliac spines.
   b. height of the crests of the ilium.
   c. vertical alignment of spinous processes.
   d. level of the inferior angle of the scapula.
   e. distances from thoracic spinous processes to vertebral border of scapula.
2. From your analysis on the skeleton of the direction of the intervertebral articulations, describe, perform, and observe on a subject the movements that predominate in the various regions of the spinal column.
3. Determine points of attachment for muscle groups of trunk and neck: flexors, extensors, and rotators. Differentiate the deep and superficial layers. Identify muscles that cross the hip and the shoulder and the shoulder girdle which may influence trunk movements. On a subject, palpate the neck and trunk musculature as described in Chapter 11.
4. Perform the following activities and movements. Analyze the muscle activity, and answer the questions.
   a. When the head is lifted up from a back-lying position, why do abdominal muscles contract? Describe movements and muscle actions required for performing a complete situp from a back-lying position.

   b. Sit on the edge of a table with legs hanging down. Shift your body weight from side to side and then forward and back as far as you can and still maintain your sitting balance. What muscle groups control the movements? What kinds of muscle contractions (i.e., shortening, lengthening, isometric) occur throughout various phases of the activity? Have someone manually resist your shifting movements and describe the muscle actions.

   c. What happens to the spine when the pelvis is tilted forward? Backward? Which muscles tilt the pelvis forward? Backward? Analyze these pelvis tilt activities in a back-lying position and in an erect standing position.

   d. Which muscles (anteriorly and posteriorly) will rotate the trunk to the right? To the left?

   e. Lie on your back and lift right leg, then left leg alternately. Now lift both legs simultaneously. Analyze muscle activity. What are some clinical implications of this activity?

UNIT 9—BALANCE AND GAIT

1. Describe the gait cycle by differentiating swing and stance phases and each sub-phase (see Chapter 12).
2. Analyze the relationship of the vertical projection of the center of gravity to the hip, knee, and ankle axes during early, mid, and late stance phase of gait.
3. Predict and simulate gait deviations that could occur as a result of the following problems.

   a. Isolated paralysis of:
      right hip extensors
      right hip abductors
      left knee extensors
      right ankle dorsiflexors

   b. Bilateral paralysis of ankle plantar flexors.

   c. Ankylosis of right knee in a completely extended position.

   d. Bilateral hip flexion contractures of approximately 35 degrees.

   e. Bilateral positive Trendelenburg sign because of bilateral congenital hip dislocations.

   f. Short leg (walk with one shoe on and one shoe off).

Explain your reasons for the deviations you simulated, with particular reference to the weight line of body masses and its relationship to the joint axes.

UNIT 10—ACTIVITY AND ANALYSIS

In preparation for observing and analyzing individuals with kinesiologic pathology, you should practice analyzing movements and muscle actions of a number of every-day activities performed by persons who have no pathology. Such analysis can be extremely complex and can encompass a multitude of social, psychologic, and physical elements. For this laboratory experience, however, focus your attention on the following basic physical components of movement emphasized in this book. You and a subject select an activity, decide how it will be performed, and then analyze it. Break down the activity so you can identify the parts. Analyze the relationships of the parts and consider the kinesiologic principles involved. In your analysis describe the:

1. Joint movements involved.
2. Muscles performing those movements—particularly those muscles that can be observed contracting or that can be palpated.
3. Synergic muscle action.
4. Kind of muscle contractions required (i.e., shortening, lengthening, isometric) throughout phases of the activity.
5. Changing effect of gravity on all body segments—especially the changing relationship of the center of gravity line to the lower limb joint axes.

Your analysis might emphasize primarily an upper limb activity, a lower limb activity, or a total body activity. Determine the selection of an activity yourself or start with these suggestions:

1. Grasp the doorknob of a heavy door. Pull the door open, walk through, and close the door behind you (analyze upper limb activity).
2. Rise to an erect standing position from a seated position in a chair and return to the seated position (analyze lower limb and trunk activity).
3. Step up and then step down one step in a flight of stairs (analyze lower limb activity).
4. Stand. Reach up to a high shelf for a book. Remove the book and place it on a table (analyze upper limb activity).
5. Sit in a wheelchair with hands on the arm rests. Perform a sitting push-up (analyze upper limb activity).
6. Crutch-walking non-weight-bearing right lower extremity (analyze upper limb activity).

REFERENCES

ABBOTT, BC, BIGLAND, B, AND RITCHIE, JM: *The physiological cost of negative work.* J Physiol (Lond) 117:380, 1952.

ADRIAN, ED AND BRONK, DW: *The discharge of impulses in motor nerve fibers, Part II.* J Physiol (Lond) 67:119, 1929.

AKERBLOM, B: *Standing and Sitting Posture.* Nordiska Bokhandeln, Stockholm, 1948.

ALTENBURGER, H: *Beitrage zur Physiologie and Pathologie des Ganges.* Z Neurol u Psychiat 148:263, 1933.

AMERICAN ACADEMY OF ORTHOPAEDIC SURGEONS: *Joint Motion—Method of Measuring and Recording.* American Academy of Orthopaedic Surgeons, Chicago, 1965.

ANDRIACCHI, TP, OGLE, JA, AND GALANTE, JO: *Walking speed as a basis for normal and abnormal gait measurements.* J Biomech 10:261, 1977.

ATKINSON, WB AND ELFTMAN, H: *The carrying angle of the human arm as a secondary sex character.* Anat Rec 91:49, 1945.

ATZLER, E AND HERBST, R: *Die Geharbeit auf horizontaler Bahn.* Pfluegers Arch 215:291, 1927.

BACKHOUSE, KM AND CATTON, WT: *An experimental study of the function of the lumbrical muscles in the human hand.* J Anat 88:133, 1954.

BACKLUND, L AND NORDGREN, L: *A new method for testing isometric muscle strength under standardized conditions.* Scand J Clin Lab Invest 21:33, 1968.

BARD, G: *Energy expenditure of hemiplegic subjects during walking.* Arch Phys Med Rehabil 44:368, 1963.

BARD, G AND RALSTON, HJ: *Measurement of energy expenditure during ambulation, with special reference to evaluation of assistive devices.* Arch Phys Med Rehabil 40:415, 1959.

BARNETT, CH AND RICHARDSON, AT: *The postural function of the popliteus muscle.* Annals of Physical Medicine 1:177, 1953.

BASLER, A: *Das Gehen und seine Veranderungen durch verschiedene Unstande auf Grund experimenteller Untersuchungen.* Abh D Med Fakultat der Sun Yatsen University, Canton, China, 1929.

BASLER, A: *Beitrage zur Physiologie des Stehens.* Arbeitsphysiol 12:105, 1942.

BASMAJIAN, JV: *Electromyography.* University of Toronto Medical Journal 30:10, 1952.

BASMAJIAN, JV: *New views on muscle tone and relaxation.* Can Med Assoc J 77:203, 1957.

BASMAJIAN, JV: *Muscles Alive: Their Functions Revealed by Electromyography,* ed 4. Williams & Wilkins, Baltimore, 1978.

BASMAJIAN, JV: *Biofeedback: Principles and Practice for Clinicians.* Williams & Wilkins, Baltimore, 1979.

BASMAJIAN, JV AND LATIF, A: *Integrated actions and functions of the chief flexors of the elbow: A detailed electromyographic analysis.* J Bone Joint Surg (Am) 39:1106, 1957.

BASMAJIAN, JV, ET AL: *Computers in Medicine Series: Computers in Electromyography.* Butterworths, Boston, 1975.

BEALS, RK: *The normal carrying angle of the elbow: A radiographic study of 442 patients.* Clin Orthop 119:194, 1976.

BEARN, JG: *An electromyographic study of the trapezius, deltoid, pectoralis major, biceps and triceps muscles, during static loading of the upper limb.* Anat Rec 140:103, 1961.

BEASLEY, WC: *Quantitative muscle testing: Principles and applications to research and clinical services.* Arch Phys Med Rehabil 42:398, 1961.

BEASLEY, WC: *Ontogenetics and Biomechanics of Ankle Plantar Flexion Force.* American Congress of Physical Medicine and Rehabilitation, Philadelphia, 1958.

BECK, O: *Die gesamte Kraftkurve des tetanisierten Froschgastrocnemius und ihr physiologisch ausgenutzter Anteil.* Pfluegers Arch Ges Physiol 193:495, 1921-22.

BEEVOR, C: *Croonian Lectures on Muscular Movement. Delivered in 1903. Edited and reprinted for the Guarantors of "Brain."* Macmillan, New York, 1951.

BELNAP, B: *Maximum Isometric Torque of the Plantar Flexors.* Unpublished Thesis, Texas Woman's University, Denton, Texas, 1978.

BELSON, P, SMITH, LK, AND PUENTES, J: *Motor innervation of the flexor pollicis brevis.* Am J Phys Med 55:122, 1976.

BENEDICT, FG AND MURSCHHAUSER, H: *Energy Transformations During Horizontal Walking.* Carnegie Institution of Washington, Publication 231, Washington, DC, 1915.

BENNETT, RL AND KNOWLTON, GC: *Overwork weakness in partially denervated skeletal muscle.* Clin Orthop 12:22, 1958.

BERNARD, BA: *Maximum Isometric Torque of the Plantar Flexors in the Sitting Position.* Unpublished Thesis, Texas Woman's University, Denton, Texas, 1979.

BETHE, A: *Beitrage zum Problem der willkurlich beweglichen Armprothesen: I. Die Kraftkurve menschlicher Muskeln und die reziproke Innervation der Antagonisten.* Munch Med Wochenschr 65:1577, 1916.

BETHE, A AND FRANKE, R: *Beitrage zum Problem der willkurlich beweglichen Armprothesen: IV. Die Kraftkurven der indirekten naturlichen Energiequellen.* Munch Med Wochenschr 66:201, 1919.

BINDER, MD AND STUART, DC: *Motor unit–muscle receptors interactions: Design features of the neuromuscular control system.* In DESMEDT, JE (ED): *Progress in Clinical Neurophysiology,* Vol 8. S Karger, Basel, 1980, p 72.

BLIX, M: *Die Lange und die Spannung des Muskels.* Skand Arch f Physiol 3:295, 1891; 4:399, 1892-3; 5:150, 175, 1895.

BLOOM, W AND FAWCETT, DW: *A Textbook of Histology,* ed 8. WB Saunders, Philadelphia, 1969.

BLOOM, W AND FAWCETT, DW: *A Textbook of Histology,* ed. 10. WB Saunders, Philadelphia, 1975.

BORELLI, GA: *De Motu Animalium.* Lugduni Batavorum, 1679.

BOYES, JH: *Bunnell's Surgery of the Hand*, ed 5. JB Lippincott, Philadelphia, 1970.

BRAUNE, W AND FISCHER, O: *Ueber den Schwerpunkt des menschlichen Korpers mit Rucksicht auf die Ausrustung des deutschen Infanteristen.* Abh d Kgl Sachs, Ges d Wissensch, Math Phys Klasse 26:562, 1889.

BRAUNE, W AND FISCHER, O: *Die Rotationsmomente der Beugemuskeln am Ellbogengelenk des Menschen.* Abh d Kgl Sachs, Ges d Wissensch, Math Phys Klasse, Vol 15, 1890.

BRAUNE, W AND FISCHER, O: *Untersuchungen uber die Gelenke des menschlichen Armes.* Abh Sachs Akad Wiss, 1887. Quoted by VON LANZ, T AND WACHSMUTH, W: *Praktische Anatomic,* Bd. I, Teil III. Julius Springer, Berlin, 1935, p 94.

BRODAL, A: *Neurological Anatomy*, ed 3. Oxford University Press, New York, 1981, p 56.

BROOKS, DM AND SEDDON, HJ: *Pectoral transplantation for paralysis of flexors of the elbow: A new technique.* J Bone Joint Surg (Br) 41:36, 1959.

BROWSE, NL: *The Physiology and Pathology of Bed Rest.* Charles C Thomas, Springfield, Ill, 1965.

BRUNNSTROM, S: *Muscle testing around the shoulder girdle.* J Bone Joint Surg (Am) 23:263, 1941.

BRUNNSTROM, S: *Some observations of muscle function: With special reference to pluri-articular muscles.* Physical Therapy Review 22:67, 1942.

BRUNNSTROM, S: *Comparative strength of muscles with similar function: Study on peripheral nerve injuries of upper extremity.* Physical Therapy Review 26:59, 1946.

BRUNNSTROM, S: *Center of gravity line in relation to ankle joint in erect standing: Application to posture training and to artificial legs.* Physical Therapy Review 34:109, 1954.

BRUNNSTROM, S: *Anatomical and physiological considerations in the clinical application of lower-extremity prosthesis.* In *Orthopedic Appliances Atlas, Vol. 2, Artificial Limbs.* JW Edwards, Ann Arbor, Mich, 1960.

BRUNNSTROM, S: *Movement Therapy in Hemiplegia: A Neurophysiological Approach.* Harper & Row, New York, 1970.

BUCHTHAL, F AND SCHMALBRUCH, H: *Motor unit of mamalian muscle.* Physiol Rev 60:90, 1980.

BUNNELL, S: *Opposition of the thumb.* J Bone Joint Surg (Am) 20:269, 1938.

BUNNELL, S: *Surgery of the intrinsic muscles of the hand other than those producing opposition of the thumb.* J Bone Joint Surg (Am) 24:1, 1942.

BUNNELL, S: *Restoring function to the paralytic elbow.* J Bone Joint Surg (Am) 33:566, 1951.

BUNNELL, S: *Surgery of the Hand*, ed 3. JB Lippincott, Philadelphia, 1956.

BURKE, RE AND EDGERTON, VR: *Motor unit properties and selective involvement in movement.* Exerc Sport Sci Rev 3:31-81, 1975.

BURKE, RE: *Motor units: Anatomy, physiology and functional organization.* In BROOKS, VB (ED): *Motor Systems (Handbook of Physiology, Section I, The Nervous System).* Williams & Wilkins, Baltimore, 1981.

CAILLIET, R: *Shoulder Pain.* FA Davis, Philadelphia, 1966.

CAILLIET, R: *Low Back Pain Syndrome*, ed 3. FA Davis, Philadelphia, 1981.

CAILLIET, R: *Foot and Ankle Pain*, ed 2. FA Davis, Philadelphia, 1983.

CAMPBELL, EJM: *An electromyographic study of the role of the abdominal muscles in breathing.* J Physiol 117:222, 1952.

CLARK, DA: *Muscle counts of motor units: A study in innervation ratios.* Am J Physiol 96:296, 1931.

CLAUSER, CE, MCCONVILLE, JT, AND YOUNG, JW: *Weight, Volume and Center of Mass of Segments of the Human Body.* AMRL-TR 69-70, Wright-Patterson Air Force Base, Ohio, 1969.

CLEMMESEN, S: *Some studies of muscle tone.* Proc R Soc Med 44:637, 1951.

CLOSE, JR: *Motor Function in the Lower Extremity: Analyses by Electronic Instrumentation.* Charles C Thomas, Springfield, Ill, 1964.

CLOSE, JR AND KIDD, C: *The functions of the muscles of the thumb, the index, and long fingers: Synchronous recording of motions and action potentials of muscles.* J Bone Joint Surg (Am) 51:1601, 1969.

CORCORAN, PJ: *Energy expenditure during ambulation.* In DOWNEY, JA AND DARLING, RC: *Physiological Basis of Rehabilitation Medicine.* WB Saunders, Philadelphia, 1971.

CORCORAN, PJ AND BRENGELMANN, GL: *Oxygen uptake in normal and handicapped subjects in relation to speed of walking beside velocity-controlled cart.* Arch Phys Med Rehabil 51:78, 1970.

CORCORAN, PJ, ET AL: *Effects of plastic and metal leg braces on speed and energy cost of hemiparetic ambulation.* Arch Phys Med Rehabil 51:69, 1970.

CRAIG, AS: *Elements of kinesiology for the clinician.* Journal of American Physical Therapy Association 44:470, 1964.

CURETON, TK: *Fitness of the feet and legs.* Res Q Am Assoc Health Phys Educ 12:368, 1941.

DANIELS, L AND WORTHINGHAM, C: *Muscle Testing: Techniques of Manual Examination,* ed 4. WB Saunders, Philadelphia, 1972.

DAVIES, GJ, WALLACE, LA, AND MALONE, T: *Mechanisms of selected knee injuries.* Phys Ther 60:1590, 1980.

DE BRUIJN, PF: *Triceps tendon transfer for paralysis of the elbow flexors.* Archives of Orthopaedic and Traumatic Surgery 96:153, 1980.

DE LACERDA, FG: *A study of anatomical factors involved in shin splints.* Journal of Orthopaedic and Sports Physical Therapy 2:55, 1980.

DEMPSTER, WT: *Space requirements of the seated operator.* WADC Technical Report 55-159, July 1955. Office of Technical Services, US Dept of Commerce, Washington, DC, 1955.

DENNY-BROWN, DE: *Histological features of striped muscle in relation to its functional activity.* Proc R Soc Med 104B:371, 1929.

DEPARTMENTS OF THE ARMY AND THE AIR FORCE: *Joint Motion Measurement.* TM 8-640/AFP 160-14, Washington, DC, 1968.

DEVINE, KL, LE VEAU, BF, AND YACK, HJ: *Electromyographic activity recorded from an unexercised muscle during maximal isometric exercise of the contralateral agonists and antagonists.* Phys Ther 61:898, 1981.

DOODY, SG, FREEDMAN, L, AND WATERLAND, JC: *Shoulder movements during abduction in the scapular plane.* Arch Phys Med Rehabil 51:595, 1970.

DOSS, WS AND KARPOVICH, PV: *A comparison of concentric, eccentric and isometric strength of elbow flexors.* J Appl Physiol 20:351, 1965.

DRILLIS, R: *Objective recording and biomechanics of pathological gait.* Ann NY Acad Sci 74:86, 1958.

DRILLIS, R, CONTINI, R, AND BLUESTEIN, M: *Body segment parameters: A survey of measurement techniques.* Artificial Limbs 8:44, 1964.

DUCHENNE, GB: *Physiologie des Mouvements.* JB Bailliere et Fils, Paris, 1867. Translated to English by EB Kaplan. JB Lippincott, Philadelphia, 1949.

EBERHART, HD AND INMAN, VI: *An evaluation of experimental procedures used in a fundamental study of human locomotion.* Ann NY Acad Sci 51:1213, 1951.

EBERHART, HD, ET AL: *Fundamental Studies of Human Locomotion and Other Information Relating to Design of Artificial Limbs: Report to National Research Council, Committee on Artificial Limbs.* University of California, Berkeley, 1947.

EDGERTON, VR, SMITH, JL, AND SIMPSON, DR: *Muscle fibre type populations of human leg muscles.* Histochem J 7:259, 1975.

EDWARDS, RHT: *Human muscle function and fatigue.* In *CIBA Foundation Symposium #82 Human Muscle Fatigue: Physiological Mechanisms.* Pittman Medical, London, 1981, p 1.

EINTHOVEN, W: *Un nouveau galvanometre.* Archives Neerlandaises des Sciences Exactes et Naturelles, Ser II. 6:625, 1901.

ELFTMAN, H: *Measurement of external force in walking.* Science 88:152, 1938.

ELFTMAN, H: *The force exerted by the ground in walking.* Arbeitsphysiol 10:485, 1939a.

ELFTMAN, H: *The function of the arms in walking.* Hum Biol 11:528, 1939b.

ELFTMAN, H: *Knee action and locomotion.* Bull Hosp Joint Dis 16:103, 1955.

ELFTMAN, H: *The transverse tarsal joint and its control.* Clin Orthop 16:41, 1960.

ELFTMAN, H: *Biomechanics of muscle with particular application to studies of gait.* J Bone Joint Surg (Am) 48:363, 1966.

EYLER, DL AND MARKEE, JE: *Anatomy and function of the intrinsic musculature of the fingers.* J Bone Joint Surg (Am) 36:1, 1954.

FEINSTEIN, B, ET AL: *Morphologic studies of motor units in normal human muscles.* Acta Anat (Basel) 23:127, 1955.

FICAT, RP AND HUNGERFORD, DS: *Disorders of the Patello-Femoral Joint.* Williams & Wilkins, Baltimore, 1977.

FICK, AE, JR AND WEBER, E: *Studien uber die schultermuskeln,* Wurzb, Verh 1872, 2. Abt, quoted by R Fick in *Anatomie und Mechanik der Gelenke: Teil II,* p 320.

FICK, R: *Anatomie and Mechanik der Gelenke: Teil II, Allgemeine Gelenk und Muskel Mechanik.* Fischer, Jena, 1910.

FICK, R: *Anatomie und Mechanik der Gelenke: Teil III, Spezielle Gelenk und Muskel Mechanik.* Fisher, Jena, 1911.

FIORENTINO, MF: *Reflex Testing Methods for Evaluating CNS Development,* ed 2. Charles C Thomas, Springfield, Ill, 1973.

FISHER, O: *Der Gang des Mesnschen.* Abh Kgl Sachs Ges d Wiss, Math Phys Klasse, Part I, Bd 21, 1895 (with W Braune). Part II, Bd 25, 1899. Part III, Bd 26, 1900. Part IV, Bd 26, 1900. Part V, Bd 28, 1904, Part VI, Bd 28, 1904.

FISHER, O: *Kinematik organischer Gelenke.* R Vierweg, Braunschweig, 1907.

FLORENCE, JM, BROOKE, MH, AND CARROLL, JE: *Evaluation of the child with muscular weakness.* Orthop Clin North Am 9:409, 1978.

FLOYD, WF AND SILVER, PHS: *Electromyographic study of patterns of activity of the anterior wall muscles in man.* J Anat 84:132, 1950.

FLOYD, WF AND WELFORD, AT (EDS): *Symposium on Fatigue.* The Ergonomics Research Society. Lewis, London, 1953.

FRANCILLION, MR: *Zur Funktion diploneurer Muskeln im Gehakt des Menschen.* Schweiz Med Wochenschr 71:419, 1941a.

FRANCILLION, MR: *Die Knieflexoren in kinetischer und phylogentischer Betrachtung.* Z Orthop 72: 122, 1941b.

FRANKE, F: *Die Kraftkurve menschlicher Muskeln bei willkurlicher Innervation und die Frage der Absoluten Muskelkraft.* Arch f d g Physiol 184:300, 1920.

FRANKEL, VH AND BURSTEIN, AH: *Orthopaedic Biomechanics.* Lea & Febiger, Philadelphia, 1970.

FRANKEL, VH, BURSTEIN, AH, AND BROOKS, DB: *Biomechanics of internal derangement of the knee: Pathomechanics as determined by analysis of the instant centers of motion.* J Bone Joint Surg (Am) 53:945, 1971.

FRANKEL, VH AND NORDIN, M: *Basic Biomechanics of the Skeletal System.* Lea & Febiger, Philadelphia, 1980.

FREEDMAN, L AND MUNRO, R: *Abduction of the arm in the scapular plane: A roentgenographic study. Scapular and glenohumeral movements.* J Bone Joint Surg (Am) 48:1503, 1966.

GARDNER, HF AND CLIPPINGER, FW: *A method for location of prosthetic and orthotic knee joints.* Artificial Limbs 13:31, 1969.

GERHARDT, JJ AND RUSSE, OA: *International SFTR Method of Measuring and Recording Joint Motion.* Distributed by Year Book Medical Publishers, Inc. Hans Huber, Bern, Switzerland, 1975.

GOLLNICK, PD, ET AL: *Enzyme activity and fiber composition in skeletal muscle of untrained and trained men.* J Appl Physiol 33:312, 1972.

GORDON, EE AND VANDERWALDE, H: *Energy requirements in paraplegic ambulation.* Arch Phys Med Rehabil 37:276, 1956.

GOSS, C (ED): *Gray's Anatomy of the Human Body,* 29th Am ed. Lea & Febiger, Philadelphia, 1973.

GRAFSTEIN, B AND FORMAN, DS: *Intracellular transport in neurons.* Physiol Rev 60:1167, 1980.

GRANT JC: *An Atlas of Anatomy,* ed 7. Williams & Wilkins, Baltimore, 1978.

GRAY, ER AND BASMAJIAN, JV: *Electromyography and cinematography of leg and foot ("normal" and flat) during walking.* Anat Rec 161:1, 1968.

GRAY, ER: *The role of leg muscles in variations of the arches in normal and flat feet.* Phys Ther 44:1084, 1969.

GRAY, H: *Anatomy of the Human Body,* ed 24. Lea & Febiger, Philadelphia, 1936.

GUTH, L: *"Trophic" influences of nerve on muscles.* Physiol Rev 48:645, 1968.

GUTMANN, E: *Neurotrophic relations.* Annu Rev Physiol 38:177, 1976.

GUTMANN, E AND HNIK, P (EDS): *The Effect of Use and Disuse on Neuromuscular Functions.* Elsevier, New York, 1963.

HAFFAJEE, D, MORITZ, U, AND SVANTESSON, G: *Isometric knee extension strength as a function of joint angle, muscle length and motor unit activity.* Acta Orthop Scand 43:138, 1972.

HAINES, RW: *On muscles of full and of short action.* J Anat 69:20, 1934.

HANAVAN, EP: *A Mathematical Model of the Human Body.* AMRL-TR-64-102, Aerospace Medical Research Laboratory, Wright-Patterson Air Force Base, Ohio, October 1964.

HANSON, J AND HUXLEY, HE: *Structural basis of the cross-striations in muscle.* Nature 172:530, 1953.

HAXTON, HA: *Absolute muscle force in the ankle flexors of man.* J Physiol 103:267, 1944.

HELFET, AJ: *Disorders of the Knee.* JB Lippincott, Philadelphia, 1974.

HELLEBRANDT, FA: *Standing as a geotropic reflex: Mechanism of asynchronous rotation of motor units.* Am J Physiol 121:471, 1938.

HELLEBRANDT, FA AND FRIES, EC: *Constancy of the oscillographic stance patterns.* Physical Therapy Review 22:17, 1942.

HELLEBRANDT, FA, ET AL: *Location of the cardinal anatomical orientation planes passing through the center of weight in young adult women.* Am J Physiol 121:465, 1938.

HENNEMAN, E: *Recruitment of motoneurones: The size principle.* In Desmedt, JE (ED): *Progress in Clinical Neurophysiology,* Vol 9. Karger, Basel, 1981, p 26.

HERMAN, R AND BRAGIN, SJ: *Function of the gastrocnemius and soleus: A preliminary study in the normal human subject.* Phys Ther 47:105, 1967.

HICKOK, RJ: *Physical therapy as related to peripheral nerve lesions.* Phys Ther Rev 41:113, 1961.

HICKS, JH: *The mechanics of the foot: I. The joints.* J Anat 87:345, 1953.

HICKS, JH: *The mechanics of the foot: II. The plantar aponeurosis and the arch.* J Anat 88:25, 1954.

HISLOP, HJ: *Response of immobilized muscle to isometric exercise.* Journal of American Physical Therapy Association 44:339, 1964.

HISLOP, HJ AND PERRINE, JJ: *The isokinetic concept of exercise.* Phys Ther 47:114, 1967.

HOGUE, RE: *Upper extremity muscular activity at different cadences and inclines during normal gait.* Phys Ther 49:963, 1969.

HOPPENFELD, S: *Physical Examination of the Spine and Extremities.* Appleton-Century-Crofts, New York, 1976.

HOUK, JC, CRAGO, PE, AND ANDRYMER, WZ: *Functional properties of the Golgi tendon organs.* In DESMEDT, JE (ED): *Progress in Clinical Neurophysiology,* Vol 8. Karger, Basel, 1980, p 33.

HSIEH, H AND WALKER, PS: *Stabilizing mechanisms of the loaded and unloaded knee joint.* J Bone Joint Surg (Am) 58:87, 1976.

HUXLEY, HE: *The mechanism of muscular contraction.* Science 164:1356, 1969.

INMAN, VT: *Functional aspects of the abductor muscles of the hip.* J Bone Joint Surg (Am) 29:2, 1947.

INMAN, VT: *The influence of the foot-ankle complex on the proximal skeletal structures.* Artificial Limbs 13:59, 1969.

INMAN, VT: *The Joints of the Ankle.* Williams & Wilkins, Baltimore, 1976.

INMAN, VT AND RALSTON, HJ: *The mechanics of voluntary muscle: Chapter 11.* In KLOPSTEG, PE AND WILSON, PD: *Human Limbs and Their Substitutes.* Hafner Publishing, New York, reprinted 1968.

INMAN, VT, SAUNDERS, JB DE CM, AND ABBOTT, LC: *Observations on function of the shoulder joint.* J Bone Joint Surg (Am) 26:1, 1944.

INMAN, VT, RALSTON, HJ, AND TODD, F: *Human Walking.* Williams & Wilkins, Baltimore, 1981.

JACOBSON, E: *Progressive Relaxation,* ed 2. University of Chicago Press, Chicago, 1938.

JARVIS, DK: *Relative strength of the hip rotator muscle groups.* Physical Therapy Review 32:500, 1952.

JENSEN, CR AND SCHULTZ, GW: *Applied Kinesiology,* ed 2. McGraw-Hill, New York, 1977, p 183.

JOHNSON, EW AND BRADDOM, R: *Over-work weakness in facio-scapulo-humeral muscular dystrophy.* Arch Phys Med Rehabil 52:333, 1971.

JOHNSON, MA, ET AL: *Data on the distribution of fibre types in thirty-six human muscles: An autopsy study.* J Neurol Sci 18:111, 1973.

JONES, DS, BEARGIE, RJ, AND PAULY, JE: *An electromyographic study of some muscles of costal respiration in man.* Anat Rec 117:17, 1953.

JONES, DS AND PAULY, JE: *Further electromyographic studies on muscles of costal respiration in man.* Anat Rec 128:733, 1957.

JOSEPH, J: *Man's Posture: Electromyographic Studies.* Charles C Thomas, Springfield, Ill, 1960.

JOSEPH, J AND NIGHTINGALE, A: *Man's posture, electromyography of muscles of posture: Thigh muscles in males.* J Physiol 126:81, 1954.

JOSEPH, J AND WILLIAMS, PL: *Electromyography of certain hip muscles.* J Anat (Lond) 91:286, 1957.

KAPANDJI, IA: *The Physiology of the Joints, Vol 1: Upper Limb,* ed 2. E & S Livingstone, London, 1970a.

KAPANDJI, IA: *The Physiology of the Joints, Vol 2: Lower Limb,* ed 2. E & S Livingstone, London, 1970b.

KAPANDJI, IA: *The Physiology of Joints, Vol 3: The Trunk and Vertebral Column.* Churchill Livingstone, Edinburgh, 1974.

KAPLAN, EB: *Functional and Surgical Anatomy of the Hand.* JB Lippincott, Philadelphia, 1953.

KAUFER, H: *Mechanical function of the patella.* J Bone Joint Surg (Am) 53:1551, 1971.

KENDALL, HO, KENDALL, FP, AND BOYNTON, DA: *Posture and Pain.* Williams & Wilkins, Baltimore, 1952.

KENDALL, HO, KENDALL, FP, AND WADSWORTH, GE: *Muscles: Testing and Function,* ed 2. Williams & Wilkins, Baltimore, 1971.

KENT, BE: *Anatomy of the trunk: A review—Part I.* Phys Ther 54:722, 1974.

KENT, BE: *Functional anatomy of the shoulder complex: A review.* Phys Ther 51:867, 1971.

KING, BG AND SHOWERS, MJ: *Human Anatomy and Physiology,* ed 6. WB Saunders, Philadelphia, 1969.

KLOPSTEG, PE AND WILSON, PD: *Human Limbs and Their Substitutes.* Hafner Publishing, New York, reprinted 1968.

KOEPKE, GH, ET AL: *An electromyographic study of some of the muscles used in respiration.* Arch Phys Med Rehabil 36:217, 1955.

KOMI, PV AND KARLSSON, J: *Physical performance, skeletal muscle enzyme activities and fibre types in monozygous and dizygous twins of both sexes.* Acta Physiol Scand (Suppl) 462:1, 1979.

KUGELBERG, E: *The motor unit: Morphology and function.* In DESMEDT, JE (ED): *Progress in Clinical Neurophysiology,* Vol 9. Karger, Basel, 1981, p 1.

LAMOREUX, LW: *Kinematic measurements in the study of human walking.* Bull Prosthet Res 10-15:3, 1971.

LANDSMEER, JM AND LONG, C: *The mechanism of finger control: Based on electromyograms and location analysis.* Acta Anat (Basel) 60:330, 1965.

LARSSON, BE, SANDLUND, B, AND OBERG, PA: *Selspot recording of gait in normals and in patients with spasticity.* Scand J Rehabil Med (Suppl) 6:21, 1978.

LARSSON, LE, ET AL: *The phases of the stride and their interaction in human gait.* Scand J Rehabil Med 12:107, 1980.

LEIB, FJ AND PERRY, J: *Quadriceps function: Electromyographic study under isometric conditions.* J Bone Joint Surg (Am) 53:749, 1971.

LEIB, FJ AND PERRY, J: *Quadriceps function: An anatomical and mechanical study using amputated limbs.* J Bone Joint Surg (Am) 50:1535, 1968.

LEHNEIS, HR, BERGOFSKY, E, AND FRISINA, W: *Energy expenditure with advanced lower limb orthoses and with conventional braces.* Arch Phys Med Rehabil 57:20, 1976.

LE VEAU, B: *Williams and Lissner: Biomechanics of Human Motion,* ed 2. WB Saunders, Philadelphia, 1977.

LICHT, S AND KAMENETZ, H: *Orthotics Etcetera.* Elizabeth Licht, Publisher, 1966.

LINDHOLM, LE: *An optical instrument for remote on-line movement monitoring.* Conference Digest for European Conference on Electrotechnics. Eurocon, Amsterdam, 1974, p E5.

LONG, C: *Intrinsic-extrinsic control of the fingers: Electromyographic studies.* J Bone Joint Surg (Am) 50:973, 1968.

LONG, C AND BROWN, ME: *Electromyographic kinesiology of the hand: Muscles moving the long finger.* J Bone Joint Surg (Am) 46:1683, 1964.

LUNNEN, JD, YACK, J, AND LE VEAU, B: *Relationship between muscle length, muscle activity and torque of the hamstring muscles.* Phys Ther 61:190, 1981.

LUSSKIN, R: *The influence of errors in bracing upon deformity of the lower extremity.* Arch Phys Med Rehabil 47:520, 1966.

MACCONAILL, MA AND BASMAJIAN, JV: *Muscles and Movements: A Basis for Human Kinesiology.* Williams & Wilkins, Baltimore, 1969.

MAITLAND, GD: *Peripheral Manipulation,* ed 2. Butterworths, Boston, 1977.

MANN, R AND INMAN, VT: *Phasic activity of intrinsic muscles of the foot.* J Bone Joint Surg (Am) 46:469, 1964.

MANTER, JT: *Movements of the subtalar and transverse tarsal joints.* Anat Rec 80:397, 1941.

MAREY, EJ: *De la locomotion terrestre chez les bipedes et les quadrupedes.* Journal d'Anatomie et de Physiologie 9:42, 1873.

MAREY, EJ: *Development de la Methode Graphique par l'emploi de la Photographie.* Paris, 1885.

MAREY, EJ: *Le Mouvement.* Paris, 1894.

MAREY, EJ AND DEMENY, G: *Etude experimentale de la locomotion humaine.* Comptes Rendus Hebdomadoires des Seances de l'Academie des Sciences 105:544, 1887.

MARGARIA, R: *Biomechanics and Energetics of Muscular Exercise.* Clarendon Press, Oxford, 1976.

MARKEE, JE, ET AL: *Two-joint muscles of the thigh.* J Bone Joint Surg (Am) 37:125, 1955.

MATTHEWS, PBC: *Proprioceptors and the regulation of movement.* In TOWE, AL AND LUSCHEI, ES (EDS): *Handbook of Behavioral Neurobiology, Vol 5: Motor Coordination.* Plenum Press, New York, 1981, p 93.

MAY, WW: *Maximum isometric force of the hip rotator muscles.* Phys Ther 46:233, 1966.

MAY, WW: *Relative isometric force of the hip abductor and adductor muscles.* Phys Ther 48:845, 1968.

MCBEATH, A, BAHRKE, M, AND BALKE, B: *Efficiency of assisted ambulation determined by oxygen consumption measurement.* J Bone Joint Surg (Am) 56:994, 1974.

MCCLUSKEY, G AND BLACKBURN, TA: *Classification of knee ligament instabilities.* Phys Ther 60:1575, 1980.

MCLEOD, WD AND HUNTER, S: *Biomechanical analysis of the knee: Primary functions as elucidated by anatomy.* Phys Ther 60:1547, 1980.

MENDLER, HM: *Knee extensor and flexor force following injury.* Phys Ther 47:35, 1967.

MENDLER, HM: *Postoperative function of the knee joint.* Journal of American Physical Therapy Association 43:435, 1963.

MENNELL, JM: *Joint Pain: Diagnosis and Treatment Using Manipulative Techniques.* Little, Brown & Co, Boston, 1964.

MERTON, PA: *How we control the contraction of our muscles.* Sci Am 226:30, 1972.

MEYER, H: *Das aufrechte Stehen.* Archiv Fuer Anatomie und Physiologie 1853, p 2.

MOFFROID, MT AND KUSIAK, ET: *The power struggle: Definition and evaluation of power of muscular performance.* Phys Ther 55:1098, 1975.

MOFFROID, MT AND WHIPPLE, RH: *Specificity of speed of exercise.* Phys Ther 50:1692, 1970.

MOFFROID, MT, ET AL: *A study of isokinetic exercise.* Phys Ther 49:735, 1969.

MOMMSEN, F: *Die Statik des gelahmten Bewegungsapparates.* Verhandl d Deutsch Orthop Gessellsch, Kong 21:302, 1927.

MOORE, ML: *The measurement of joint motion: Part II. The technique of goniometry.* Physical Therapy Review 29:256, 1949.

MORRIS, JM, LUCAS, DB, AND BRESLER, B: *Role of the trunk in stability of the spine.* J Bone Joint Surg (Am) 43:327, 1961.

MORRIS, JM, BRENNER, G, AND LUCAS, DB: *An electromyographic study of the intrinsic muscles of the back in man.* J Anat 96:509, 1962.

MORRISON, JB: *The mechanics of the knee joint in relation to normal walking.* J Biomechan 3:51, 1970.

MORTON, DJ: *Human Locomotion and Body Form: A Study of Gravity and Man.* Williams & Wilkins, Baltimore, 1952.

MOSSBERG, K AND SMITH, LK: *Axial rotation of the knee in adult females* (submitted for publication).

MULLI, A: *Myokinesiographische Feststellung der Grenzwerte in der Automatie des physiologischen Geh-Aktes.* Inaugural Dissertation, University of Zurich, 1940.

MURRAY, MP: *Gait as a total pattern of movement.* Am J Phys Med 46:290, 1967.

MURRAY, MP AND CLARKSON, BH: *The vertical pathways of the foot during level walking: I. Range of variability in normal men.* Phys Ther 46:585, 1966a.

MURRAY, MP AND CLARKSON, BH: *The vertical pathways of the foot during level walking: II. Clinical examples of distorted pathways.* Phys Ther 46:590, 1966b.

MURRAY, MP, DROUGHT, AB, AND KORY, RC: *Walking patterns of normal men.* J Bone Joint Surg (Am) 46:335, 1964.

MURRAY, MP, KORY, RC, AND CLARKSON, BH: *Walking patterns in healthy old men.* J Gerontol 24:169, 1969.

MURRAY, MP, KORY, RC, AND SEPIC, SB: *Walking patterns of normal women.* Arch Phys Med Rehabil 51:637, 1970.

MURRAY, MP, SEPIC, SB, AND BARNARD, EJ: *Study of normal man during free and fast speed walking: Patterns of sagittal rotation of the upper limbs in walking.* Phys Ther 47:272, 1967.

MURRAY, MP, GORE, DR, AND CLARKSON, BH: *Walking patterns of patients with unilateral hip pain due to osteo-arthritis and avascular necrosis.* J Bone Joint Surg (Am) 53:259, 1971.

MURRAY, MP, ET AL: *Comparison of free and fast speed walking patterns of normal men.* Am J Phys Med 45:8, 1966.

MUSTARD, WT: *Iliopsoas transfer for weakness of the hip abductors: A preliminary report.* J Bone Joint Surg (Am) 34:647, 1952.

MUYBRIDGE, E: *The Human Figure in Motion.* Dover, New York, plate 190, reprinted in 1955 from original volume published in 1887.

NAPIER, JR: *The prehensile movements of the human hand.* J Bone Joint Surg (Br) 38:902, 1956.

New York University Manual on Upper Extremity Prosthetics. New York University, Post-Graduate Medical School, Prosthetics and Orthotics, New York, 1971.

OLSON, VL, SMIDT, GL, AND JOHNSTON, RC: *The maximum torque generated by the eccentric, isometric and concentric contractions of the hip abductor muscles.* Phys Ther 52:149, 1972.

O'SULLIVAN, SB, CULLEN, KE, AND SCHMITZ, TJ: *Physical Rehabilitation: Evaluation and Treatment Procedures.* FA Davis, Philadelphia, 1981.

OUELLET, R, LEVESQUE, HP, AND LAURIN, CA: *The ligamentous stability of the knee: An experimental investigation.* Can Med Assoc J 100:45, 1969.

PARTRIDGE, MJ AND WALTERS, CE: *Participation of the abdominal muscles in various movements of the trunk in man: An electromyographic study.* Physical Therapy Review 39:791, 1959.

PASSMORE, R AND DURNIN, JVGA: *Human energy expenditure.* Physiol Rev 35:801, 1955.

PERRY, J: *Kinesiology of lower extremity bracing.* Clin Orthop 102:18, 1974.

PERRY, J, EASTERDAY, CS, AND ANTONELLI, DJ: *Surface versus intramuscular electrodes for electromyography of superficial and deep muscles.* Phys Ther 61:7, 1981.

PETTER, CK: *Methods of measuring the pressure of the intervertebral disc.* J Bone Joint Surg (Am) 15:365, 1933.

POORE, GV: *Nervous affections of the hand.* Lancet 2:405, 1881.

POCOCK, GS: *Electromyographic study of the quadriceps during resistive exercises.* Journal of American Physical Therapy Association 43:427, 1963.

RADAKOVICH, M AND MALONE, T: *The superior tibiofibular joint: The forgotten joint.* Journal of Orthopaedic and Sports Physical Therapy 3:129, 1982.

RALSTON, HJ: *Energy-speed relation and optimal speed during level walking.* Internationale Zeitschrift fur Angewandte Physiologie Einschliesslicn Arbeitsphysiologie 17:277, 1958.

RALSTON, HJ: *Uses and limitation of electromyography in the quantitative study of skeletal muscle function.* Am J Orthod 47:521, 1961.

RALSTON, HJ AND LIBET, B: *The question of tonus in skeletal muscle.* Am J Phys Med 32:85, 1953.

RALSTON, HJ, ET AL: *Dynamic features of human isolated voluntary muscle in isometric and free contractions.* J Appl Physiol 1:526, 1949.

RAMSEY, RW AND STREET, SF: *Isometric length-tension diagram of isolated skeletal muscle fibers of frog.* J Cell Comp Physiol 15:11, 1940.

RASCH, PJ AND BURKE, RK: *Kinesiology and Applied Anatomy: The Science of Human Movement*, ed 6. Lea & Febiger, Philadelphia, 1978.

RECKLINGHAUSEN, N VON: *Gliedermechanik and Lahmungsprothesen*. J Springer, Berlin, 1920.

REDFORD, JB (ED): *Orthotics Etcetera*, ed 2. Williams & Wilkins, Baltimore, 1980.

REILLY, DT AND MARTENS, M: *Experimental analysis of the quadriceps muscle force and patellofemoral joint reaction force for various activities.* Acta Orthop Scand 43:126, 1972.

RESNICK, R AND HALLIDAY, D: *Physics for Students of Science and Engineering*. John Wiley & Sons, New York, 1960.

REULEAUX, F: *Theoretische Kinematik*. Braunschweigh, 1875.

REYS, JHO: *Uber Die Absolute Kraft Der Muskeln Im Menchlichenn Korper*. Pfleugers Arch 160:183, 1915.

ROSS, RF: *A quantitative study of rotation of the knee joint in man*. Anat Rec 52:209, 1932.

ROSSE, C AND CLAWSON, K: *The Musculoskeletal System in Health and Disease*. Harper & Row, Hagerstown, Md, 1980.

RUSSE, OA AND GERHARDT, JJ: *International SFTR Method of Measuring and Recording Joint Motion*. Hans Huber, Bern, Switzerland, 1975.

SALTER, N AND DARCUS, HD: *The effect of the degree of elbow flexion on the maximum torques developed in pronation and supination of the right hand*. J Anat 86:197, 1952.

SAUNDERS, JB DE CM, INMAN, VT, AND EBERHART, HD: *The major determinants in normal and pathological gait*. J Bone Joint Surg (Am) 35:543, 1953.

SCHEDE, F: *Theoretische Grundlagen fur den Bau von Kunstbeinen*. Ferdinand Enke Verlag, Stuttgart, 1941.

SCHERB, R: *Ein Vorschlag zur kinetischen Diagnostik in der Orthopadie*. Verhandl d Deutsch Orthop Gesellsch, Kong 21:462, 1927.

SCHERB, R: *Keinetisch-Diagnostische Analyse von Gehstorungen: Technik und Resultate der Myokinesiographie*. Z Orthop 82 (Suppl), 1952.

SCHERB, R AND ARIENTI, A: *Ist die Myokinesigraphie als Untersuchungsmethode objectiv zuverlassig?* Schweiz Med Wochenschr 75:1077, 1945.

SCHLESINGER, G: *Der mechanische Aufbau der kuntslichen Glieder. In Ersatzglieder und Arbeitshilfen*. J Springer, Berlin, 1919.

SCHLESINGER, G: *Technische Ausnutzung der kinoplastischen Armstumpfe*. Dtsch Med Wochenschr 46:262, 1920.

SCHMIDT, RF (ED): *Fundamentals of Neurophysiology*, ed 2. Springer-Verlag, New York, 1978.

SCHOTTELIUS, BA AND SCHOTTELIUS, DD: *Textbook of Physiology*, ed 17. CV Mosby, St Louis, 1973.

SCHWINDT, PC: *Control of motoneuron output by pathways descending from the brain stem.* In TOWE, AL AND LUSCHEI, ES (ED): *Handbook of Behavioral Neurobiology, Vol 5: Motor Coordination*. Plenum, New York, 1981, p 139.

SHEFFER, DB, LEHMKUHL, LD, AND HERRON, RE: *Stereometric analysis of static equilibrium in CNS disorders.* In *Proceedings, NATO Symposium on Applications of Human Biostereometrics, Paris, July 9–13, 1978*. Society of Photo-Optical Instrumentation Engineers, Bellingham, Wash, 1978.

SHEFFIELD, FJ: *Electromyographic study of the abdominal muscles in walking and other movements*. Am J Phys Med 41:142, 1962.

SKOGLUND, S: *Anatomical and physiological studies of knee joint innervation in the cat*. Acta Physiol Scand (Suppl) 124:1, 1956.

SMIDT, GL: *Biomechanical analysis of knee flexion and extension*. Biomechanics 6:79, 1973.

SMITH, JW: *The forces acting at the human ankle joint during standing*. J Anat 91:545, 1957.

SODERBERG, GL AND GABEL, RH: *A light-emitting diode system for the analysis of gait.* Phys Ther 58:426, 1978.

STAUFFER, RN, CHAO, EYS, AND BREWSTER, RC: *Force and motion analysis of the normal, diseased and prosthetic ankle joint.* Clin Orthop 127:189, 1977.

STEEL, FL AND TOMLINSON, JD: *The 'carrying angle' in man.* J Anat 92:315, 1958.

STEINDLER, A: *Kinesiology of the Human Body under Normal and Pathological Conditions.* Charles C Thomas, Springfield, Ill, 1955.

STRONG, CL AND PERRY, J: *Function of the extensor pollicis longus and intrinsic muscles of the thumb: An electromyographic study during interphalangeal joint extension.* Phys Ther 46:939, 1966.

STUDER, F: *Der Sauerstoffverbrauch beim Gehen auf horizontaler Bahn.* Pfluegers Arch 212:105, 1926.

SUNDERLAND, S: *Actions of the extensor digitorum communis, interosseous and lumbrical muscles.* Am J Anat 77:189, 1945.

SWANSON, AB, MATEV, IB, AND DEGROOT, G: *The strength of the hand.* Bull Prosthet Res BPR 10-14:145, 1970.

TAKEBE, K AND HIROHATA, K: *EMG biofeedback in tendon transplantation for foot drop.* Archives of Orthopaedic and Traumatic Surgery 97:77, 1980.

TAYLOR, A: *The contribution of the intercostal muscles to the effort of respiration in man.* J Physiol (Lond) 151:390, 1960.

TAYLOR, A AND PROCHAZKA, A (EDS): *Muscle Receptors and Movement.* Oxford University Press, New York, 1981.

TAYLOR, CL AND SCHWARZ, RJ: *The anatomy and mechanics of the human hand.* Artificial Limbs 2:22, 1955.

THORSTENSSON, A: *Muscle strength, fibre types and enzyme activities in man.* Acta Physiol Scand (Suppl) 443:1, 1976.

TICHAUER, ER: *Biomechanics sustains occupational safety and health.* Ind Eng Feb:46, 1976.

TOEWS, JV: *A grip-strength study among steelworkers.* Arch Phys Med Rehabil 45:413, 1964.

TORNVALL, G: *Assessment of physical capabilities.* Acta Physiol Scand (Suppl) 201:1, 1963.

TOURNAY, A AND FESSARD, A: *Etude electromyographique de la Synergie entre l'Abducteur du Pouce et le Muscle Cubital Posterieur.* Rev Neurol (Paris) 80:631, 1948.

VAN LINGE, B AND MULDER, JD: *Function of the supraspinatus muscle and its relation to the supraspinatus syndrome: An experimental study in man.* J Bone Joint Surg (Br) 45:750, 1963.

VARON, SS AND BUNGE, RP: *Trophic mechanisms in the peripheral nervous system.* Annual Review of Neuroscience 1:327, 1978.

VON LANZ, T AND WACHSMUTH, W: *Praktische Anatomie, Band I, Teil III.* J Springer, Berlin, 1935, p 94.

VON RECKLINGHAUSEN, N: *Gliedermechanik und Lahmungsprothesen.* J Springer, Berlin, 1920.

WATERS, RL, ET AL: *The energy cost of walking of amputees: The influence of level of amputation.* J Bone Joint Surg (Am) 58:42, 1976.

WEATHERSBY, HT, SUTTON, LR, AND KRUSEN, UL: *The kinesiology of muscles of the thumb: An electromyographic study.* Arch Phys Med Rehabil 44:321, 1963.

WEBER, EF: *Ueber die Langeverhaltnisse der Muskeln im Allgemeinen.* Verh Kgl Sach Ges d Wiss, Leipzig, 1851.

WEBER, W AND WEBER, E: *Mechanik der menschlichen Gehwerkzeuge.* Gottingen, 1836.

WILKIE, DR: *The relation between force and velocity in human muscle.* J Physiol (Lond) 110:249, 1949.

WILLIAMS, M AND LISSNER, HR: *Biomechanics of Human Motion.* WB Saunders, Philadelphia, 1962.

WILLIAMS, M AND STUTZMAN, L: *Strength variation through the range of joint motion.* Physical Therapy Review 39:145, 1959.

WILLIAMS, M, TOMBERLIN, J, AND ROBERTSON, KJ: *Muscle force curves of school children.* Phys Ther 45:539, 1965.

WILLIAMS, M AND WESLEY, W: *Hip rotator action of the adductor longus muscle.* Physical Therapy Review 31:90, 1952.

WINTER, DA: *Biomechanics of Human Movement.* John Wiley & Sons, New York, 1979, p 12.

WOODRUFF, G: *Maximum Isometric Torque of the Hip Rotator Muscles in Four Positions of Hip Flexion-Extension.* Unpublished Thesis, Texas Woman's University, Denton, Tex, 1976.

WYATT, MP AND EDWARDS, AM: *Comparison of quadriceps and hamstring torque values during isokinetic exercise.* Journal of Orthopaedic and Sports Physical Therapy 3:48, 1981.

WYNN-PARRY, CB: *Rehabilitation of the Hand,* ed 4. Butterworths, London, 1981.

ZOHN, DA AND MENNELL, J: *Musculoskeletal Pain: Diagnosis and Physical Treatment.* Little, Brown & Co, Boston, 1976, p 123.

INDEX

Numbers in *italics* refer to illustrations; numbers followed by a (t) indicate tables.

437